ANTIBIOTICS IN OBSTETRICS AND GYNECOLOGY

DEVELOPMENTS IN

PERINATAL MEDICINE 2

SERIES EDITOR: WILLIAM J. LEDGER

Also in this series:

1. De Meyer R, ed., Metabolic Adaptation to Extrauterine Life. 1981. XXII + 372 pp., ISBN 90-247-2484-8.

Series ISBN 90-247-2443-0

ANTIBIOTICS IN OBSTETRICS AND GYNECOLOGY

Edited by

WILLIAM J. LEDGER

The New York Hospital – Cornell Medical Center,
New York, N.Y., U.S.A.

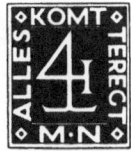

1982

MARTINUS NIJHOFF PUBLISHERS

THE HAGUE / BOSTON / LONDON

Distributors:

for the United States and Canada

Kluwer Boston, Inc.
190 Old Derby Street
Hingham, MA 02043
USA

for all other countries

Kluwer Academic Publishers Group
Distribution Center
P.O. Box 322
3300 AH Dordrecht
The Netherlands

Library of Congress Cataloging in Publication Data   CIP

Main entry under title:

Antibiotics in obstetrics and gynecology.

    (Developments in perinatal medicine ; v. 2)
    Includes index.
    1. Antibiotics.   2. Generative organs, Female – Infections – Chemotherapy.
3. Communicable diseases in pregnancy – Chemotherapy.   I. Ledger, William J., 1932-
II. Series. [DNLM: 1. Genital diseases, Female – Drug therapy.   2. Pregnancy complications ·
Drug therapy.   3. Antibiotics – Therapeutic use. W1 DE998NI v. 2 / WQ 240 A629]
RG129.A56A57   618   81-18915
           AACR2

ISBN-13:978-94-009-7466-1   e-ISBN-13:978-94-009-7464-7
DOI: 10.1007/978-94-009-7464-7

CONTENTS

FOREWORD

The motive to prepare this volume on antibiotics for the physician caring for women was based upon the editor's perception that the subject matter had never been fully developed for the obstetrician-gynecologist. Most textbooks of infectious disease have a small section devoted to antibiotics, which has little relevance for the physician caring for post-operative or post-partum infections. Basic antibiotic pharmacology is described and there is a reflex prohibition of antibiotics for the pregnant woman. Correctly, the reader assumes that the authors themselves do not care for women with bacterial infections of the pelvis. Recent texts in infectious disease in obstetrics-gynecology have been little better. Although the focus has been more clinically oriented, space requirements have too often kept the discussions at a superficial level. A total focus upon antibiotics in this volume eliminates the restraints of space in prior publications.

The greatest reward in my task as editor of this volume is related to the quality of the individual authors. They range from former students, to contemporary colleagues, to respected peers in infectious disease. Since the quality of this volume is related to the sum total of the individual chapters, I wish to comment about each of the contributors. Philip Mead from the University of Vermont is an old friend, who brings to the question of prophylactic antibiotics, his wide clinical experience and encyclopedic knowledge. His chapter will be a reference source for clinicians for years to come. Agneta Philipson from Stockholm, Sweden is a highly respected investigator internationally. Her original research on the pharmacokinetics of antibiotics in the pregnant woman has brought the light of knowledge to a formerly dark area of obstetrical practice. This chapter is a classic. Robert Harris from San Antonio, Texas is a renaissance man. In addition to this exhaustive research into urinary tract infections, he still has time to read fiction and be articulate about the arts. Perhaps this is the reason that his chapter, filled with academic nuggets, is so enjoyable to read. His love of the language shines through every page. Lynn Yonekura's contribution from the University of Southern California fills me with delight. It is excellent, well written, and justifies my faith in this former student. How pleasing it is for a teacher to see a young mind grow and develop. David Eschenbach's contribution from the University of Washington in Seattle is stunning. David is a respected colleague who had the courage to investigate pelvic infection in the non-pregnant female, unfettered by the established biases of our specialty. This chapter is well worth the reader's close examination. I first met Richard Schwarz in the late 1960's, and I was impressed with the extent of productivity of a counterpart in academic obstetrics and gynecology. Our careers are parallel with our interest in infectious disease, as well as his recent assumption of chair of Obstetrics-Gynecology at Downstate Medical Center in Brooklyn in New York. I was happy to gain his agreement to write this chapter, and the reader may share in the experience of a master. David Charles, the chairman of Obstetrics-Gynecology at Marshall University in West Virginia, is my friend and mentor. He was a leader in the investigation of infectious disease, before it was respectable academically, and he has always been a learned counsel. His chapter is must reading for any physician dealing with a soft tissue infection of the pelvis in which anaerobic bacteria are involved, and is skillfully written. The work of Richard Sweet from the University of California in San Francisco gives me great pride. He is my student, who has subsequently grown beyond his mentor. His discussion of the newer cephalo-sporins is important for it represents the observations of an excellent clinical investigator. Finally, I found great satisfaction in preparing my own chapter on tetracyclines and the penicillins.

A final word of advice for the reader. Some books remain beautiful in their bound form on the bookshelf. This will not be the fate of *Antibiotics in Obstetrics and Gynecology*. It is readable, and may be read with profit from cover to cover by the practicing physician. The importance of the subject matter will make it a valuable source of reference for many years.

WILLIAM J. LEDGER

LIST OF CONTRIBUTORS

David Charles, M.D., Department of Obstetrics and Gynecology, Marshall University School of Medicine, Huntington, West Virginia 25701

David Eschenbach, M.D., Department of Obstetrics and Gynecology RH-20, University of Washington School of Medicine, Seattle, Washington 98195

Robert Harris, M.D., University of Texas, San Antonio, 6402 Red Jacket, San Antonio, Texas 78238

Philip Mead, M.D., Associate Professor of Obstetrics and Gynecology, University of Vermont, College of Medicine, Given Building, Burlington, Vermont 05405

Dr. Agneta Philipson, Department of Infectious Diseases, Danderyd Hospital, S-182 88 Danderyd, Sweden

Richard Schwarz, M.D., Professor and Chairman, Department of Obstetrics and Gynecology, Downstate Medical Center, 450 Clarkson Avenue, Brooklyn, New York 11203

Richard L. Sweet, M.D., Department of Obstetrics and Gynecology, San Francisco General Hospital, 1001 Potrero Avenue, San Francisco, California 94110

Lynn Yonekura, M.D., George Washington University Medical Center, Department of Obstetrics and Gynecology, The H.B. Burns Memorial Building, 2150 Pennsylvania Avenue, N.W., Washington, D.C. 20037

PART I

PREVENTIVE ANTIBIOTICS AND ANTIBIOTIC TREATMENT IN PREGNANCY

1. PROPHYLACTIC ANTIBIOTICS IN GYNECOLOGY

PHILIP B. MEAD, M.D.

PREVENTION OF BACTERIAL ENDOCARDITIS

Perhaps the least controversial area of chemoprophylaxis involves the use of antibiotics to prevent subacute bacterial endocarditis. Accordingly, we will begin this chapter with a discussion of the employment of prophylactic antibiotics for this infection.

Development of bacterial endocarditis remains one of the most serious complications of cardiac disease with significant morbidity and mortality despite advances in antimicrobial therapy and cardiovascular surgery. This infection occurs most often in patients with structural abnormalities of the heart or great vessels who undergo transient bacteremias.

Patients at risk of the development of bacterial endocarditis are those with valvular heart disease, congenital heart disease, a previous episode of infective endocarditis, and particularly those with prosthetic heart valves. The presence of an uncomplicated atrial septal defect of the secundum type probably does not indicate an increased risk, and there is probably no need for endocarditis prophylaxis following six months of healing after surgical closure of an atrial septal defect or patent ductus.

What procedures regularly result in transient bacteremia? Many workers have investigated the rate of transient bacteremia following various procedures and manipulations including those involving the genitourinary tract [26]. Unfortunately, the results of these studies have often been confusing because of diversity in blood culture timing, technique, and bacteriologic methods. Bacteremia may be caused by surgery or instrumentation of the genitourinary tract, especially urethral manipulations including urethral catheterization whether the urine is infected or not. Bacteremia has been associated with septic abortion, hysterectomy, and other major gynecologic surgery. Documented cases of bacterial endocarditis have been recorded following these procedures and antibiotic prophylaxis to prevent this infection should be employed. Endocarditis following uncomplicated dilatation and curettage of the uterus is extremely rare and has not been considered an indication for endocarditis prophylaxis by the American Heart Association. This author has seen endocarditis following uncomplicated D & C in predisposed patients, and at this institution we continue to utilize endocarditis

W.J. Ledger (ed.), Antibiotics in Obstetrics and Gynecology, 3–36. All rights reserved.
Copyright © 1982 by Martinus Nijhoff Publishers, The Hague/Boston/London. ISBN-13:978-94-009-7466-1

prophylaxis for patients undergoing D & C who have underlying cardio-vascular lesions. Although endocarditis has been attributed to infected intra-uterine contraceptive devices by Cobbs [20] and De Swiet [23], Everett found no bacteremia at 1 to 3, 15 or 30 min following their insertion in 84 and their removal in 16 women [27]. Since none of these women had pelvic infection or endometritis, the incidence of bacteremia following removal of infected de-vices is unknown. Regatz reported 40 patients undergoing biopsies from two to seven areas of the cervix [76]. Blood cultures were obtained from 1–5 min following the procedure. All cultures were negative, although aerobic and anaerobic bacteria grew from most of the cervical swabs taken before the procedure. A Schiller's test using Lugol's iodine solution done just before the biopsy may have killed the cervical flora, however. Harris performed endo-cervical and endometrial biopsies in 101 women [104]. A blood culture was obtained immediately prior to and 5 min after the biopsy in each patient. No growth occurred in any of the 202 blood cultures, again suggesting that bacteremia is rare following these procedures.

It should be mentioned that since the patient with a prosthetic valve appears to be at such high risk of the development of endocarditis, it may be wise to administer antibiotic prophylaxis with any genitourinary proce-dure in such a patient. This recommendation is not based upon definitive data. Enterococci (*Streptococcus fecalis*) are one of the most frequent causes of endocarditis after genitourinary procedures. Gram negative organisms are a frequent cause of bacteremia and even of sepsis, but are a rare cause of endocarditis. Thus, prophylaxis after these procedures must be directed mainly against enterococci. The most recent recommendations by the Ameri-can Heart Association for the prevention of bacterial endocarditis following genitourinary tract surgery are as follows [49, 63, 95]: Aqueous crystalline penicillin G 2 million units intramuscularly or intravenously or ampicillin 1 g intramuscularly or intravenously plus gentamicin 1.5 mg/kg (not to exceed 80 mg) intramuscularly or intravenously or streptomycin 1 g intramuscularly, giving initial doses 30 min to one hour prior to procedure. If gentamicin is used then give a similar dose of streptomycin and penicillin or ampicillin every 12 h for two additional doses. For patients who are allergic to penicillin, vancomycin 1 g intravenously given over 30 min to 1 h plus streptomycin 1 g intramuscularly. A single dose of these antibiotics begun 30 min to 1 h prior to the procedure is probably sufficient, but the same dose may be repeated in 12 h. During prolonged procedures, or in the case of delayed healing, it may be necessary to provide additional doses of antibiotics.

Several points in regard to endocarditis prophylaxis should be stressed: First, the above recommendations apply only to patients with the underlying, predisposing cardiovascular lesions described. They are designed to prevent infective endocarditis in these patients and their use is not concerned with nor directed against the development of postoperative pelvic infection. Second, it must be admitted that no proof exists that antibiotics given prior to procedures causing bacteremia prevent endocarditis in humans. However, recent experimental evidence in rabbits supports their use; [49] therefore, in situations where bacteremia is highly predictable, it would seem wise to administer prophylactic antimicrobials. Third, it must be admitted that only 40% of patients who develop enterococcal endocarditis have a history of a predisposing event. Thus, meticulous adherence to the above protocols will not prevent all cases of infective endocarditis.

PROPHYLACTIC ANTIBIOTICS IN GYNECOLOGIC SURGERY

Background

It was probably inevitable that the successful introduction of therapeutic antibiotics in the early 1940's would soon be followed by attempts at the prevention, as well as treatment, of infection. Trials using antibiotics in a preventive or prophylactic manner were not long in coming. In 1946 Falk published the first paper evaluating the use of prophylactic antimicrobials in gynecologic surgery [28]. In this study of 500 vaginal hysterectomies, febrile morbidity was 23% in patients receiving prophylactic sulfonamides as compared with 18% in control patients not given sulfonamides. Falk concluded that prophylactic antibiotics were not effective in reducing febrile morbidity following vaginal hysterectomy. The next published report concerned morbidity in 1000 consecutive hysterectomies performed during 1949 and 1950 as reported by Cron et al. [22]. The authors concluded that the use of prophylactic intramuscular penicillin did not appreciably alter the incidence of febrile morbidity. In 1952 Blahey described the use of oral terramycin in 44 patients undergoing vaginal hysterectomy or repair [7]. He noted a decrease in infectious morbidity in patients undergoing vaginal hysterectomy but this was not true in the patients who had only a vaginal repair. Additionally, he found that patients receiving the prophylactic antibiotic were less likely to need therapeutic parenteral penicillin therapy later in their course. These studies are of historical interest only. Although they represent the first attempts to answer questions relating to the efficacy of prophylactic antibiotics in gynecologic surgery, they were poorly designed and do not allow valid conclusions to be drawn.

It was Burke, a surgeon at Harvard, whose work paved the way for the modern use of antibiotic prophylaxis. In a series of simple yet revealing experiments first published in 1961, he showed that prophylaxis was effective if given within three hours of bacterial inoculation, but was most efficacious when instituted before the wound was made. He concluded that there was a limited period of time when the operative site would benefit from the effect of antibiotic prophylaxis and, that to be most effective in suppressing infection, antibiotics had to be given before bacteria were introduced into tissue [11]. In separate clinical studies published in the late 1960's Alexander and Altemeier [1] and Polk and Lopez-Mayer [72] independently confirmed Burke's observations that a short perioperative course of antibiotics was effective in decreasing the incidence of operative site infection. In 1973, Burke reemphasized the rationale for the use of prophylactic antibiotics and described additional experiments that delineated the delicate interaction between host-defense mechanisms and systemic antimicrobial prophylaxis [13].

In 1969, Goosenberg published the first modern series describing the use of antibiotic prophylaxis in vaginal hysterectomy [35], and in 1972 Allen published similar data for abdominal hysterectomy [2]. The decade of the 1970's saw the publication of 36 separate clinical studies evaluating the effectiveness of antimicrobial prophylaxis in vaginal or abdominal hysterectomy.

In 1975 Ledger published suggested guidelines for antibiotic prophylaxis in gynecology, recommendations which have stood the test of time [52].

To conclude these opening comments on the historical perspective of antibiotic prophylaxis in gynecologic surgery, it would seem that at the time of the preparation of this review (August 1980) the use of prophylactic chemotherapy for vaginal hysterectomy has won firm acceptance. It is likely that studies in the 1980's will consider the value of chemoprophylaxis in other procedures, clarification of the optimal antimicrobial regimen, elucidation and clarification of potential hazards, and efforts to delineate the mechanism of action of this undeniably beneficial clinical strategy.

Mechanism of Action

Before discussing the probable mechanism of action of prophylactic antibiotics in preventing infections following gynecologic surgery, it is useful to review the pathophysiology of such infections. The normal vagina contains a rich and diverse flora of both facultative and anaerobic bacteria [3, 34]. Importantly, a similar flora is present in the endocervix as well. During hysterectomy, relatively large clamps are applied and heavy sutures used, thus creating large pedicles of devitalized tissue which subsequently undergo avascular necrosis. During vaginal hysterectomy, each clamp and suture applied to a tissue pedicle must first pass through the bacteria-laden vagina. In this way microorganisms are crushed into these devitalized pedicles. Swartz and Tanaree have shown that an average of 40 cm^3 (range 10–200 cm^3) of a serosanguinous fluid can be suctioned from the retroperitoneal space following hysterectomy [89]. This fluid is composed of blood, serum, lymph, and the breakdown products of devitalized tissue by enzymatic activity distal to the suture ligatures. This retroperitoneal collection of devitalized tissue fluids provides an ideal culture medium. These two factors – the presence of a suitable culture medium plus its routine contamination with sufficient numbers of virulent bacteria present contiguously in the normal vaginal and endocervical flora – provide the likely explanation for the high incidence of pelvic infection associated with hysterectomy.

Two observations suggest that the endocervical flora may be the most important source of bacteria contaminating the retroperitoneal fluid collection. Osborne has shown that a preoperative vaginal scrub, as commonly performed prior to hysterectomy, was capable of rendering the vagina bacteria free in 92% of cases while the endocervix was bacteria free in only 8% [69]. In a later study he was able to dramatically reduce postoperative febrile morbidity following vaginal hysterectomy with the use of preoperative hot conization of the cervix [70].

It appears likely, then, that prophylactic antibiotics work by the following mechanism: Following administration of antibiotics, effective levels are established in blood and tissues. If antibiotics are administered preoperatively, before the placement of clamps and sutures, high tissue levels of antibiotics will be established in tissue prior to devitalization. These high antibiotic levels, present in the devitalized tissue pedicles and resultant retroperitoneal fluid collection, prevent the proliferation of organisms seeded during surgery from the vagina and endocervix, thus preventing the development of pelvic infection. This explanation is consistent with the results of experimental and clinical studies which demonstrate that antibiotics are most effective when administered preoperatively. It is also consistent with the observation of Swartz that suction drainage used alone (preventing the retroperitoneal collection from forming), *or* prophylactic antibiotics used alone (preventing proliferation of organisms in the retroperitoneal fluid collection) are equally effective in preventing postoperative infectious morbidity, with no further reduction achieved if both methods are combined [88].

It is probably unnecessary that all organisms introduced into the tissues at surgery be killed by the previously established antibiotic levels. As long as the inoculum size is maintained below a critical level, host defenses will be sufficient to prevent the development of overt infection.

Prophylactic antibiotics clearly do not result in sterilization of the endocervix and vagina. Although the number of organisms is reduced, all studies employing pre- and post-therapy cultures have confirmed the continued presence of organisms in the vagina and endocervix following the use of prophylactic antibiotics [36]. Similarly, it is clear that prophylactic antibiotics do not have as their mechanism of action the treatment of infection. Multiple studies (see below) have shown that a short, 12 h perioperative course of

8

antibiotics or even a single preoperative dose have regularly been as effective as longer courses of therapy in preventing postoperative infectious morbidity. Such brief antimicrobial usage could only be considered a preventive, and not a therapeutic mechanism.

Guidelines for Use

Risk of infection
If one is to justify the routine administration of prophylactic antibiotics for any given surgical procedure the risk of postoperative infectious morbidity must be significantly great. The exact definition of a significant risk of postoperative infectious morbidity is illusive. A judgement as to what constitutes excessive postoperative infectious morbidity must be made by each individual service after prospectively monitoring patients on their own service so that accurate rates of infectious morbidity for each surgical procedure in question can be calculated. The use of prophylactic antibiotics in gynecology is justified only for serious postoperative pelvic infections which will require systemic antibiotics or operative drainage. Indirect measures such as technical febrile morbidity should not be the sole criterion for the widespread use of antibiotics. Moreover, there is little evidence that postoperative urinary tract infections or respiratory infections are rational targets for prophylactic antibiotic therapy.

Choice of antibiotic
For reasons which are not entirely clear, antimicrobials of widely varying spectra have been shown to be equally efficacious when utilized for prophylaxis in gynecologic surgery. Reference to Table 1 shows that all of the antimicrobials shown to be effective for chemoprophylaxis in gynecologic surgery fail to cover one or more of the organisms known to be associated with the development of postoperative infection. It has been postulated that prophylactic antibiotics prevent postoperative pelvic infection by both decreasing the absolute number of vaginal bacteria ('decreasing inoculum size') and killing organisms which are integral members of synergistic bacterial groups. Either of these mechanisms would explain the clinical observation that most antibiotics are successful chemoprophylactic agents for pelvic surgery regardless of their antibacterial spectrum.

Despite the proven efficacy of the majority of antibiotics in preventing postoperative pelvic infection, choice of a chemoprophylactic agent should be limited to those antimicrobials which are not commonly used for the treatment of infected gynecologic patients. Antibiotics such as the penicillins, aminoglycosides, chloramphenicol, and clindamycin should be reserved for treatment and not used for prophylaxis. Use of these agents for prophylaxis

Table 1. Antimicrobials used successfully for prophylaxis in gynecologic surgery.

Antimicrobial	Organisms inadequately covered
Ampicillin	*B. fragilis*, many gram negative enterics, many staphylococci
Carbenicillin or ticarcillin	Klebsiella sp., some enterococci, many staphylococci
Penicillin	*B. fragilis*, many gram negative enterics, many staphylococci
Cephalothin, cefazolin, cephaloridine, cephalexin or cephradine	*B. fragilis*, Enterobacter sp., enterococci
Cefoxitin	Enterobacter sp., enterococci
Tetracycline or doxycycline	Enterococci, some gram negative enterics, many *B. fragilis*, some other anaerobes, many staphylococci
Sulfamethoxazole – trimethoprim	Some entereococci, some anaerobes, Clostridia sp.
Metronidazole	All gram negative enteric aerobes, enterococci, staphylococci, some anaerobes
Chloramphenicol	Few enterococci, few staphylococci

will result in no greater chemoprophylactic effectiveness than use of other antibiotics, and, through selection pressure, will render these valuable agents less effective when needed to treat infected patients. In view of these considerations, cephalosporins, agents which are not commonly employed for the primary treatment of pelvic infections, appear to be the ideal choice for prophylaxis in gynecologic surgery.

There is one situation where prophylactic antibiotic choice may have important bearing on subsequent efficacy. Stone has shown that, for an antimicrobial to successfully prevent abdominal wound infection, the agent must be effective against the contaminating bacteria [85, 86]. This would suggest that the choice of chemoprophylaxis for the prevention of abdominal wound infections should be an antibiotic effective against *Staphylococcus aureus*. Cephalosporins are active against most *Staphylococcus aureus*, another reason for selecting them as ideal agents for prophylactic use in gynecology.

Timing

The period of time between bacterial contamination of tissue and the delivery of a prophylactic antibiotic appears to be enormously important to antibiotic effectiveness. Definitive animal model studies, first reported by Burke in 1961, demonstrated conclusively that antibiotics given one hour before or at the same time as bacterial contamination occurred protected against the infection, but the longer the time after contamination the antibiotic was given the less effect it had [11]. If the antibiotic was administered 4 h after contamination it had no effect at all on the eventual size of the bacterial lesions. Burke postulated that bacterial contamination resulting from a surgical incision triggers a period of intense biochemical activity on the part of the host. This is the time when the host's own defenses have the opportunity to eliminate the bacteria before a lesion has developed. This also seems the most logical time for an effective antibiotic concentration to be able to augment the host's natural resistance. Further, prevention of a bacterial lesion must be accomplished shortly after bacterial contamination, for within a matter of 2–3 h, sufficient biochemical damage has taken place to make the development of an anatomic lesion inevitable. Thus, Burke's studies established the fact that to be maximally effective the antibiotic must be in the tissue before the contaminating bacteria arrive [12]. Moreover, since his evidence indicated that antibiotics delivered 3–4 h after contamination occurs will be useless, it appeared, on theoretical grounds, that the continuation of prophylactic antibiotics beyond the immediate postsurgery period was unnecessary. The clinical studies to be discussed below have repeatedly documented the validity of Burke's initial observation in his animal model.

Efficacy of Prophylactic Antibiotics: Specific Surgical Procedures

Several authors [4, 5, 17, 18, 24, 43] have recently reviewed the current literature dealing with prophylactic chemotherapy in surgical procedures including gynecologic procedures. All agree that some of these studies fail to meet the minimal standards of sound experimental design and therefore allow no valid conclusions. Many studies fail to define clear outcome endpoints, leaving the reader with vague descriptions of 'infectious morbidity' without further defining the infectious complications. While most trials have demonstrated that prophylaxic decreases morbidity (defined as number of infections or febrile morbidity), many have failed to address the clinical significance of these observed differences between experimental and control groups. Thus, studies may show a statistically significant difference in the rate of wound infections, but if they fail to grade the severity of these infections, it is often difficult to determine their impact on the patient's ultimate clinical course.

Although adherence to methodological standards has improved over the past decade, new problems may be emerging. In a recent study evaluating prophylactic antibiotics in vaginal hysterectomy the authors report that the Joint Committee on Clinical Investigation for their institution felt it was unethical to use a placebo group and therefore concurrent controls were not used [39]. If these concerns become widespread it may soon become extremely difficult to design methodologically acceptable studies of prophylactic chemotherapy in those clinical situations where there is already some evidence of patient benefit [14].

Despite all of the above, the experimental evidence in support of antimicrobial prophylaxis in gynecologic surgery has generally been of a prospective and controlled nature and the studies have been carried out at the same level of proficiency as have similar studies in other branches of surgery. While variability exists in almost all of the areas of design, most studies are in general agreement as to the value of prophylaxis for specific gynecologic procedures.

Vaginal hysterectomy

Tables 2 and 3 summarize the modern English literature concerning the use of prophylactic antibiotics in vaginal hysterectomy through August of 1980. Several comments are necessary regarding these summary tables. Since the studies reviewed did not always provide uniform definitions of infection related morbidity, the general categories of technical febrile morbidity and pelvic infection were chosen to represent infectious morbidity. The most common definition of febrile morbidity in these studies was an oral temperature of 38° C or greater on two separate occasions exclusive of the first 24 postoperative hours. However, other definitions were used as well. Pelvic infection refers to the entire group of operative site infections including pelvic cellulitis, cuff cellulitis, septic pelvic thrombophlebitis, pelvic abscess, and adnexal abscess. Urinary tract infections were excluded from this category. As Duff and Park have noted, differences in definition of postoperative morbidity between studies make interstudy comparisons somewhat difficult [24].

When appropriate statistical analysis was carried out by the authors of each report, it was utilized in the summary tables. When such data were not present, statistical analyses were performed utilizing the data presented in each paper. For these calculations, antibiotic treated and control groups were compared by a chi-square analysis without Yates correction. Probability values less than 0.05 were taken to represent statistically significant differences.

Between 1965 and 1980, 32 human studies concerning the use of prophylactic antibiotics in vaginal hysterectomy were reported in the English literature. Ninety-one percent of these studies were prospective, 81% were randomized and 60% were double-blinded. A multiplicity of antimicrobials were used with no clear superiority of any agent.

Of the 32 studies, 30 showed that antibiotic prophylaxis successfully decreased the incidence of postoperative febrile morbidity. In two studies, febrile morbidity was halved in the treated group but this decrease did not reach statistical significance.

Twenty-four studies evaluated the effect on pelvic infection. In 18 there was a statistically significant decrease in pelvic infection among treated patients,

Table 2. Clinical studies of antibiotic prophylaxis in vaginal hysterectomy – experimental design.

Authors	Dates of study	Total no. of patients	Study design	Antibiotic	Duration of therapy
Goosenberg et al. [35]	1965–1966	120	Prospective, randomized, not blinded	Penicillin and streptomycin vs. Chloramphenicol	5 days
Thomsen [93]	1970	95	Prospective, not randomized, not blinded	Cephaloridine (1 gm bid)	Night preop until discharge
Allen et al. [2]	1970–1971	98	Prospective, randomized, double blinded	Cephalothin	5 days
Bolling and Plunkett [8]	1970–1972	296	Prospective, randomized, not blinded	Ampicillin vs. tetracycline	7 days 7 days
Breeden and Mayo [10]	1970–1972	120	Prospective, randomized, double-blinded	Cephaloridine	3 perioperative doses
Hedican and Sarto [41]	1971–1972	70	Prospective, randomized, blinded	Cefazolin and cephalexin	Until Foley out 24 h
Harralson et al. [40]	1971–1973	200	Prospective, randomized, not blinded	Penicillin and streptomycin	3 days
Bivens Neufeld et al. [6]	1973–1974	60	Prospective, randomized, double-blinded	Cephalothin and cephalexin	4–5 days

	Year	Number	Study design	Antibiotic	Duration
Ohm and Galask [65]	1973	48	Prospective, randomized, double-blinded	Cephaloridine and cephalexin	5 days
Ledger et al. [52]	1973	96	Prospective, randomized, double-blinded	Cephaloridine vs. cephaloridine and cephalexin	3 perioperative doses; Duration of hospitalization
Mayer et al. [58]	1974–1975	44	Prospective, randomized, not blinded	Cephalothin and kanamycin	2 days
Boyd and Garceau [9]	1969–1974	264	Prospective, not randomized, not blinded	Ampicillin	5 days
Glover and Nagell [33]	1971–1975	200	Prospective, randomized, not blinded	Ampicillin (started in recovery room)	1.5 days
Forney et al. [29]	1972–1975	32 conization, TVH	Prospective, randomized, double-blinded	Cephaloridine and cephalexin	6 (from preconization to 4 days after TVH)
Osborne et al. [70]	1971–1976	242	Not prospective, not randomized, not blinded	Cephalothin and cephalexin	3 perioperative doses; 5 days
Peterson et al. [71]	1972–1976	930	Prospective, not randomized, not blinded	Cephalothin	3 days
Clement [19]	1973	80	Not prospective, not randomized, not blinded	A cephalosporin	10 days

Table 2. (continued)

Authors	Dates of study	Total no. of patients	Study design	Antibiotic	Duration of therapy
Jackson and Amstey [46]	Not stated	147	Not prospective, not randomized, not blinded	Ampicillin or tetracycline	Immediately postop until discharge
Jennings [47]	1974–1975	91	Prospective, randomized, blinded	Cefazolin and cephalexin	Until foley out 24 h
Matthews et al. [59]	1975–1978	50	Prospective, randomized, blinded	Sulfamethoxazole-trimethoprim	1 dose IV
Holman et al. [45]	1975–1976	84	Prospective, randomized, double-blinded	Cefazolin	3 perioperative doses
Swartz and Tanaree [90]	1974–1975	96	Prospective, randomized, not blinded (excludes patients treated with suction drainage)	Cefazolin	3 perioperative doses
Lett et al. [54]	1974–1975	153	Prospective, randomized, double-blinded	Cefazolin vs cephaloridine	Single preop dose 3 perioperative doses
Ledger et al. [53]	1973	100	Prospective, randomized, double-blinded	Cephaloridine	3 perioperative doses

Roberts and Homesley [79]	1975–1977	52	Prospective, randomized, double-blinded	Carbenicillin	1 day
Wheeless et al. [96]	1973–1975	90	Prospective, randomized, double-blinded	Doxycycline	3 days
Mendleson et al. [61]	1977	66	Prospective, randomized, double-blinded	Cephradine vs. cephradine	Single preop dose / 1 preop dose and 4 postop doses
Grossman et al. [38]	1975–1977	78	Prospective, randomized, double-blinded	Penicillin vs. cefazolin	2 days / 2 days
Polk et al. [73]	1976–1978	86	Prospective, randomized, blinded	Cefazolin	3 perioperative doses
Hamod et al. [39]	Not stated	79	Prospective, randomized, not blinded	Cephalothin 3 gm IV / Cephalothin / Metronidazole	Single preop dose / 2 days / Preop night
Collins et al. [21]	1978–1979	50	Prospective, randomized, blinded	Cefazolin / ticarcillin	1 gm preop / 6 gm preop
Mickal et al. [103]	Not stated	125	Prospective, randomized, blinded	Cefoxitin	3 perioperative doses

Table 3. Clinical studies of antibiotic prophylaxis in vaginal hysterectomy – Effect on infectious morbidity.

Authors	Febrile morbidity			Pelvic infection			Comment
	Control	Drug	p Value	Control	Drug	p Value	
Goosenberg et al. [35]	31/40 (78%)	3/40 (8%) / 21/40 (53%)	<0.005 / <0.025				
Thomsen [93]	47/75 (63%)	3/95 (3%)	<0.005				'Infectious morbidity'
Allen et al. [2]	25/50 (50%)	2/48 (4%)	<0.001	19/50 (38%)	2/48 (4%)	<0.005	
Bolling and Plunket [8]	57/177 (32%)	9/119 (8%)	<0.005	48/177 (27%)	5/119 (4%)	<0.005	
Breeden and Mayo [10]	29/56 (52%)	6/64 (9%)	<0.001	11/56 (20%)	3/64 (5%)	<0.025	
Hedican and Sarto [41]				9/32 (28%)	8/38 (8%)	<0.05	'Vaginal cuff inflammation'
Harralson et al. [40]				19/100 (19%)	1/100 (1%)	<0.01	
Bivens et al. [6]	13/30 (43%)	4/30 (13%)	<0.01	6/30 (20%)	4/30 (13%)	NS	
Ohm and Galask [65]	11/23 (48%)	0/25 (1%)	≤0.005	8/23 (35%)	1/25 (4%)	<0.01	
Ledger et al.[52]		10/48 (21%) / 15/48 (31%)			5/48 (10%) / 8/48 (17%)		Cephaloridine / Cephaloridine cephalexin
Mayer et al. [58]	9/21 (43%)	2/23 (9%)	<0.05	5/21 (24%)	1/23 (4%)	NS	
Boyd and Garceau [9]	61/190 (32%)	2/74 (2%)	<0.001				
Glover and Nagell [33]	Not given		<0.001	18/100 (18%)	3/100 (3%)	<0.01	
Forney [29]	6/14 (43%)	0/18 (0%)	<0.05	4/14 (29%)	0/18 (0%)	<0.025	
Osborne et al. [70]	53/108 (49%)	3/35 (8.6%)	<0.001	46/108 (43%)	3/35 (8.6%)	<0.001	Cephalothin – 3 peri-operative doses
		10/99 (10%)	<0.001		10/99 (10%)	<0.001	Cephalothin and cephalexin × 5 days
Peterson [71]	189/597 (32%)	34/333 (10%)	<0.001	– (2%)	– (2%)	NS	

Study			p			p	
Clement [19]	14/16 (87%)	6/20 (30%)	<0.005				With repair
	12/24 (50%)	5/30 (24%)	NS				No repair
Jackson and Amstey [46]	72/106 (68%)	66/41 (39%)	<0.005				
Jennings [47]	32/43 (74%)	10/48 (21%)	<0.005	14/43 (33%)	1/48 (2%)	<0.005	
Mathews et al. [55]	16/50 (32%)	8/50 (16%)	NS				
Holman et al. [45]	13/44 (30%)	2/40 (5%)	<0.005	10/44 (23%)	0/40 (0%)	<0.005	
Swartz and Tanaree [90]	28/54 (52%)	10/42 (24%)	<0.005	9/54 (17%)	2/42 (5%)	NS	
Lett et al. [54]	25/51 (49%)	4/52 (8%)	<0.005				Single dose cefazolin
		6/50 (12%)	<0.005				3 doses cephaloridine
Ledger et al. [53]	23/50 (46%)	12/50 (24%)	<0.025	17/50 (34%)	4/50 (8%)	<0.005	
Roberts and Homesley [79]	9/26 (35%)	2/26 (8%)	<0.05	3/26 (12%)	0/26 (0%)	NS	
Wheeless et al. [96]	11/31 (36%)	4/59 (7%)	<0.005				
Mendleson [61]	16/22 (73%)	2/32 (9%)	<0.0005	14/22 (64%)	1/23 (4%)	<0.0005	Single dose
		0/21 (0%)	<0.0005		0/21 (0%)	<0.0005	Multidose
Grossman [38]	17/24 (71%)	5/26 (19%)	<0.005	6/24 (25%)	2/26 (8%)	NS	Penicillin
		5/28 (18%)	<0.005		1/28 (4%)	<0.025	Cefazolin
Polk et al [73]	13/42 (31%)	6/44 (14%)	<0.05	9/42 (21%)	1/44 (2%)	0.006	
Hamod and Spence [39]		0/23 (0%)			0/23 (0%)		Cephalothin – 1 dose
		2/30 (7%)			2/30 (7%)		Cephalothin – 2 days
		2/26 (8%)			1/26 (4%)		Metronidazole
Collins et al. [21]		6/50 (12%)			1/23 (4%)		Cefazolin
					1/27 (4%)		Ticarcillin
Mickal et al. [103]				17/57 (30%)	7/68 (10%)	<0.01	

NS not significant (p > .05)

while in six studies such a beneficial effect on pelvic infection was not seen. Interestingly, in the six studies where a statistically significant decrease in pelvic infection was not shown, antibiotic treatment *had* been shown to result in a significant decrease in febrile morbidity.

Five studies [39, 52, 54, 61, 70] compared short-term chemoprophylaxis (three perioperative doses or less) versus long-term therapy. All of these studies found no significant differences in clinical response between short-term and long-term regimens. Additionally, four studies evaluated single dose chemoprophylaxis. In three studies [39, 54, 61] where a single dose was compared to a multidose regimen, the single dose regimen was equally effective in preventing infectious morbidity. In the one study [55] where a single dose of antibiotic was compared with an untreated control group a statistically significant decrease in febrile morbidity was not found although febrile morbidity was halved.

It is currently popular to recommend prophylactic antibiotics for vaginal hysterectomy in premenopausal as opposed to postmenopausal women. One expects that the basis for this philosophy is probably the traditional view among gynecologists that the young premenopausal patient is at highest risk for increased operative blood loss and infectious morbidity [16, 91]. In 1966 Ledger published a review of adnexal abscesses at the Wayne County General Hospital in Michigan [101, 102] A startling finding was the observation that all of the postoperative adnexal abscesses included in their review had occurred in premenopausal women undergoing vaginal hysterectomy. These postoperative adnexal abscesses were not found in women undergoing total abdominal hysterectomy nor were they found in postmenopausal women undergoing vaginal hysterectomy. In response to these findings, Ledger designed a study of prophylactic chemotherapy in vaginal hysterectomy to include only premenopausal patients in the hope of preventing these serious infections. It is likely that these events initiated the presently held belief that prophylactic antibiotics are of a greater benefit to the premenopausal patient. It is, however, difficult to substantiate this belief in reviewing the published literature. Of the 32 studies summarized in Tables 2 and 3, 17 do not even address the variable of menopausal status, in six the number of postmenopausal patients studied are too few to allow statistical comparison to be made, and in eight only premenopausal patients were studied. In only one study was the variable of menopausal status considered, and in this paper it was not associated with either a difference in the incidence of infection in control patients, nor in the ability of the prophylactic antibiotic to prevent infection [9]. However, based on Ledger's initial observations, perhaps it would be of greater value to review the frequency of adnexal or pelvic abscesses (vaginal cuff abscesses not included) as a function of menopausal status. Of the 32 papers, 18 fail to mention postoperative adnexal or pelvic abscesses, apparently including them under the general category of pelvic infections. In seven papers, precise diagnoses were given but no abscesses were found. In the remaining seven studies, a total of 12 postoperative adnexal or pelvic abscesses were identified. Bivens noted a pelvic abscess in a 54-year-old control patient [6]; Ohm records a pelvic abscess in a 37-year-old patient who received antibiotics; Glover noted a right ovarian abscess in a patient who received antibiotics (menopausal status not given) [33]; Osborne found two pelvic abscesses in 108 control patients as compared to one pelvic abscess in 99 patients receiving antibiotics (all premenopausal) [70]: Holman found a single adnexal abscess in a control patient (menopausal status was not given) [45]; Ledger found three postoperative adnexal abscesses in 50 control patients as compared to 1 out of 50 drug patients (all premenopausal) [53]; and Roberts found one pelvic abscess out of 26 control patients [79]. Thus, there were eight pelvic abscesses recorded in control patients with one patient being postmenopausal, five premenopausal, and two with menopausal age not stated. There was a total of four abscesses in the patients who received antibiotics, three in premenopausal women, and one with menopausal age not stated. These data suggest that while postoperative adnexal and pelvic abscesses are more common in premenopausal women they can occur in the postmenopausal woman. Moreover, there appears presently to be no definitive data to support the concept that premenopausal women derive greater benefit from prophylactic antibiotics for vaginal hysterectomy than their postmenopausal sisters. In this context, Sprague and Van Nagell have noted in a large series from Kentucky that morbidity caused by pelvic infection was found to be more closely correlated with errors in operative technique than with the age or endometrial histology of the patient [100].

Perhaps the most striking finding in reviewing Table 3 is the close agreement between studies when incidence of pelvic infections for control groups or drug groups is compared. The 'reproducibility' of these data from study to study lends added weight to their significance. In summary, a global assessment of the presently published English literature would suggest that prophylactic antibiotics are able to effect a significant reduction in the rates of febrile morbidity and pelvic infection following vaginal hysterectomy. A short perioperative course, or even a single dose, is as effective as long-term prophylaxis and will reduce cost, risk of toxicity, and rate of emergence of resistant organisms. Whether premenopausal women benefit more than postmenopausal women is presently unclear.

Abdominal hysterectomy

Tables 4 and 5 present the studies concerning antibiotic prophylaxis for total abdominal hysterectomy published in the English literature between 1968 and 1980. Eighty-seven percent of these studies were prospective, 87% were

20

Table 4. Clinical studies of antibiotic prophylaxis in total abdominal hysterectomy – Experimental design.

Authors	Dates of study	Total no. of patients	Study design	Antibiotic(s)	Duration of therapy
Rosenheim [80]	1968–1970	200	Not prospective, not randomized, not blinded	Ampicillin (85) or tetracycline (15)	5 days
Allen et al. [2]	1970–1971	168	Prospective, randomized, blinded	Cephalothin	5 days
Clement [19]	1973	66	Not prospective, not randomized, not blinded	A cephalosporin	10 days
Ohm and Galask [67]	1973–1974	93	Prospective, randomized, blinded	Cephaloridine and cephaloxin	5 days
Wheeless et al. [96]	1973–1975	52	Prospective, randomized, blinded	Doxycycline	3 days
Swartz and Tanaree [90]	1974–1975	135	Prospective, randomized, not blinded	Cefazolin	3 perioperative doses
Jennings [47]	1974–1975	102	Prospective, randomized, not blinded	Cefazolin and cephalexin	'Until Foley out 24 h'
Holman et al. [45]	1975–1976	80	Prospective, randomized, blinded	Cefazolin	3 perioperative doses

Mathews et al. [57]		59	Prospective, randomized, blinded	IV sulfamethoxazole-trimethoprim	1 dose
Mayer et al. [58]	1974–1975	56	Prospective, randomized, not blinded	Cephalothin and Kanamycin	2 days
Mathews et al. [56]	1975–1977	100	Prospective randomized blinded	Cephaloridine	3 perioperative doses
Roberts and Homesley [79]	1975–1977	47	Prospective randomized blinded	Carbenicillin	1 day
Grossman et al. [38]	1975–1977	239	Prospective randomized blinded	Penicillin vs.	2 days
				Cefazolin	2 days
Polk et al. [73]	1976–1978	429	Prospective randomized blinded	Cefazolin	3 perioperative doses
Applebaum et al. [99]		94	Prospective randomized blinded	Metronidazole	7 days

Table 5. Clinical studies of antibiotic prophylaxis in total abdominal hysterectomy – Effect on infectious morbidy.

Authors	Febrile morbidity			Pelvic infection			Wound infection			Hospital stay	
	p Value	Control	Drug	p Value	Control	Drug	p Value	Control	Drug	Control	Drug
Rosenheim [80]	11/100(11%)	3/100(3%)	<0.05	3/100(3%)	2/100(2%)	NS	0/100(0%)	1/100(0%)	NS	5.7	6.6
Allen et al. [2]	34/83(41%)	12/185(14%)	<0.001	11/83(13%)	7/85(8%)	NS	7/83(8%)	0/85(0%)	<.01		
Clement [19]	12/30(40%)	13/36(36%)	NS							5.8	5.9
Ohm and Galask [67]	18/46(39%)	7/47(15%)	<0.01	5/46(11%)	3/47(6%)	NS	2/46(4%)	3/47(0%)	NS	7.4	7.2
Wheeless et al. [96]	2/15(13%)	0/37(0%)	<0.025								
Swartz and Tanaree [90]	18°/78(23%)	9°/57(16%)	<0.05	6°/78(8%)	2/57(4%)	NS	1/78(1%)	0/78(0%)	NS		
Jennings [47]	24/52(46%)	12/50(24%)	<0.04							9.1	8.0
Holman et al. [45]	17/38(45%)	6/42(14%)	<0.005	7/38(18%)	1/42(2%)	<.025	6/38(16%)	1/42(2%)	<0.05	8.5	6.9
Mathews et al. [57]	12/29(41%)	12/30(40%)	NS	4/29(14%)	1/30(3%)	NS	7/29(24%)	7/30(23%)	NS		
Mayer et al. [58]	14/28(50%)	8/28(8%)	NS	2/28(7%)	0/28(0%)	NS	7/28(25%)	8/28(28%)	NS		
Mathews et al. [56]	9/49(18%)	2/51(4%)	<0.025	7/49(14%)	2/51(4%)	NS	11/49(22%)	0/51(0%)	<0.005		
Roberts et al. [79]	12/22(54%)	1/25(4)	<0.025	1/22(5%)	0/25(0%)	NS	2/22(9%)	1/25(4%)	NS	10.5	7.7
Grossman et al. [38]	22/84(26%)	24/76(32%)	NS	5/84(6%)	2/76(3%)	NS	4/84(5%)	2/76(3%)	NS	6.9	7.2
		28/79(35%)	NS		5/79(6%)	NS		4/79(5%)	NS	6.9	7.1
Polk et al. [73]	45/223(20%)	29/206(14%)	<0.05	14/223(6%)	11/206(5%)	NS	14/223(6%)	4/206(2%)	<0.05	8.6	8.2
Applebaum et al. [99]				4/50(8%)	1/54(2%)	NS	21/50(42%)	7/54(13%)	<0.005		

NS not significant (p > 0.05)

randomized and 67% were double-blinded. Failure to provide uniform definitions of infection-related morbidity is a problem with this series of cases as it was for the vaginal hysterectomy series. For these abdominal hysterectomies, I have used three parameters of infectious morbidity: technical febrile morbidity, pelvic infection (cuff abscess, pelvic cellulitis, pelvic abscess, adnexal abscess, septic pelvic thrombophlebitis), and abdominal wound infection. Additionally, the duration of the hospitalization is given as another indirect measure of the efficacy of chemoprophylaxis.

Prophylactic antibiotics successfully decreased the incidence of febrile morbidity in 10 of 15 studies, pelvic infection in only one of 13 studies, and abdominal wound infection in five of the 13 studies.

In eight studies where the incidence of febrile morbidity was significantly decreased, pelvic infection and wound infection data were recorded. In four cases, febrile morbidity was decreased but neither the incidence of pelvic infection nor wound infection was decreased. In one case febrile morbidity decreased and the incidence of both pelvic infection and wound infection decreased. In no cases in which febrile morbidity decreased did the incidence of pelvic infection alone decrease. These data suggest to me that prophylactic antibiotics for total abdominal hysterectomy are most effective at decreasing technical febrile morbidity and have little effect on the prevention of pelvic infection. There seems to be an intermediate effect upon the prevention of wound infection.

In the nine studies where information was available concerning the duration of hospitalization, five patients who received prophylactic antibiotics had a shorter stay while four were hospitalized for a longer period of time than those patients not receiving chemoprophylaxis. Reference to Table 5 shows little difference between duration of hospital stay for control or drug treated patients, and the true clinical significance of these slight differences is open to question.

Table 6 compares duration of chemoprophylaxis against the results from each of the 15 studies relative to successful prevention of the various parameters of infectious morbidity. Review of these data suggests that, when chemoprophylaxis was found to be effective for reducing morbidity of total abdominal hysterectomy, a short perioperative course lasting no longer than one day was optimal.

In regard to menopausal status as a predictor of benefit from prophylactic antibiotics in total abdominal hysterectomy, 13 of the 15 studies failed to address the question. Holman found a decrease in the infection rate among postmenopausal women from 37% to 20%; this was not statistically significant [45]. Jennings had too few patients in his postmenopausal group to achieve statistical significance but again a trend toward fewer infections was observed [47] As with vaginal hysterectomy, the question of menopausal status awaits further evaluation.

Table 6. Successful reduction of infectious morbidity vs. duration of chemoprophylaxis (TAH).

Duration of chemoprophylaxis	Studies where infectious morbidity prevented		
	Febrile morbidity	Pelvic infection	Wound infection
1 dose	0/1	0/1	0/1
≤ 1 day	5/5	1/5	3/5
2–3 days	1/4	0/3	0/3
5–10 days	3/4	0/4	2/4

To summarize, the data suggesting a beneficial effect of prophylactic antibiotics in total abdominal hysterectomy are considerably less compelling than those for vaginal hysterectomy. A majority of studies have found a decrease in the incidence of febrile morbidity but this does not seem to be achieved through prevention of specific pelvic infection. There does seem to be a modest decrease in abdominal wound infection when prophylactic antibiotics are utilized. It is this author's belief that the value of prophylactic antibiotics for total abdominal hysterectomy is still unproven. Until more definitive studies appear, each institution must individualize their decision to use prophylactic antibiotics for total abdominal hysterectomy, and this decision must be based on their past experience with the infectious morbidity associated with this surgical procedure.

In many of the studies reported diagnostic categories are too imprecise to allow one to judge the impact of 'infectious morbidity' on the patient. An exception to this is the report of Swartz where infectious morbidity was carefully defined [88]. Minor morbidity was defined as a temperature greater than 100.4 for two days, while major infection was defined as a hospital stay more than 14 days, re-operation or re-admission for the management of pelvic abscess or pelvic thrombophlebitis. After a retrospective analysis of some 668 consecutive cases using T-tube suction drainage and/or prophylactic antibiotics as infection prophylaxis for hysterectomy. Swartz concluded the following: (1) minor febrile morbidity as defined frequently followed abdominal hysterectomy (incidence of 20–30%) and vaginal hysterectomy (incidence of 30–50%): (2) minor febrile morbidity had temporary but significant consequences in the form of increased patient discomfort, medical staff effort, and financial cost; (3) major infections were rare following abdominal hysterectomy (less than 0.5%) and uncommon following vaginal hysterectomy (1–4%). This paper raises an interesting question. Should the value of prophylactic antibiotics be judged solely by their ability to prevent serious infections, or should their ability to reduce minor febrile morbidity and its consequences be a consideration as well? Swartz, and others, have shown that major infectious morbidity occurs predominantly following vaginal hysterectomy as opposed to total abdominal hysterectomy. Thus, if the prevention of major infectious morbidity was the sole criterion for choosing prophylactic antibiotics, one might exclude their use for total abdominal hysterectomy. However, Swartz has further demonstrated that the prevention of minor febrile morbidity can result in identifiable gains in terms of patient comfort, decreased medical staff effort, and financial costs. Ultimately, this decision must be based on a comparison of the risks of chemotherapy versus the benefits described.

Radical pelvic surgery

Gynecologic oncological procedures including anterior, posterior, and total exenteration, as well as radical hysterectomy with lymph node dissection, are commonly accompanied by serious postoperative infectious morbidity. In the case of posterior and total exenteration in which bowel resection and colostomy are involved, studies in the general surgical literature are supportive of the use of antibiotic prophylaxis. Although antibiotic prophylaxis is commonly used in patients undergoing radical hysterectomy and pelvic and paraaortic lymph node dissection, there are no controlled studies which have evaluated chemoprophylaxis in this setting. Gall has recently reported a prospective, randomized, double-blind, placebo controlled investigation of cefamandol prophylaxis in patients undergoing total abdominal hysterectomy, bilateral salpingo-oophorectomy, and pelvic and paraaortic lymph node sampling. There were 25 patients in each of the drug and placebo groups. Sixty percent in the placebo group developed postoperative febrile morbidity and 36% were judged to have serious infections. Twenty percent in the cefamandol group developed febrile morbidity and only 8% were diagnosed as having serious infections. Although the surgery described in this report is not particularly extensive or 'radical,' this represents the first effort to apply a sound methodological approach to the study of antibiotic prophylaxis in gynecologic patients undergoing extended surgical procedures [30].

Infertility surgery

Postoperative infection in the patient undergoing tuboplasty has grave consequences with regard to subsequent fertility. Moreover, some surgeons utilize antiinflammatory agents to prevent adhesions following tubal surgery and are concerned that such use may increase the frequency or severity of postoperative infection. Accordingly, infertility patients undergoing tubal surgery commonly have received prophylactic antibiotics. Until recently there have been no controlled, scientifically valid studies to support the use of prophylactic antibiotics in this clinical situation. However, an unpublished report by Seigler et al., quoted by Schwarz [81], is said to show that in a controlled series of tubal surgical procedures without the use of antiinflammatory agents, febrile morbidity was not only very low but was, in fact, no different in controls than in patients receiving prophylactic antibiotics. Based on this preliminary information, prophylaxis in infertility surgery cannot be supported.

Elective abortion

Although never officially advocated, it is likely that prophylactic antibiotics are commonly used at the time of elective first trimester abortion. Only one published study bears upon this problem. Hodgson studied 4000 women undergoing first trimester abortions [44]. Alternate subgroups of 1000 consecutive patients were given oral tetracycline and complications associated with abortion were analyzed in those receiving antibiotics and in the 2000 controls. Major complications were defined as all instances of hospitalization or fever of 38° C or greater for three days or longer. Minor complications included fever of 38° C for more than 24 but less than 72 h and complaints of cramps and bleeding. Minimal complications consisted of reported temperature elevations of 38° C or higher and were of less than 72 h duration. Both major, minor, and minimal complications were reduced in those phases of the study when patients were receiving prophylactic tetracycline. Corroboration of this report of beneficial effects of prophylactic antibiotics for patients undergoing elective first trimester abortion awaits the appearance of additional controlled and double-blinded studies.

There are also no firm guidelines for SBE prophylaxis in women with underlying cardiovascular lesions undergoing elective out-patient abortion. For these brief out-patient procedures, two approaches have been suggested although the value of neither has been subjected to controlled evaluation. One approach has been to give a single dose of antibiotics 30 min prior to the procedure, omitting the two additional doses usually prescribed (see p. 4). Since enterococci are the most frequent causes of endocarditis after these procedures, a second approach has been to utilize oral ampicillin begun approximately two hours prior to the procedure and continued for 2 or 3 doses following the abortion.

Late hematogenous infection in total joint replacement

Joint replacement has become so commonplace that gynecologists can soon expect to be performing gynecologic surgical procedures on patients who have prosthetic joints. Transient asymptomatic bacteremia may lead to metastatic infection at the site of the prosthetic joint with serious results requiring subsequent surgery or resulting in loss of function and even mortality [105] At present, no guidelines or recommendations for administration of prophylactic antibiotics for patients with prosthetic joints undergoing procedures associated with transient bacteremia have been promulgated. However, guidelines similar to those used for SBE prophylaxis may be useful in preventing infection in these prosthetic joints.

Prophylactic antibiotics for hysterosalpingography

Stumpf and March have reviewed the subject of febrile morbidity following hysterosalpingography [87]. In their uncontrolled retrospective series, prophylactic ampicillin or tetracycline failed to prevent pelvic infection after HSG in 9 of 140 patients. Traditional laboratory tests such as ESR's did not predict patients at risk. The authors developed a scoring system to evaluate patients for the risk of post HSG infection and suggest that the procedure be avoided in high risk patients but that prophylactic antibiotics with anaerobic coverage be considered for patients with intermediate risk. One can question whether these infections following HSG represent new infections or exacerbations of chronic disease. If the latter is true, treatment regimens are probably called for rather than prophylaxis.

Useless or Harmful Chemoprophylaxis

Indwelling catheters

Although antibiotics protect against transient bacteremia at the time of urethral manipulation, they cannot prevent the development of bacteriuria after the insertion of an indwelling catheter. Whether or not one employs a systemic antibiotic or constantly irrigates the bladder with an antibiotic solution, the incidence of bacteriuria remains the same if the catheter stays in the bladder for any period of time. Thus, almost all workers agree that prophylactic systemic antimicrobial therapy is of little value for the patient with an indwelling catheter except in very unusual circumstances [50]. Moreover, the use of prophylactic antibiotics to 'cover' a catheter may well result in the selection of more virulent and antibiotic-resistant bacteria.

Hospital acquired pneumonia

The administration of antibiotics by any route for prolonged periods not only will not decrease the likelihood that a patient will develop a hospital-acquired pneumonia, but will select our antibiotic resistant organisms that pose great therapeutic difficulties [75].

COMPLICATIONS OF PROPHYLACTIC ANTIBIOTIC THERAPY

It should be clear that the decision to employ antibiotic prophylaxis cannot be based solely upon the ability of this therapy to prevent serious postoperative infectious morbidity. One must also consider the potential risks of such therapy. As we have shown above, prophylactic antibiotics correctly utilized can do much good. Unfortunately, harm can result from their use as well. When it is recognized that from one-fourth to one-half of all use of anti-microbial agents in hospitals is for the prevention rather than the treatment of infection [48, 51, 78, 82], the importance of considering chemoprophylactic toxicity becomes readily apparent. We will consider four theoretical concerns relating to prophylactic antibiotic therapy: Alteration of hospital flora, alte-ration of microflora of treated patients, antimicrobial toxicity, and cost.

The development of bacterial resistance is presently a subject of great concern, especially as regards transfer of resistance between bacteria by means of R factors (also called episomes, resistance transfer factors or plas-mids) [60]. While transfer of resistance is important in continually widening the range of organisms resistant to antibiotics, it is selection pressure that maintains the high incidence of these strains in the environment. There is abundant evidence that once a resistant cell has emerged, the selective pres-sure of antibiotic therapy will lead to displacement of the sensitive population by the resistant [32, 74, 77, 83, 92]. Since selection is a direct result of, and proportional to, antibiotic usage, it is inevitable that increased usage of antibiotics for any reason, including prophylaxis, will increase the resevoir of resistant bacteria by increasing selection pressure. The clinical consequences of this are twofold: (1) The emergence of resistant resident strains of or-ganisms within a hospital; (2) the occurrence of clinically significant alte-rations of flora within individual patients (superinfection).

Alteration of Hospital Flora

Two examples serve to illustrate the effect of selection pressure on the resident flora of a hospital. Moellering and associates, using a computerized system, found a significant increase in the prevalence of gentamicin resistance, and increase in nosocomial infections due to gentamicin resistant organisms, with increasing use of the agent at Massachusetts General Hospital [62]. Mc-Gowan and associates showed an increased prevalence of antibiotic re-sistance among gram negative bacilli isolated from the bloodstream of pa-tients with nosocomial infection when compared with organisms isolated from blood of patients with community acquired infection [59]. Many other examples have been recorded as well.

Despite the obvious importance of careful epidemiologic surveillance of clinical trials of antibiotic prophylaxis in pelvic surgery, only one such study has appeared in the literature [37]. In an attempt to assess adverse selection pressures upon resident flora exposed to prophylactic antibiotics at the Yale-New Haven Hospital, Grossman reviewed cephalothin susceptibility of all isolates of *E. coli* in adult and pediatric in-patients for selected quarters of the years 1973 through 1976. A clinical trial of prophylactic penicillin or cefazolin for hysterectomy had been started in early 1975. Over 5000 first site isolates were tabulated, of which approximately 10% came from the gynecologic service. Cephalothin susceptibility of isolates from the gynecologic service was compared with isolates from the nongynecologic service. *E. coli* was selected as the index organism because it was the most frequent gram negative nosocomial isolate. The results of this study were equivocal. Large scale antibiotic prophylaxis was not in effect on the gynecological service during the initial phases of the study but the number of *E. coli* resistant to cephalothins in both gynecologic and nongynecologic patients increased significantly at this time, probably secondary to the widespread use of cephalothins in the hospital population. During the last four quarters of the study, with the antibiotic study in progress, *E. coli* cephalothin resistant appeared to stabilize with the exception of one quarter where it was significantly increased in the gynecologic service. Although no firm conclusions were drawn from the study, it represents the first realistic effort to monitor the effect of a large prophylactic antibiotic protocol on susceptibility patterns of resident flora in a single hospital.

Institutions considering prophylactic antibiotic programs for any service should conduct epidemiologic surveillance of resident flora and patterns of infection. Susceptibilities of hospital flora to antibiotics in frequent use should be determined and reviewed on a regular basis. Grossman has correctly emphasized the fact that antibiotic prophylaxis must be beneficial to its recipients without being detrimental to others [37].

Alteration of Microflora of Treated Patients

A second concern associated with the selection pressure of prophylactic antibiotic therapy involves the risks of clinically significant alterations of flora within individual patients. Several examples from the Obstetric Gynecologic literature can be cited to illustrate this potential complication of prophylactic antibiotic therapy. Gibbs and Weinstein noted significant alterations in the flora of febrile patients who received clindamycin-gentamicin prophylaxis for cesarean section [31]. When patients were given only two doses of this combination for prophylaxis, the endometrial flora samples 48–96 h later consisted almost entirely of enterococci and *E. coli*. Work and Ledger found that in women receiving prophylactic cephalothin who nevertheless developed a serious post-cesarean section infection, *Bacteroides* was consistently recovered from the infection site [97]. *Bacteroides* was not recovered from those women with serious post-section infections who had received a placebo. Ohm and Galask, utilizing meticulous bacteriologic techniques, reported on alterations of microbial flora in patients undergoing abdominal [68] and vaginal [66] hysterectomy. Changes in cervical-vaginal flora occurred following surgery with or without the use of prophylactic cephalosporins. In the abdominal hysterectomy group, aerobic gram negative rods which were generally susceptible to cephalosporins were isolated from the post-operative patients who received placebo, while species of *Pseudomonas* and *Enterobacter* increased in patients receiving active drugs. In the vaginal hysterectomy series there were similar findings of an increased frequency of isolation of cephalosporin resistant gram negative rods (*Enterobacter* and *Pseudomonas* species) in the patients receiving cephalosporins, as well as an increased isolation of *Bacteroides fragilis* and group D streptococci from both groups.

Grossman has reported on the vaginal flora of women undergoing hysterectomy with cefazolin or penicillin prophylaxis [36]. Although he concluded that the changes in pre-operative versus post-operative flora were similar among antibiotic treated and placebo treated groups, reference to his paper shows an increase in the isolation of group D streptococci from the treated patients. Phelan, reporting on a double blind study of cefazolin prophylaxis for cesarean section, found the group D streptococcus to be the predominant organism in postoperative cultures from the cefazolin treated group [106]. Finally, Hill evaluated perioperative changes in the vaginal flora of patients undergoing vaginal hysterectomy with cephalosporin prophylaxis. She found an increased rate of isolation of *Klebsiella, Enterobacter* species, *Bacteroides bivius*, and *Bacteroides fragilis* in the discharge cultures as compared with admission cultures. Moreover, antibiotic susceptibility of the anaerobic gram negative rods to cephalothins and ampicillin decreased from approximately 75% on admission cultures to 50% on discharge cultures. Her conclusion was that the vaginal flora in patients receiving cephalosporin prophylaxis change in composition to more closely reflect the species commonly found in infection [42].

To summarize, virtually all authors have shown that changes in the cervical-vaginal flora occur following surgery with or without the use of prophylactic antibiotics. It is important, however, to note a difference between the placebo and active drug groups in regard to the change in flora. In the placebo groups most authors have documented an increased isolation rate of antibiotic susceptible aerobic gram negative rods. In the active drug groups, the shift in flora has been toward a potentially more virulent and antibiotic resistant group, namely *Enterobacter* species, *Pseudomonas aeruginosa, Bacteroides* species, and group D streptococci. In some cases this shift in flora represents only asymptomatic colonization, while in others it has resulted in clinical infectious morbidity. Clearly, these studies showing a shift of flora in patients receiving prophylactic antibiotics toward potentially dangerous organisms argue at the very least for short courses of chemoprophylaxis, and may even raise questions of the wisdom of using prophylactic antibiotic therapy in situations other than those unequivocally proven to be of unquestioned benefit.

ANTIMICROBIAL TOXICITY

Two cases have recently been reported in which prophylactic intraoperative administration of cephalothin was associated with anaphylactoid reactions and death [84]. Both of these patients were undergoing orthopedic procedures under general anesthesia and received the cephalothin intravenously. I am aware of an additional case (unreported) again involving anaphylactoid reaction and death in a woman undergoing a gynecologic procedure under general anesthesia who received prophylactic intravenous cephalothin intraoperatively. Whether these cases represent delayed recognition of an immediate drug allergy or are a unique manifestation of intravenous cephalothin in patients under general anesthesia is presently unknown. Until this is further clarified, it would seem prudent to avoid giving the initial dose of any antibiotic intravenously to a patient under general anesthesia. Other deaths from antibiotic prophylaxis have been reported as well [15].

Aside from the question of mortality, even brief courses of antimicrobial agents for prophylaxis are capable of resulting in anaphylaxis, renal failure, hemolysis, jaundice, hearing loss, aplastic anemia, etc. All of these risks must be weighed carefully before one embarks upon a program of antibiotic prophylaxis for any given surgical procedure.

Costs

Although cost is commonly mentioned as an issue of concern in the use of prophylactic antibiotics, it is readily evident that the prevention of even minor degrees of infectious morbidity, with consequent decrease in hospital costs, will usually result in savings much greater than the expense of the prophylactic antibiotics themselves. A relatively simple evaluation of the cost of prophylaxis, and one which is rarely performed, is an assessment of the total use of antimicrobial agents. Routine prophylaxis may reduce the number of infections to the point that the total amount of antimicrobial agents used (both for prophylaxis and for the treatment of infections that do occur) is less when such prophylaxis is used. If routine prophylaxis results in less total antimicrobial use than would occur without it, both the financial and ecologic costs are decreased. As Hirschmann has pointed out, the demonstration of such a reduction would provide compelling evidence for the net benefits of prophylaxis [43].

CONCLUSIONS

Conclusions concerning the benefits of antimicrobial prophylaxis in gynecologic surgery must remain somewhat tentative. The effectiveness of chemoprophylaxis for vaginal hysterectomy seems now to be unequivocally documented. Efficacy in other situations is considerably less clear due to both a paucity of available studies and/or methodological inadequacies in those studies which have been performed. Whether the reduction of postoperative infectious morbidity achieved with prophylactic antibiotics can be equalled or surpassed by other techniques designed to reduce these complications (e.g. pre-operative hot conization [70], interoperative application of an aerosolized antibiotic [98], or postoperative suction drainage [90]) remains to be seen.

The risks of prophylactic antibiotic therapy thus far appear to be small, but diligent monitoring for such toxicity remains essential. More studies assessing the total use of antibiotics on a service, and those performing meticulous epidemiologic surveillance are urgently needed.

Finally, it should be stressed that antibiotic prophylaxis is only one component of the care of the gynecologic patient, and certainly not the most important one. Our goal should be the performance of indicated surgery, skillfully carried out in the operating room, in patients whose pre- and postoperative courses are managed by intelligent, conscientious, compassionate physicians. In certain situations, antibiotic prophylaxis can complement such care, but it can never replace any portion of it.

ACKNOWLEDGEMENT

The author wishes to acknowledge the assistance of Tahamura Ashikaga, Ph.D. who performed the statistical analyses.

REFERENCES

1. Alexander JW, Altemeier WA: Penicillin prophylaxis of experimental staphyloccal wound infections. Surg Gynecol Obstet 120:243, 1965
2. Allen JL, Rampone JF, Wheeless CR: Use of a prophylactic antibiotic in elective major gynecologic operations. Obstet Gynecol 39:218, 1972
3. Bartlett JG, Onderdonk AB, Durde E: Quantitative bacteriology of the vaginal flora. J Infect Dis 136:271, 1977.
4. Berger SA, Nagar H, Gordon M: Antimicrobial prophylaxis in obstetric and gynecologic surgery – a critical review. J Reprod Med 24:185, 1980.
5. Berger SA, Nagar H, Weitzman S: Prophylactic antibiotics in surgical procedures. Surg Gynecol Obstet 146:469, 1978
6. Bivens MD, Neufeld J, McCartly WC: The prophylactic use of Keflex and Keflin in vaginal hysterectomy. Am J Obstet Gynecol 122:169, 1975

7. Blahey P: Experiences with terramycin in urinary and genital tract infections. Can Med Assoc 66:151, 1952

8. Bolling DR, Plunkett GD: Prophylactic antibiotics for vaginal hysterectomies. Obstet Gynecol 41:689, 1972

9. Boyd ME, Garceau R: The value of prophylactic antibiotics after vaginal hysterectomy. Am J Obstet Gynecol 125:581, 1976

10. Breeden JT, Majo JE: Low dose prophylactic antibiotics in vaginal hysterectomy. Obstet Gynecol 43:379, 1974

11. Burke JF: The effective period of preventive antibiotic action in experimental incisions and dermal lesions. Surgery 50:161, 1961

12. Burke JF: Preoperative antibiotics. Surg Clin North Am 43:665, 1963

13. Burke JF: Preventive antibiotic management in surgery. Ann Rev Med 24:289, 1973

14. Byar OB, Simon RM, Friedwald WT, et al.: Perspectives on some recent issues. N Engl J Med 295:74, 1976

15. Carter ET: Possible role of streptomycin in postoperative deaths of two patients. Q Bull Northwest Univ M School 23:27, 1949

16. Chehab HE: Decreasing the morbidity of vaginal hysterectomy. Obstet Gynecol 31:198, 1968

17. Chodak GW, Plaut ME: Use of systemic antibiotics for prophylaxis in surgery. A critical review. Arch Surg 112:326, 1977

18. Chodak GW, Plaut ME: Wound infections and systemic antibiotic prophylaxis in gynecologic surgery. Obstet Gynecol 51:123, 1978

19. Clement JE: Prophylactic antibiotics in hysterectomy. NC Med J 36:542, 1975

20. Cobbs CG: IUD and endocarditis. Ann Intern Med 78:451, 1973

21. Collins MS, Kreutner AK, DelBene VE: Single dose prophylaxis for vaginal hysterectomy. Presented at George Washington University, Washington, D.C., May 31, 1980

22. Cron RS, Stauffer J, Paegel H, Jr: Morbidity studies in one thousand consecutive hysterectomies. Am J Obstet Gynecol 63:344, 1952

23. DeSwiet, MD, Ramsey ED, Rees GM: Bacterial endocarditis after insertion of intrauterine contraceptive device. Br Med J 3:76, 1975

24. Duff P, Park RC: Antibiotic prophylaxis in vaginal hysterectomy: a review. Obstet Gynecol 55:193S, 1980

25. (Editorial) Antibiotic accountability. N Engl J Med 301:380, 1979

26. Everett ED, Hirshmann JF: Transient bacteremia and endocarditis prophylaxis: A review. Medicine 56:61, 1977

27. Everett ED, Reller LB, Droegemueller W, et al.: Absence of bacteremia after insertion or removal of intrauterine devices. Obstet Gynecol 47:207, 1976

28. Falk HC, Bunkin IA: A study of 500 vaginal hysterectomies. Am J Obstet Gynecol 52:623, 1946

29. Forney JP, Morrow CP, Townsend DE, et al.: Impact of cephalosporin prophylaxis on conization-vaginal hysterectomy morbidity. Am J Obstet Gynecol 125:100, 1976

30. Gall SA, Hill GB, Creasman WT: The efficacy of prophylactic antibiotic in radical gynecologic surgery. Presented at George Washington University, Washington, D.C., May 31, 1980

31. Gibbs RS, Weinstein AJ: Bacteriologic effects of prophylactic antibiotics in cesarean section. Am J Obstet Gynecol 126:226, 1976

32. Gibson CD, Jr, Thompson WC, Jr: The response of burn wound staphylococci to alternating programmes of antibiotic therapy. Antibiot Annu 1955–56, p. 32

33. Glover MW, Nagell JR: The effect of prophylactic ampicillin on pelvic infection following vaginal hysterectomy. Am J Obstet Gynecol 126:385, 1976

34. Gorback SL, Menda KB, Thadepalli H, et al.: Anaerobic microflora of the cervix in healthy women. Am J Obstet Gynecol 117:1053, 1973

35. Goosenberg J, Emich JP, Schwarz RH: Prophylactic antibiotics in vaginal hysterectomy. Am J Obstet Gynecol 105:503, 1969

36. Grossman JH, Adams RL: Vaginal flora in women undergoing hysterectomy with anti-

biotic prophylaxis. Obstet Gynecol 53:23, 1979
37. Grossman JH, Adams RL, Hierholzer WJ: Epidemiologic surveillance during a clinical trial of antibiotic prophylaxis in pelvic surgery. Am J Obstet Gynecol 128:690, 1977
38. Grossman JH, Greco TP, Minikin MJ, et al.: Prophylactic antibiotics in gynecologic surgery. Obstet Gynecol 53:537, 1979
39. Hamod KA, Spence MR, Rosenshein NB, et al.: Single-dose and multidose prophylaxis in vaginal hysterectomy: a comparision of sodium cephalothin and metronidazole. Am J Obstet gynecol 136:976, 1980
40. Harralson JD, Van Nagell JR, Roddick JW, et al.: The effect of prophylactic antibiotics on pelvic infection following vaginal hysterectomy. Am J Obstet Gynecol 120:1046, 1974
41. Hedican RE Jr, Sarto GE: Use of prophylactic antibiotic and vaginal cuff inflammation. J Iowa Med Assoc 66:374, 1976
42. Hill GB, Kohan AO, Ayers OM, et al.: Peri-operative changes in the vaginal flora. Presented at George Washington University, Washington, D.C., May 31, 1980
43. Hirschmann JF, Invi TS: Antimicrobial prophylaxis: a critique of recent trials. Reviews Inf Dis 2:1, 1980
44. Hodgson JE, Major B, Portmann K, et al.: Prophylactic use of tetracycline for first trimester abortions. Obstet Gynecol 45:574, 1975
45. Holman JF, McGowan JE, Thompson JD: Perioperative antibiotics in major elective gynecologic surgery. South Med J 71:417, 1978
46. Jackson C, Amstey MS: Prophylactic ampicillin therapy for vaginal hysterectomy. Surg Gynecol Obstet 141:755, 1975
47. Jennings RH: Prophylactic antibiotics in vaginal and abdominal hysterectomy. South Med J 71:251, 1978
48. Jones, SR, Barks J, Bratton T, McRee E, Pannell J, Yanchick VA, Browne R, Smith JW: The effect of an educational program upon hospital antibiotic use. Am J Med Sci 273:79, 1977
49. Kaplan EL, Anthony BR, Bisno A, et al.: Prevention of bacterial endocarditis. Circulation 56:139A, 1977
50. Kunin CM: *Detection, Prevention and Management of Urinary Tract Infections*, Lea & Febiger, Phila., 1974, p. 147
51. Kunin CM, Tupasi T, Craig WA: Use of antibiotics: a brief exposition of the problem and some tentative solutions. Ann Intern Med 79:555, 1973
52. Ledger WJ, Gee C, Lewis WP: Guidelines for antibiotic prophylaxis in gynecology. Am J Obstet Gynecol 121:1038, 1975
53. Ledger WJ, Sweet RL, Headington JT: Prophylactic cephaloridine in the prevention of postoperative pelvic infections in premenopausal women undergoing vaginal hysterectomy. Am J Obstet Gynecol 115:766, 1973
54. Lett WJ, Ansbacher R, Davison BL, et al.: Prophylactic antibiotics for women undergoing vaginal hysterectomy. J Reprod Med 19:51, 1977
55. Mathews DD, Agarwal V, Gordon AM, Cooper J: A double-blind trial of single-dose chemoprophylaxis with co-trimoxazole during vaginal hysterectomy and repair. Br J Obstet Gynecol 86:717, 1979
56. Mathews DD, Agarwal V, Ross H: A randomized controlled trial of a short course of cephaloridine in the prevention of infection after abdominal hysterectomy. Br J Obstet Gynaecol 85:381, 1978
57. Mathews DD, Ross H, Cooper J: A double blind trial of single-dose chemoprophylaxis with co-trimoxazole during total abdominal hysterectomy. Br J Obstet Gynaecol 84:894, 1977
58. Mayer W, Gordon M, Rothbard MJ: Prophylactic antibiotics: use in hysterectomy. NYS J Med 76:2144, 1976
59. McGowan JE, Garner C, Wilcox C, et al.: Antibiotic susceptibility of gram-negative bacilli isolated from blood cultures. Am J Med 57:225, 1974
60. Mead PB: Prophylactic antibiotics and antibiotic resistance. Seminars in Perinatol 1:101, 1977

35

61. Mendleson J, Portnoy J, Victor JR, et al.: Effect of single and multidose cephradine prophylaxis on infectious morbidity of vaginal hysterectomy. Obstet gynecol 53:31, 1979
62. Moellering RC, Jr, Wennersten C, Kunz LJ, et al.: Patterns of emerging resistance in gentamicin among bacteria in a general hospital. 15th Interscience Conference on Antimicrobial Agents and Chemotherapy, 1975 (Abstr)
63. Murillo J, Standiford H, Tatem B, et al.: Parenteral antibiotic combinations for prophylaxis against enterococcal endocarditis (abstr). 17th Interscience Conference on Antimicrobial Agents and Chemotherapy, 1977
64. O'Grady FW: Chemoprophylaxis in medicine and surgery. J R Coll Physicians Lond 6:203, 1972
65. Ohm JM, Galask RP: The effect of antibiotic prophylaxis on patients undergoing vaginal operations – I. Am J Obstet Gynecol 123:590, 1975
66. Ohm MJ, Galask RP: The effect of antibiotic prophylaxis on patients undergoing vaginal operations – II. Am J Obstet Gynecol 123:597, 1975
67. Ohm MJ, Galask RP: The effect of antibiotic prophylaxis on patients undergoing total abdominal hysterectomy. I. Effect on morbidity. Am J Obstet Gynecol 125:442, 1976
68. Ohm MJ, Galask RP: The effect of antibiotic prophylaxis on patients undergoing total abdominal hysterectomy. II. Alterations of microbial flora. Am J Obstet Gynecol 125:448, 1976
69. Osborne NG, Wright RC: Effect of preoperative scrub on the bacterial flora of the endocervix and vagina. Obstet Gynecol 50:148, 1977
70. Osborne NG, Wright RC, Dubay M: Preoperative hot conization of the cervix. Am J Obstet Gynecol 133:374, 1979
71. Peterson LF, Justema EJ, Wiersma AF, et al.: Comparative efficacy of preoperative and postoperative cephalothin therapy in vaginal hysterectomy. Curr Ther Res 22:792, 1977
72. Polk HC, Lopez-Mayor JF: Postoperative wound infection. Surgery 66:97, 1969
73. Polk BF, Shapiro M, Goldstein P, et al.: Randomized clinical trial of perioperative cefazolin in preventing infection after hysterectomy. Lancet 1:437, 1980
74. Price DJE, Sleight JD: Control of infection due to Klebsiella aerogenes in a neurosurgical unit by withdrawal of all antibiotics. Lancet 2:1213, 1970
75. Quintiliani R: Modern approaches to antibiotic chemophrophylaxis. Infectious Disease Practice 3:(3)8, 1979
76. Regetz MJ, Starr SE, Dowell VR, Jr, et al.: Absence of bacteremia after diagnostic biopsy of the cervix. Chemoprophylactic implications. Chest 65:223, 1974
77. Richmond MH: Some environmental consequences of the use of antibiotics: Or 'What goes up must come down.' J Appl Bacteriol 35:155, 1972
78. Roberts AW, Visconti JA: The rational and irrational use of systemic antimicrobial drugs. Am J Hosp Pharm 29:828, 1972
79. Roberts JM, Homesley HD: Low-dose carbenicillin prophylaxis for vaginal and abdominal hysterectomy. Obstet Gynecol 52:83, 1978
80. Rosenheim GE: Prophylactic antibiotics in elective abdominal hysterectomy. Am J Obstet Gynecol 119:335, 1974
81. Schwarz RH: Antibiotic prophylaxis in obstetrics and gynecology. Postgrad Obstet Gynecol 1:1, 1979, Williams and Wilkins Co., Baltimore, Md
82. Shapiro M, Townsend TR, Rosner B, Kass EH: Use of antimicrobial drugs in general hospitals. Patterns of prophylaxis. N Engl J Med 301:351, 1979
83. Shulman JA, Terry PM, Hough CE: Colonization with gentamicin-resistant Pseudomonas aeruginosa, pyocine type 5, in a burn unit. J Infect Dis 124:S18, 1971
84. Spruill FG, Minette CJ, Sturner WQ: Two surgical deaths associated with cephalothin. JAMA 229:440, 1974
85. Stone HH, Haney BB, Kolb LD, et al.: Prophylactic and preventive antibiotic therapy. Ann Surg 189:691, 1979
86. Stone HH, Hooper CA, Kolb LD, et al.: Antibiotic prophylaxis in gastric, biliary, and colonic surgery. Ann Surg 184:443, 1976
87. Stumpf PG, March CM: Febrile morbidity following hysterosalpingography: identifi-

36

cation of risk factors and recommendations for prophylaxis. Fertil Steril 33:487, 1980

88. Swartz WH: Prophylaxis of minor febrile and major infectious morbidity following hysterectomy. Obstet Gynecol 54:285, 1979

89. Swartz WH, Tanaree P: Suction drainage as an alternative to prophylactic antibiotics for hysterectomy. Obstet Gynecol 45:305, 1975

90. Swartz WH, Tanaree P: T-tube suction drainage and/or prophylactic antibiotics. Obstet Gynecol 47:665, 1976

91. Taylor ES, Hansen RR: Morbidity following vaginal hysterectomy and colpoplasty. Obstet Gynecol 17:346, 1961

92. Thomas FE, Leonard JM, Alford RM: Serious infections due to hospital-acquired multiple-resistant Serratia marcescens. Clin. Res 23:53A, 1975

93. Thomsen RJ: Prophylactic antibiotics for vaginal surgery: a historical addendum. Am J Obstet Gynecol 125:270, 1976

94. Turner SJ: The effect of penicillin vaginal suppositories on morbidity in vaginal hysterectomy and on the vaginal flora. Am J Obstet Gynecol 60:806, 1950

95. Weinstein L: Infective endocarditis prophylaxis in penicillin-sensitive patients. JAMA 240:2485, 1978

96. Wheeless CR, Dorsey JH, Wharton LR: An evaluation of prophylactic doxycycline in hysterectomy patients. J Reprod Med 21:146, 1978

97. Work B, Ledger WJ: The use of prophylactic cephalothin in women undergoing emergency cesarean section (abstr). 9th International Congress of Chemotherapy, 1975

98. Wright VC, Lanning NM, Natale R: Use of a topical antibiotic spray in vaginal surgery. Can Med J 118:1395, 1978

99. Appelbaum PC, Moodley J, Chatterton SA, et al.: Metronidazole in the prophylaxis and treatment of anaerobic infection. S Afr Med J 54:703, 1978

100. Sprague AD, Van Nagell JR: The relationship of age and endometrial histology to blood loss and morbidity following vaginal hysterectomy. Am J Obstet Gynecol 118:805, 1974

101. Ledger WJ, Campbell C, Willson JR: Postoperative adnexal infections. Obstet Gynecol 31:83, 1968

102. Ledger WJ, Campbell C, Taylor D, Willson JR: Adnexal abscess as a late complication of pelvic operations. Surg Gynec Obstet 129:973, 1969

103. Mickal A, Curole D, Lewis C: Cefoxitin sodium – Double blind vaginal hysterectomy prophylaxis in premenopausal patients. Obstet Gynecol 56:222, 1980

104. Harris G, Marraro RV, Ugenas AJ: Bacteremia or pelvic infection – a consequence of gynecologic biopsies? Am J Obstet Gynecol 136:408, 1980

105. Lattimer G, Keblish PA, Dickson TB, Vernick CG Finnegan WJ: Hematogenous infection in total joint replacement – recommendations for prophylactic antibiotics. JAMA 242:2213, 1979

106. Phelan JP, Pruyn SC: Prophylactic antibiotics in cesarean section – a double blind study of cefazolin. Am J Obstet Gynecol 133:474, 1979

Author's address:
Department of Obstetrics and Gynecology,
University of Vermont, College of Medicine,
Burlington, Vermont 05405
U.S.A.

2. PHARMACOKINETICS OF ANTIBIOTICS IN THE PREGNANT WOMAN

AGNETA E.L. PHILIPSON, M.D.

Dosage schedules for antibotics should be based upon pharmacokinetic studies. Such studies provide knowledge about serum, tissue, and urine levels which may be obtained in a patient with various dose sizes or with different routes of administration of an antibiotic. The dosage schedule should also take into account the sensitivity pattern of the infecting organism. Thus, the appropriate dosage for each patient should be the one which will produce antibiotic levels in serum and tissues sufficiently high to combat an infection caused by microorganisms with a sensitivity pattern that renders them amenable to treatment with the antibiotic in question. The pharmacokinetic studies on which dosage recommendations are based have been carried out in healthy volunteers as well as in patients with various diseases, but for obvious reasons they are never carried out in pregnant women.

However, it is well known that infections which require antibiotic treatment are far from uncommon during pregnancy. The infection may be confined to maternal tissues only as with pharyngitis, pyclonephritis, pneumonia, or, as in the case of syphilis, involve the fetus as well. In the first case the main concern in the choice of dose and route of administration should be to obtain adequate serum and tissue levels of antibiotic in the infected maternal tissue, not so low to be ineffective in which case the patient's suffering from the infection will be prolonged, and not too high which might increase the risk of adverse effects and unduly expose the fetus. In the case where the fetus is infected as well it is vital that sufficiently high levels of antibiotic are reached and maintained in fetal tissues in order for the infection to be cured effectively. If, on the other hand, the pregnant woman has a genital infection which may rise and reach the amniotic fluid it is crucial that a satisfactory level of antibiotic is reached in the amniotic fluid following administration to the pregnant patient without any unnecessary delay.

When infections that require treatment occur during pregnancy most physicians will prescribe antibiotics in the same dosage as is used in the treatment of nonpregnant patients, or possibly they will even lower the dosage because of fear of harmful effects either to the pregnant woman or to the fetus. However, it is quite clear that the same ratio between the minimum inhibitory concentration (MIC) of the infecting organism and the tissue level of antibiotic is desirable in pregnant as in nonpregnant patients. Thus, if the

W.J. Ledger (ed.), Antibiotics in Obstetrics and Gynecology, 37–60. All rights reserved.
Copyright © 1982 by Martinus Nijhoff Publishers, The Hague/Boston/London. ISBN-13:978-94-009-7466-1

pharmacokinetics of an antibiotic is altered during pregnancy, thereby increasing or decreasing serum and tissue levels that result from a certain dose size, the dosage schedule will have to be adjusted accordingly as to size of the dose or route of administration, in order not to make the treatment of a pregnant woman less satisfactory than had she not been pregnant.

Considering the great physiological changes, that occur within most organ systems during the course of pregnancy, some very early and some progressing with time [1] it seems obvious that several pharmacokinetic parameters will be influenced, the reasons being the same for antibiotics as for other drugs [2, 3], and hence that dosage requirements will not be the same for pregnant as for nonpregnant women.

What is said above will hopefully illustrate why it is extremely important to gain extensive knowledge of pharmacokinetics of antibiotics in pregnancy, i.e. serum and tissue levels, excretion, as well as transplacental passage and possibly acumulation. Data obtained from studies carried out in men and nonpregnant women may not be applicable to pregnant women without thorough investigation and monitoring.

In spite of the obvious need for knowledge about the behaviour of antibiotics in pregnancy little has been published on this subject compared to what is known about pharmacokinetics of antibiotics in man by and large. Many articles on antibiotics in pregnancy fall into either of the three categories: 1) Retrospective studies of possible or definite harmful effects of an antibiotic to the pregnant woman or to the fetus, or 2) Prospective treatment studies, usually on urinary tract infections or 3) Studies that qualitatively demonstrate the transplacental passage of an antibiotic. Only rather few studies concern themselves with pharmacokinetics. The most extensive encyclopedia on antibiotics, the Antibiotika-Fibel by Walter and Heilmeyer [4] provides very little help as to dosage of antibiotics for the phycisian who wants to treat an infection in a pregnant patient.

The use of most new antibiotics is discouraged during pregnancy due to lack of knowledge of possible harmful effects, and some of the older ones are known or suspected of such effects. Therefore it is essential that the antibiotics which have either been in use for a long time without suspicion of increased toxicity during pregnancy or are known to be safe are handled and prescribed in such a skilled way as to compensate for the decreased antibiotic armamentum and provide optimal cure and protection of infections during pregnancy. This can be achieved only by gaining detailed knowledge of pharmacokinetics. The whole concept of pharmacokinetics as such is fairly new and the shortage of pharmacokinetic data in pregnancy is of course due to technical as well as to ethical problems related to such studies.

TECHNICAL PROBLEMS

Conclusions on the pharmacokinetics of a drug in humans must be based on data from several individuals who should all be healthy, in the same condition, or suffering from the same disorder, the possible influence of which on one or more of the pharmacokinetic parameters is known or possible to evaluate. Also, meaningful information can only be obtained for antibiotics which may be accurately measured, are not metabolized, or have metabolites which can be assayed. Thus, when pharmacokinetics in pregnancy is studied and antibiotic levels in serum or plasma are assayed standards should preferably be prepared in plasma or serum from pregnant women. A minimal requirement is to confirm that a standard prepared in such serum – because of possible differences in protein content which may imply an alteration in the protein binding – does not perform differently in the assay than the actual standard to be used. Likewise, studies which involve the determination of fetal plasma levels of an antibiotic appropriately call for standards prepared in fetal plasma, as drugs may bind differently to fetal and adult plasma [5, 6]. When bioassays are used to determine antibiotic levels, the activity in the assay is produced by the free fraction. However, the result of the assay is expressed as the total level of drug, i.e. free as well as unbound, because the sample is read against a standard which has been made up in the same kind of body fluid and consequently has the same degree of protein binding as the sample. A lower degree of protein binding in fetal serum or plasma will give falsely high values for fetal levels if read against a standard with a higher degree of protein binding and vice versa. The technical problems involved in the monitoring of fetal tissue levels of antibiotic are innumerable; freeing the tissue from blood, extracting the antibiotic from the tissue in order to make it measurable, and selecting proper standards being a few.

Animal studies will not provide pertinent data due to differences between species in duration of pregnancy, in anatomy, in histology, and in physiology.

To enable an adequate comparison between pharmacokinetics of a drug in pregnant and in nonpregnant individuals the need for a control group is indisputable as variations in antibiotic serum levels between pregnant women may be tremendous. The controls must be matched for age, weight, sex, and possibly for medical condition as well. Samples to be assayed have to be treated in an identical way as certain antibiotics will deteriorate within weeks even when stored at $-20°$.

ETHICAL PROBLEMS

Over the last ten years ethical aspects on human as well as on animal studies righfully have more and more been brought into focus. This is particularly true for studies on pregnant women. It is considered unethical to give to a pregnant woman, especially if she wants to proceed with her pregnancy, any antibiotic solely for study purposes. The medication has to be medically indicated. Certain accurate methods for determination of excretory capacity, metabolism, or volumes of distribution which are carried out with radioactive substances clearly should not be employed in pregnant women, and the use of radioactively labeled antibiotics is evidently out of question for the same reasons.

However, there is another ethical aspect that can be argued on drug studies during pregnancy. Is it ethical *NOT* to perform such studies? Can it be considered ethical to give to a pregnant woman any drug for which the pharmacokinetics during pregnancy is not known? Many drugs that might have been beneficial in the treatment of pregnant women may not be considered for such treatment because of lack of knowledge of performance in pregnancy, thus depriving the pregnant woman of as good a treatment as someone who is not pregnant.

In view of the fact that pharmacokinetics of many drugs most likely will have changed, the pregnant patient may be either undertreated or overtreated if a dosage is used that has been calculated from studies performed on men or nonpregnant women.

PHARMACOKINETICS IN PREGNANCY

Several reasons for alternations in drug kinetics in pregnancy have been discussed [2]. Dose requirements of certain drugs are known to change when the patient becomes pregnant and as pregnancy proceeds [3]. Even for antibiotics, pharmacokinetics will most likely change as pregnancy advances, and the changes may successively become more pronounced. The gradual improvement of renal function will probably increase the elimination rate and thus lower the serum levels of antibiotics which are renally excreted, although this change may be reversed during the last six weeks of gestation when the creatinine clearance decreases significantly [7]. Altered drug metabolism [8] may well influence pharmacokinetics of antibiotics which are metabolized and as a consequence increase or decrease the serum levels. Serum levels may also be altered in pregnant patients, the extent depending on the distribution properties of each antibiotic and on the increase of blood volume at each stage of pregnancy. For antibiotics with a small volume of distribution levels may be affected differently than for antibiotics with a large volume of distribution.

Little precise data are available on pharmacokinetics of antibiotics during pregnancy. Most studies intended to provide such data include investigations of the transplacental passage and have been carried out at the time of abortion, labor and delivery, or caesarean section. When evaluating the results derived from such studies it must be borne in mind that the data may not be representative for any stage of pregnancy except precisely abortion, labor, or caesarean section.

Abortion – by surgery or otherwise – as well as labor and caesarean section will most likely affect renal excretion, blood perfusion through various organs, as well as other mechanisms which regulate drug pharmacokinetics. The stress involved for most patients may be an important factor as such. Gastrointestinal absorption of antibiotics administered orally at such occasions may be impaired as well. Other pharmaceutical compounds which are often administered during labor or surgery may affect the pharmacokinetics of an antibiotic and this influence is difficult to evaluate.

Antibiotic levels found in amniotic fluid and fetal serum, plasma, or fetal tissues following administration of the drug to a woman in labor must be evaluated with precaution. Pronounced changes of the haemodynamics due to contractions of the uterus will most likely impair the placental transfer of a drug.

PRESENT KNOWLEDGE OF PHARMACOKINETICS OF ANTIBIOTICS IN PREGNANCY

In spite of the numerous problems involved, several investigations of pharmacokinetics of antibiotics in pregnancy have been carried out according to various protocols. Maternal levels of antibiotic in plasma or serum have been studied following single or multiple doses, mostly prior to abortion, delivery, or caesarean section. In some studies serial serum levels have been studied in the same patients whereas in other studies only the serum level at the time of delivery was studied. In the latter type of studies serum concentration versus time curves have been constructed from single values from a great number of patients through variations of the dose-delivery interval. Also, the presentation of data is widely diverging, thus making comparisons between results obtained in different studies difficult. Evaluation of whether or not serum levels, excretion, or other parameters for a particular antibiotic differ during pregnancy from what may be known for nonpregnant individuals or from what could be expected is difficult or often impossible. However, several antibiotics have been studied and some interesting information has accumulated. That more studies have been carried out on β-lactam antibiotics than on aminoglycosides and other antibiotics probably reflects the more frequent need for such antibiotics during pregnancy. In the review below the author assumes that the reader is familiar with terms such as area under the serum level versus time curve (AUC), apparent volume of distribution (V_D), bioavailability, and half-life of elimination (T 1/2). The values for T 1/2, when not available in the original publication, have been deduced from the terminal slope of the plotted serum level versus time curves, i.e. the part of the curve which follows the distribution phase in a two compartment model.

β-LACTAM ANTIBIOTICS

Isoxazolyle Penicillins

Serum levels of methicillin following a single i.v. dose have been studied in women 32–40 weeks pregnant or in labor [9, 10]. Similar studies have been published for dicloxacillin where a dose of 500 mg was administered to women in labor [9, 11]. According to MacAulay et al. T 1/2 for dicloxacillin was 2 h. The maternal serum levels reported in these studies of dicloxacillin differ considerably. On the basis of these two studies it is not possible to determine if the pharmacokinetics of methicillin or dicloxacillin is altered in pregnancy. However, after administration of methicillin, serial serum levels were reported to be generally lower in three women in active labor than in one man and one nonpregnant woman who were used as controls [9].

Pharmacokinetic parameters for oxacillin have been studied in 12 women 38–41 weeks pregnant at the time of amniocenteses [12]. Following a single i.v. dose of 2 g the calculated serum level at time zero (C_0) was 79 μg/ml, the elimination constant was 1.044 h^{-1}, T 1/2 was 40 min, V_D was 25.31, and the total clearance of drug 441 ml/min. The authors point out that in their study the values for V_D and clearance are higher than those found in other studies performed in nonpregnant individuals. The calculations were based on observations during the first 2 h. following dose administration.

Ampicillin

Ampicillin in pregnancy has been subjected to more studies than any other antibiotic, most often though with regard to its transplacental passage. When comparing studies where the same size of dose and route of administration have been used it is obvious that the mean serum levels differ widely from one study to another (Table 1). The actual figures for serum levels are not always given but have then been interpolated from graphs.

In one of these studies T 1/2 is approximately 46 min as calculated from the graph [15]. It has also been reported to be 30 min at caesarean section [17], 40 min at delivery [18], and 40 min in the 8th month of gestation as opposed to 58 min in women in labor [19]. These discrepancies may in part be due to a difference in the study groups, for instance eight months pregnancy versus

Table 1. Mean values reported in various publications for levels of ampicillin in serum and plasma (μg/ml) in pregnant women at 1, 2 and 3 h following a single i.v. dose of 500 mg. Figures within brackets represent the number of patients for which the mean was calculated. Standard deviations (SD) are given when available (50).

Time after dosage						Reference
1 h	SD	2 h	SD	3 h	SD	
6.3 (4)	2.2	1.0 (2)	0.1	0.6 (1)		13
7.9 (13)		4.5 (13)		3.4 (13)		14
15.0 (8)		6.0 (4)		2.8 (3)		15
6.2 (26)	2.14	1.9 (26)	0.9	0.7 (26)	0.4	16

labor, but also to different protocols and methods for calculations of T 1/2. V_D for ampicillin during labor or surgery in late pregnancy was found to be 0.23 l/kg [18].

That certain pharmacokinetic parameters of ampicillin change in pregnancy has been demonstrated in a crossover study in 26 women, 9–36 weeks pregnant, with lower urinary tract infections [16]. Ampicillin was administered as a single dose of 0.5 g i.v. as well as orally. Each woman served as her own nonpregnant control and received identical doses after pregnancy when lactation had ceased and normal menstruations reappeared. Plasma levels were found to be 50% lower in pregnant women than in the same women when they were not pregnant. Some other relevant data are shown in Table 2. These findings have been confirmed in a study where ampicillin was given intramuscularly to 14 pregnant and to six healthy nonpregnant controls in a dose of 10 mg/kg [20]. Also in this study a significant difference was found in several pharmacokinetic parameters. In the pregnant women the values for V_D and clearance were larger and the values for serum levels and AUC lower than in the nonpregnant women, whereas there was no significant difference in the absorption rate. Further studies have shown that subsequent doses of ampicillin 0.5 g during a ten days course of oral therapy give similar levels in plasma and urine as the initial oral dose and that no accumulation of drug occurs [21]. By increasing the dose of ampicillin to 1.0 g the plasma levels in pregnant women were brought up to levels somewhat exceeding those produced in nonpregnant women by a dose of 0.5 g. In the same study pivampicillin was found to produce plasma levels of the same magnitude during pregnancy as those produced by twice the equimolar dose of oral ampicillin, thus indicating lower serum levels in pregnant than in nonpregnant women following administration of pivampicillin as well. Following the onset of labor, however, attained blood levels could not be maintained despite repeated administration of pivampicillin [22]. This finding was interpreted as a result of impaired absorption from the intestine and stomach.

Table 2. Mean values and SD for apparent volume of distribution (V_D), T 1/2, bioavailability, renal clearance (Cl_R), and recovery in urine of ampicillin in 26 women during and after pregnancy, following identical doses (16).

	V_D (1/kg)	T 1/2 (min.)	Bio- availability (%)	Cl_R ml/min.	Recovery in urine % of i.v. dose
in urine					
During pregnancy	0.55	39	45.6	330	79.4
SD	0.28	8.1	20.2	(137–535)*	24.7
After pregnancy	0.41	44	48.1	238	79.5
SD	0.20	6.8	19.3	(85–425)*	30.6
P-value	<0.05	<0.05	Not significant	<0.01	Not significant

* Range within which 90% of the values were found

CEPHALOSPORINS

Over the last ten years several cephalosporins have been studied in pregnant women. Rarely though has any cephalosporin been subjected to more than one study.

Cephalexine levels in serum were studied in 15 women following a single oral dose of 1 g administered at the time of caesarean section [23]. The peak serum level was found 1.75 h after drug administration, which is later than has been reported in nonpregnant individuals, and the mean serum levels reported were lower than those found in other subjects following the same dose [4]. The later peak may well be attributed to delayed absorption, caused by pregnancy itself or by the preoperative state of the patients.

Cephaloridine was administered in single i.m. dose of 1 g to 70 women and 2 g to 35 women with ruptured membranes and produced serum levels that appeared to be similar to those which have been found in other studies in nonpregnant individuals [24].

Cephalothin administered i.v. or i.m. as a single dose of 1 g to women at term [25, 26] produced serum levels that are considerably lower than one would expect [4].

Studies on the pharmacokinetics of cephalothin at term or at the time of delivery have been carried out by MacAulay and Charles [27] and by Bastert et al. [28]. In the first study an i.v. dose of 1 g was administered to 54 women. Maternal serum was sampled at delivery which took place 9–810 min later. A serum concentration versus time curve was constructed from the 54 individual observations. The elimination constant was calculated to be 86×10^{-4} which gives a T 1/2 of 1.3 h. This value is different from the value of approximately 40 min which is found in nonpregnant populations [4]. C_0 was

30.2 μg/ml. Calculations of clearance from plasma give a value of 285 ml/min.

In the study by Bastert et al. [28] cephalothin was given as a single i.v. dose of 2 g to 25 women 38–41 weeks pregnant at the time of amniotomy. Serum levels were assayed and a regression line was made up based only on the serum levels during the first 2 h following dose administration. C_0 was 63.8 μg/ml, T 1/2 31 min., V_D 0.31 l/kg, and total clearance from serum 687 ml/min. Even in these two studies the mean serum levels of cephalothin in pregnant women appear to be lower than what would be expected [4].

Cefazolin serum levels have been studied at the time of interruption of pregnancy in 40 women who were 8–20 weeks pregnant. The drug was administered as a single i.m. dose of 14 mg/kg body weight. Serum levels were measured and they were found to be 23–55% lower than what had earlier been reported for nonpregnant adults following a similar dose [29]. T 1/2 in this study was 1.5 h which is 25% shorter compared to the T 1/2 of 2 h found in nonpregnant individuals [4].

In a study of cefatrizin, a single oral dose of 1 g was administered prior to abortion and was found to produce a wide range of serum levels at 1 h in women who were 8–20 weeks pregnant. Less variation was found at 2, 4, and 8 h [30]. T 1/2 was 2.4 h. The authors state that this is 1 h longer than in healthy adult males but similar to what has been found in infected hospitalized patients. The authors believe that the difference in T 1/2 is due more to an ambulatory or hospitalized state of the patient than to pregnancy itself. This may be true, although it would be interesting to have the corresponding data for pregnant women who are *not* undergoing surgery.

Cefacetrile has been studied in women in labor. The drug was given i.v. to 13 patients as a continuous infusion of 500 mg/h or i.v. as repeated bolus doses of 1 g every 2 h to 15 women. The continuous infusion gave a serum level of about 30 μg/ml. This was lower than the calculated level which was aimed at with the chosen dosage [31].

Cephradine 1.0 g was given as a single i.v. dose to seven women at the time of delivery and the resulting serum levels were studied. The mean serum levels at 1 h and 2 h were 6 μg/ml and 1.8 μg/ml respectively which was found to be lower than one would have expected [32]. In another study, cephradine was administered as a single dose of 0.5 g i.v. as well as orally to ten women who were 12 to 19 weeks pregnant and to the same women after pregnancy when the normal menstrual cycle had been reestablished and breast-feeding had ceased. Plasma levels were found to be 25–50% lower in pregnant than in nonpregnant women, T 1/2 was 29 min in pregnancy as opposed to 41 min after pregnancy. V_D was larger and plasma clearance significantly higher in pregnancy whereas there was no difference in bioavailability [33].

When Cefoxitin was given as a single dose of 2 g i.v. to five women 38–41 weeks pregnant or with premature rupture of the membranes [34] it produced serum levels which were similar to those which were produced in healthy adult males by half that dose [35].

Cefuroxime, when given as a single i.m. injection of 750 mg to 16 women who were either in labor or undergoing caesarean section [36], produced mean serum levels which are much lower than have been found in other populations following administration of the same dose [37, 3]. In another study cefuroxime was given as a single i.v. dose of 750 mg to seven women when they were 11–35 weeks pregnant and to the same women when they were in labor as well as after pregnancy when they served as their own nonpregnant controls. In this study significant differences in certain pharmacokinetic parameters were observed for pregnant as compared to nonpregnant women. Plasma levels were lower and consequently AUC as well. The values of V_D, plasma clearance, and recovery in urine were larger but T 1/2 was significantly shorter. Differences in the same direction although less consistent and less pronounced were observed in some of these parameters at delivery as compared to earlier in pregnancy [39].

CLINDAMYCIN

Maternal serum levels of clindamycin following administration of a single i.v. dose of 600 mg have been studied in 54 women undergoing caesarean section [40]. In another study the same drug was given as single or multiple oral doses of 450 mg to 22 women who were undergoing abortion, and the resulting levels in serum and urine were assayed [41]. In the first study T 1/2 can be estimated to approximately 1.3 h from the serum concentration versus time plot. This is shorter than 1.5–3. h which has been found in nonpregnant individuals [4]. It was pointed out in these two studies that the serum levels of clindamycin in pregnant women were similar to those which had been reported by other authors from studies in nonpregnant populations.

ERYTHROMYCIN

Serum levels of erythromycin were studied in 17 women at the time of abortion. The drug was given as single or muliple doses of erythromycin estolate 500 mg. The variation in serum levels between individuals after single as well as after multiple doses was found to be more than tenfold. The mean serum levels were considerably lower than those that had previously been reported in men following administration of the same or similar doses [41].

AMINOGLYCOSIDES

Very few studies have been published on aminoglycosides that enable any pharmacokinetic parameters to be calculated, a fact that most probably reflects the rare need for these antibiotics during pregnancy.

Gentamicin

Eighty mg of gentamicin was administered as a single i.m. injection to 58 women at the time of caesarean section. The mean serum level at 30 min was low, only 2 μg/ml. Subsequent serum levels during 8 h following dose administration were also consistantly lower than those observed in nonpregnant individuals [40]. An estimation of T 1/2 from the serum concentration versus time plot gives a value of 2 h. This is within the range of what has been found in nonpregnant individuals [4]. Serum levels of gentamicin were found to be lower than had been expected from the calculated dose per kg body weight also when a constant infusion of the antibiotic was given to women in late pregnancy [42].

Kanamycin

Serum levels of kanamycin after administration of a single i.m. dose of 500 mg to 27 women at term or in labor have been reported [43]. The levels are low in comparison to what has been found in other subjects. T 1/2 estimated from the serum concentration versus time curve is approximately 2 h which is in accordance with what is found in other populations [4].

Amikacin

Amikacin in a dose of 7.5 mg/kg body weight and administered i.m., was found to give lower serum levels than in nonpregnant adults when administered at the time of hysterectomy to 30 women 6–20 weeks pregnant. T 1/2 was 2 h which was somewhat shorter than had been expected [44].

Tobramycin

Tobramycin in a dose of 2 mg/kg body weight was administered i.m. to 35 women prior to therapeutic abortion. T 1/2 was found to be 1.54 h and the mean peak serum level was 4.0 μg/ml at 1 h after injection [45]. The authors state that these data are within the ranges reported by others for nonpregnant adults. However, they are definitely on the low side [4].

THIAMPHENICOL

In an interesting study by Plomp et al. [46]. thiamphenicol was given as a single i.v. dose of 500 mg to 29 women at term. Plasma levels of the antibiotic were determined at the time of delivery in samples drawn synchronously from a maternal artery and a maternal vein. T 1/2, as estimated from the maternal venous plasma concentration versus time curve, is approximately 1.3 h, a low value compared to those reported in other populations [4]. However, the authors find the plasma levels in their study comparable to those observed by others in nonpregnant individuals. A very interesting observation in this study is that maternal thiamphenicol levels were higher in arterial plasma than in venous plasma. The difference probably reflects the size of the loss in the capillary bed from diffusion, metabolism, binding to tissues, and renal excretion.

NITROFURANTOIN

Levels of nitrofurantoin in serum and urine following an oral dose of 100 mg were measured during 10 h in 16 nonpregnant women and in 30 pregnant women undergoing abortion [47]. In half of the pregnant women but only in three of the 16 nonpregnant women the serum levels were too low to be measurable. This fact indicates that nitrofurantoin serum levels are generally lower in pregnancy. The recovery of drug in urine was somewhat higher for pregnant than for nonpregnant women.

SULFAMETHOXAZOLE/TRIMETHOPRIM

Before entering a discussion of the actual data for pharmacokinetics of sulfamthoxazole/trimethoprim (SMX/TMP) it should be noted that the optimal antimicrobial effect of the combination SMX/TMP is generally considered to be achieved when the drugs are present in a ratio of approximately 20:1. The recommended dosage in the combined therapy has a ratio of 5:1 and is chosen so as to give the 20:1 ratio after absorption and distribution.

Also, it is well worth pointing out that studies in which the combination SMX/TMP is given are actually to be regarded as crossover studies in the sense that two different drugs with independent pharmacokinetics are given to the same subjects under identical conditions. Thus, such studies provide very special information.

Following a single oral dose of TMP 80 mg and SMX 400 mg serum levels of both drugs were studied in ten women, 8–20 weeks pregnant, at the time of abortion [48]. The mean peak serum level was found 4 h after dose administration. The mean SMX/TMP ratio was reported to be about 35:1. T 1/2 of TMP was 11 h which was found to agree well with what had been found in nonpregnant subjects. If, however, T 1/2 is calculated for the elimination phase only, and not from the time of the peak, after which abortion continues, the value is slightly over 6 h. The similarly extrapolated value for SMX is just over 9 h which should be compared with a mean value of 10.7 h found in nonpregnant individuals [4]. Urinary recoveries of TMP and SMX were not reported in this study. However, it is likely that the shorter T 1/2 of the drugs is due to an increased renal clearance during pregnancy, although altered metabolism of TMP cannot be excluded as part of the cause. The faster net disappearance from maternal serum of TMP than of SMX found in this study will help to explain the high SMX/TMP ratio. The ratio is actually 34:1 at 2 h following dose administration and has increased to 42:1 at the time of the last observation at 12 h. There is no evidence in this study that pregnant women differ from other populations in respect to mean serum levels of either drug.

In a study by Reid et al. [49] seven pregnant women were given a total oral dose of SMX 4.6 g and TMP 960 mg in divided doses every 12 h over 36 to 48 h prior to abortion (9–22 weeks of gestation). Levels of both drugs were measured in serum and urine at the time of the operation which took place 8 to 12 h following administration of the last dose.

The ratio between mean maternal serum levels of SMX and TMP at the time of operation was 23:1 but between individuals the ratio at that time varied from 10:1 to 58:1. The ratio between mean levels in maternal urine was 4:1 with variations from 1:1 to 14:1.

The mean SMX/TMP ratio in maternal serum at the time of operation was close to the ideal of 20:1 in contrast to the less favourable mean ratio in maternal urine. The great difference in SMX/TMP ratio of serum levels between pregnant women may be caused by individual alterations in distribution volume during pregnancy, more pronounced for one of the drugs than for the other. Also, both drugs are mainly eliminated through renal excretion and due to surgery, pregnancy, or both, the rate of excretion of one drug may be more altered than of the other, thus contributing to shifting the ratio in serum as well as in urine either way.

Renal excretion may also be influenced by possible alterations during pregnancy in the protein binding of the two drugs. In nonpregnant individuals the degree of protein binding of TMP is 42 to 46% and of SMX 68%. If the binding is altered differently for TMP and SMX as to quality or quantity the renal excretion is likely to be influenced, since only unbound drug is available for excretion. If the metabolism of TMP is altered during pregnancy, increased or decreased, this would also affect the serum levels and ratios.

Only a limited number of studies have been published in which it is suggested or from which it can be suspected that serum levels of antibiotics in pregnant women deviate from those found in other populations. Table 3, a revision from an earlier publication [50], summarizes these studies. The overall impression from available data is that the serum levels of many antibiotics are lower during pregnancy.

It is tempting to assume that lower serum levels are caused by an increased renal clearance of drug, due to improved renal function in pregnancy. Another apparent explanation for lower serum levels in pregnant women than in other individuals is the increased volumes of plasma and body water which will be reflected in a larger V_D during pregnancy, as has been shown for some antibiotics. Most antibiotics have been shown to pass the placenta and to be distributed to the fetus and amniotic fluid, thus possibly contributing to lowering the maternal serum levels. The transplacental passage, however, will not substantially lower maternal serum levels or augment the value for V_D, at least not up to the time of mid-pregnancy, since the uterus with its content at this stage of pregnancy accounts for only 18% *of the increase* in body weight [51]. At term the corresponding figure is of course higher, but still, a substantial part of the weight increase is due to larger volumes of plasma and body water.

NEED FOR STUDIES INCLUDING CONTROLS

Proper judgement of possible differences in pharmacokinetic parameters due to pregnancy must be based on drug studies which include adequate controls. Actual discrepancies due to pregnancy may not be revealed when results obtained in studies on pregnant women are compared with results obtained in other studies performed on nonpregnant individuals, unless observed parameters are strikingly different. However, some authors have pointed out for certain antibiotics that individual variations in serum levels are greater among pregnant women than among other individuals.

The hazards of comparing results obtained in different and small study populations are apparent from the SMX/TMP study by Reid referred to above. Antibiotic levels and ratios obtained for two groups of women who received either drug alone are distinctly different from values obtained in a third group of women who received the same doses of both drugs in combination. Evidently, the ideal control subject for a pregnant woman is the very same woman after pregnancy, thus eliminating the influence of the variations in pharmacokinetic parameters which are mainly genetically determined [52].

Badly needed information on pharmacokinetics of antibiotics in pregnancy can be obtained from a limited number of patients if a protocol is used where pregnant women who are treated with antibiotics volunteer to serve as their

Table 3. A summary of studies of antibiotics in pregnancy in which alterations in one or more pharmacokinetic parameters were originally suggested (uninterrupted arrow) or where the results in retrospect (interrupted arrow) suggest such deviations. When available, data are given for length of gestation, condition of patients, number of patients or observations in the study, levels in serum or plasma, half-life in serum or plasma (T 1/2) apparent volume of distribution (V_D), and clearance (50).

Antibiotic	Length of gestation (weeks)	Condition of patient	No. of patients	Serum levels	T 1/2	V_D	Clearance	Reference
dicloxacillin	32–40	delivery	57		↑			11
methicillin	40	labor	3	↓				10
oxacillin	38–41	amniocenteses	12			↑	↑	12
ampicillin	38–41	labor	14	↓				13
ampicillin		labor	16	↑	↓			15
ampicillin	28–32	healthy	13		↓			19
ampicillin		labor	10		↑			
ampicillin	38–41	amniocenteses	34	↓				18
ampicillin	9–33	healthy	26	↓	↓	↑	↑	16
ampicillin	21–40	UTI*	14	↓			↑	20
pivampicillin	10–23	healthy	10	↓				21
pivampicillin	>36	labor	8	↓				22
cephalexine		caesarean section	15	↓				23
cephaloridine		ruptured membrane	105	→				24
cephalothin		labor	30	↓				26
cephalothin		labor	43	↓				25
cephalothin		labor	54	↓	↑			27
cephalothin	38–41	amniocenteses	25	↓	↓			28
cefazolin	8–20	surgery	40	↓	↓			29
cefatrizine	8–20	surgery prostaglandin	33	↓	↑			30
cephacetril		labor	15	↓	↓			31
cephradine		labor	7	↓				32
cephradine	12–29	healthy	10	↓	↓	↑	↑	33
cefoxitine	38–41	prem rupt membrane caesarean section	13	↓				34
cefuroxime		labor or caesarean section	16	↓				36
cefuroxime	11–35 and 37–42	UTI* labor	7	↓	↓	↑	↑	39
clindamycin		caesarean section	54	→	↓			40
clindamycin	10–22	surgery saline infusion	22	→				41
erythromycin	10–19	surgery saline infusion	17	↓				41
gentamicin		caesarean section	58	↓	→			40
gentamicin		labor	24	↓				42
kanamycin	38–42	labor	27	↓	→			43
amikacin	6–20	surgery	30	↓	↓			44
tobramycin	1st and 2nd trimester	surgery	35	↓	→			45
thiamphenicol		labor	29	→	↓			46
nitrofurantoin	5–16	abortion	30	↓				47
trimethoprim	8–20	surgery	10	→	↓			48
sulfa-methoxazole	8–20	surgery	10	→	↓			48

* UTI = urinary tract infection

own controls after pregnancy, thereby enabling all statistical analysis to be based on paired observations if test conditions are identical [53]. Provided medication is medically required such a protocol does not involve any undue risks to the pregnant woman or to the fetus. According to the above mentioned protocol plasma levels of cloxacillin were studied in one woman following a single i.v. test dose of 1.0 g. The patient was 21 weeks pregnant and her weight was 69 kg. Four weeks earlier she had been treated during ten days with i.v. benzyl penicillin and cloxacillin for an acute infection. Following the test dose the cloxacillin levels in plasma and urine were studied during 6 h. After pregnancy she served as her own control weighing 65.4 kg and received again an i.v. test dose of cloxacillin of 1.0 g. The plasma levels are shown in Fig. 1. The recovery in urine of cloxacillin during the same 6 h was 62.5% of the dose when she was pregnant and 36.8% after pregnancy. Note that during pregnancy no cloxacillin could be detected in plasma after 2 h following dose administration and that the plasma levels after pregnancy were strikingly higher. In this patient the values for AUC, V_D, T 1/2, and plasma clearance were 33.8, 14.3 l, 21 min, and 472 ml/min during pregnancy and 85.1, 9.5 l, 35 min, and 186 ml/min, respectively afterwards.

Fig. 2 shows the serum levels of isoniazid (INH) in one woman following a

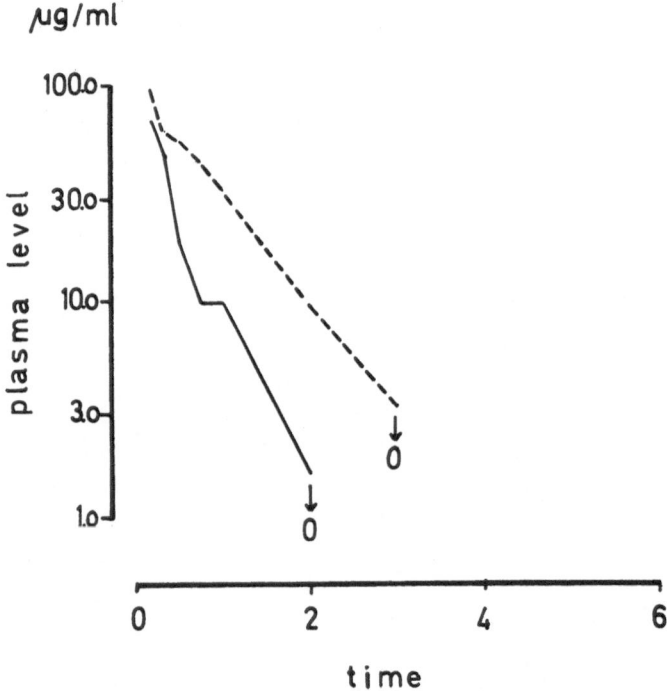

Fig. 1. Plasma levels versus time in semilog scale of cloxacillin in one woman following administration of a single i.v. dose of 1.0 g during (————) and after (----) pregnancy.

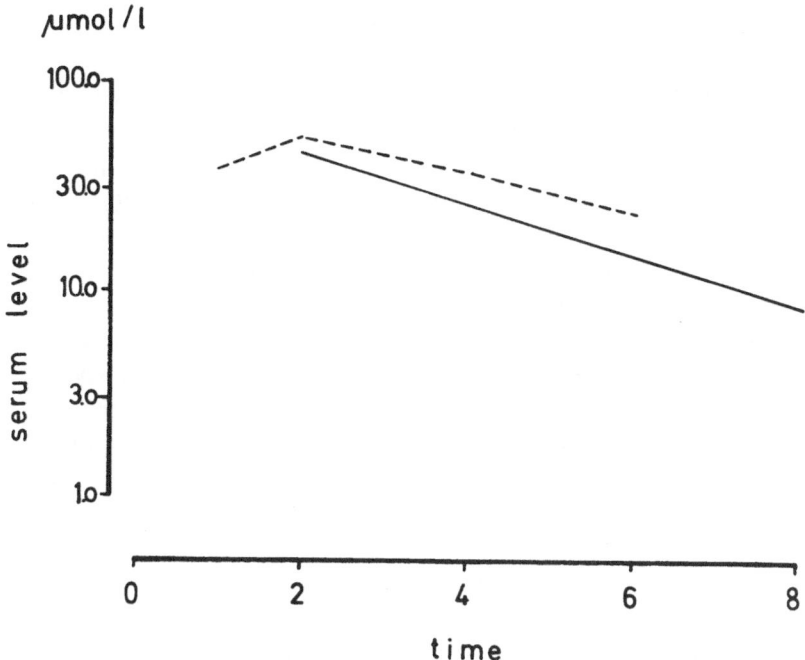

Fig. 2. Serum levels versus time in semilog scale of isoniazid in one woman following administration of an oral dose of 250 mg during (————) and 300 mg after (- - - -) pregnancy.

250 mg dose given when she was 26 weeks pregnant and of 300 mg 10 months after delivery. At the time of the 250 mg test dose the patient weighed 51.5 kg and had been treated for five weeks with INH 250 mg and para-aminosalicylic acid 10 g once daily for a newly discovered pulmonary tuberculosis from which she recovered uneventfully. At the time of the 300 mg test dose she was being treated with INH, 300 mg once daily and ethambutol 400 mg b.i.d. and her weight was 55 kg. T 1/2 during pregnancy was 2.4 h as opposed to 3.4 h after pregnancy.

Although these data by no means permit extensive conclusions on the pharmacokinetics of cloxacillin and INH in pregnancy, they may illustrate the necessity for further controlled studies of these and other compounds and how such studies can be accomplished.

By studying a few patients thoroughly i.e. assaying antibiotic levels in serum or plasma as well as in urine and when possible following oral as well as parenteral, preferably i.v., administration, more precise information can be gained than by doing a few assays on a large number of patients, or by studying just serum levels following oral administration only. Assays of antibiotic levels in amniotic fluid, cord serum, fetal tissues, and fetal urine may provide additional information.

54

About half of the studies listed in Table 3 which suggest altered pharmaco-kinetics of antibiotics in pregnant women have been carried out in early or mid-pregnancy, when the influence of the passage on various pharmacokinetic parameters – as mentioned earlier – is likely to be negligible. In late pregnancy, however, it must be assumed that the 'escape' of drug into the uterus and fetus affects the pharmacokinetics, although the exact extent of that influence is very difficult to estimate. The effect of the transplacental passage on various pharmacokinetic parameters is impossible to separate from the influence of other factors and alterations due to pregnancy. Also, the impact of transplacental passage on various pharmacokinetic parameters at term will not necessarily be the same for single as for repeated doses of an antibiotic. It may well be that the kinetics of the first dose is affected differently than that of subsequent doses.

Numerous studies carried out on a great number of antibiotics administered to pregnant women at different stages of pregnancy clearly demonstrate that antibiotics may pass from the maternal to the fetal circulation. As for most other drugs the placenta is no strict barrier, although the speed and the facility of the transfer, its quantity or quality may differ between drugs. The transplacental transfer of a drug will be ruled by the same laws of diffusion which apply to diffusion across any biological membrane, i.e. lipid solubility, molecular weight, degree of ionization, and protein binding, as well as the size of the surface available for diffusion [54]. Other transport mechanisms than simple diffusion may exist as well. Only the free fraction of a drug is available for diffusion. The speed of the diffusion process also depends on the concentration gradient. Most likely the passage of a drug does not remain the same throughout pregnancy but increases or decreases as the pregnancy proceeds.

The further intrauterine 'fate' of an antibiotic depends on whether the drug is metabolized by the fetus or excreted by the fetus. Metabolites may be excreted into the amniotic fluid or diffuse back to the maternal circulation. Drug, as well as metabolites, may also be deposited in various tissues according to their ability to adhere to or enter into fetal mammalian cells. Whenever the level of free antibiotic in fetal serum exceeds that in maternal serum, diffusion back to maternal circulation will take place. The level of total antibiotic at which equilibrium takes place varies with the degree of protein binding in fetal as compared to in maternal serum. Observed differences between maternal and fetal serum levels of an antibiotic may actually partially be due to a difference in the degree of protein binding in fetal as opposed to in maternal blood, the free fractions in fact being more similar than the levels of total drug. However, the levels of free antibiotic are very rarely measured and compared.

A further discussion of the transplacental passage as such is beyond the scope of this chapter, but a few points will be made, either because they may be relevant in treatment or prophylaxis of pregnant women or because they are interesting from a pharmacokinetic point of view.

Levels of antibiotic in fetal serum, tissues, and amniotic fluid will most probably increase following repeated doses of an antibiotic to the mother, unless the interval between doses is long enough for the fetus to rid itself from active drug. When antibiotic levels in fetal tissues have been compared following single as well as multiple doses, levels have been higher following multiple doses [55].

High bolus doses of ampicillin and cephacetrile administered i.v. every 2 h have been shown to give higher levels of antibiotic in fetal serum and amniotic fluid than continous i.v. infusion of the same amount of drug [31, 56].

Initially increasing and later decreasing levels in fetal serum and amniotic fluid as a function of time between dose administration and sampling have been demonstrated for many β-lactam antibiotics but also for aminoglycosides, thiamphenicol, clindamycin and erythromycin. Overall, the antibiotics start to appear in fetal serum at varying intervals following the appearance of drug in maternal serum, and begin to be present in measurable levels in the amniotic fluid still later. However, the levels in amniotic fluid continue to increase for some time after fetal serum levels have started to decline and are no longer detectable, most likely reflecting fetal excretion of antibiotic into the amniotic fluid.

In the study by Plomp et al. [46] levels of thiamphenicol were found to be higher in plasma from the umbilical vein than in plasma from the umbilical artery. It is tempting to believe that this difference reflects disappearance from the fetal circulation by means of diffusion to and possibly binding to fetal tissues, metabolism, and excretion by the term fetus. On the other hand, this hypothesis is not substantiated by the study by Craft and Forster [57] on cephradine. These authors reported the antibiotic level in serum from the umbilical artery and vein to be similar, whereas a higher level in serum from the vein would have been expected if excretion by the fetal kidneys and distribution to fetal tissues were of any significance.

That drugs may pass the placenta differently according to their individual properties is well illustrated in studies of the combination TMP/SMX. The transplacental passage of TMP is most probably facilitated in comparison to that of SMX. TMP has a molecular weight of 290.32, a protein binding of 42–46%, a pKa of 6.6, and it is only slightly soluble in water. Corresponding data for SMX is 314.35, 68%, 5.8–6.1 and highly soluble in water at ph 7.45 [4]. These differences may explain why, in the study by Reid et al. [49], fetal levels of TMP were higher and levels of SMX were lower than what would be expected on the basis of maternal serum levels, had the transplacental passage been similar for both drugs. Thus the SMX/TMP ratios in fetal serum and tissues were different from those in maternal serum. It can be assumed that in late and mid pregnancy SMX as well as TMP mainly reach the amniotic fluid via excretion by the fetal kidneys. Consequently the levels and ratios of SMX/TMP in amniotic fluid will be depending on the fetal serum levels of both drugs as well as on the fetal renal capacity.

CLINICAL IMPLICATIONS OF ALTERED PHARMACOKINETICS IN PREGNANCY

Treatment with antibiotics is usually short but intense. The target for treatment is not the patient but the microorganisms which have caused the infection to be treated. Once the microorganisms are killed or their multiplication at least inhibited the normal host will heal by itself.

For each strain of microorganisms there are two clinical 'threshold' levels for antibiotic concentration: The MIC and the MBC (*M*inimum *I*nhibitory *C*oncentration and *M*inimum *B*actericidal *C*oncentration). The latter is 2–10 times higher than the former but more elaborate to determine, which is the reason why in routine laboratory work only MIC values are given, although MBC values are more pertinent to dosage and treatment. MIC and MBC values express the levels of *free*, unbound antibiotic necessary to inhibit or kill one particular bacterial strain with one particular antibiotic. On the other hand serum and tissue levels are usually measured against a standard prepared in serum or plasma and will thus be expressed as the *total* levels of antibiotic, i.e. free *and* protein bound, although in bioassays only the free fraction is active. The level of the free fraction – which is what should be compared to the MIC value – can be estimated from the total level through knowledge of the degree of protein binding for the antibiotic in question. Tissue levels of free antibiotic below the MIC will probably not affect the infection at all. In order to reach the MBC of free antibiotic at the site of infection – which is rarely located to the blood stream – the level of free antibiotic available for diffusion must exceed the MIC by severalfold. In severe infections, especially if they are encapsulated or surrounded by any kind of diffusion barrier, the height and duration of the peak serum level are crucial for obtaining optimal diffusion from the blood stream to the site of infection.

Altered pharmacokinetics during pregnancy may be clinically important. Lower antibiotic levels in serum or plasma have been documented during pregnancy for some antibiotics and suspected for others. Thus, if a certain ratio between plasma or serum levels of an antibiotic and the MIC value of the infecting organism is aimed at with a particular dosage, resulting lower serum levels in pregnant women than in other individuals must be regarded as unsatisfactory. Lower antibiotic levels will then also be reached where the antibiotic is needed, i.e. at the site of infection, and treatment may fail. This, however, does apparently not apply to treatment of lower urinary tract infections if antibiotics with renal excretion are used. The levels of such antibiotics in urine seem to be unchanged in pregnancy.

When common dosage is used in pregnancy, antibiotic treatment failure may well be falsely blamed on a wrong choice of antibiotic rather than on insufficient dosage. This is possibly the case with the failures that have been reported with erythromycin in the treatment of syphilis during pregnancy [58, 59, 60]. Inadequate dosage may also be at least one part of the explanation for the failure of oral penicillin to eradicate group B streptococcal colonization in pregnant women reported by Gardner et al. [61]. In contrast, the same authors found ampicillin 500 g administered i.v. to be highly effective in preventing the intrapartum transmission of group B streptococcus when ampicillin was given to pregnant women after they were admitted for delivery [62]. The success recorded in the latter study may be ascribed to the fact that the i.v. route was used, which gives a bioavailability of 100% as opposed to 45% by the oral route [16], and thus corresponds to a higher oral dose. The considerably higher dose of ampicillin than of penicillin may more than compensate for differences in MIC values for ampicillin and penicillin V, especially when the protein binding of the two drugs is taken into account, approximately 20% for ampicillin and 65% for penicillin.

If the first antibiotic when used in routine dosage during pregnancy is considered ineffective it is likely to be substituted for another which is often less good an alternative to the patient, time will be wasted and the patient's infection prolonged. Also, the patient will unduly be exposed to additional antibiotics, each of them carrying a certain sensitizing risk. The selective pressure towards more resistant strains in the patient's own bacterial flora will also unnecessarily be increased.

If the usual dosage – expressed as mg per kg body weight – is not valid when a patient is pregnant, because the resulting serum levels are too low, such a fact must be taken into consideration when dosage schedules are calculated or routes of drug administration selected. If the antibiotic therapy fails or in the case of a serious infection in a pregnant patient it is advisable to measure the serum levels. This comparatively cheap and easy procedure may be of great help as guidance of therapy and improve the quality of antibiotic treatment during pregnancy.

Only by increasing the knowledge of pharmacokinetics of antibiotics in healthy as well as ill pregnant women can the quality of antibiotic treatment in pregnancy be ameliorated.

58

REFERENCES

1. Hytten FE, Leitch I: The physiology of human pregnancy. Sec ed, Oxford, London, Edinburgh: Blackwell Scientific Publications, 1977
2. Krauer B, Krauer F: Drug kinetics in pregnancy. Clin Pharmacokinet 2:167–181, 1977
3. Eadie MJ, Lander CM, Tyrer JH: Plasma drug level monitoring in pregnancy. Clin Pharmacokinet 2:427–436, 1971
4. Walter AM, Heilmeyer L: Antibiotika-Fibel 4. Auflage, Stuttgart: Georg Thieme Verlag, 1975
5. Ehrnebo M, Agurell S, Jalling B, Boréus LO: Age differences in drug binding by plasma proteins: Studies on human foetuses, neonates and adults. Eur J Clin Pharmacol 3:189–193, 1971
6. Pruitt AW, Dayton PG: A comparison of the binding of drugs to adult and cord plasma. Eur J Clin Pharmacol 4:59–62, 1971
7. Davison JM, Dunlop W, Ezimokhai M: 24-hour creatinin clearance during the third trimester of normal pregnancy. Br J Obstet Gynaecol 87:106–109, 1980
8. Feuer G, Karaish R: Hormonal regulation of drug metabolism during pregnancy. Int J Clin Pharmacol 11:336–374, 1975
9. Depp R, Kind AC, Kirby WMM, Johnson WL: Transplacental passage of methicillin and dicloxacillin into the fetus and amniotic fluid. Am J Obstet Gynecol 107:1054–1057, 1970
10. MacAulay MA, Molloy WB, Charles D: Placental transfer of methicillin. Am J Obstet Gynecol 115:58–65, 1973
11. MacAulay MA, Berg SR, Charles D: Placental transfer of dicloxacillin at term. Am J Obstet Gynecol 102:1162–1168, 1968
12. Bastert G, Müller WG, Wallhäuser KH, Hebauf H: Pharmakokinetische Untersuchungen zum Übertritt von Antibiotika in das Fruchtwasser am Ende der Schwangerschaft. 3. Teil: Oxacillin. Z Geburtshilfe Perinatal 179:346–355, 1975
13. Bray RE, Boe RW, Johnson WL: Transfer of ampicillin into fetus and amniotic fluid from maternal plasma in late pregnancy. Am J Obstet Gynecol 96:938–942, 1966
14. MacAulay MA, Abou-Sabe M, Charles D: Placental transfer of ampicillin. Am J Obstet Gynecol 96:943–950, 1966
15. Perry JE, Leblanc AL: Transfer of ampicillin across the human placenta. Tex Rep Biol Med 25:547–551, 1967
16. Philipson A: Pharmacokinetics of ampicillin during pregnancy. J Infect Dis 136:370–376, 1977
17. Boréus LO: Placental transfer of ampicillin in man. Acta Pharmacol Toxicol 3 (Suppl): 250–254, 1976
18. Bastert G, Wallhäuser KH, Wernicke K, Müller WG: Pharmakokinetische Untersuchungen zum Übertritt von Antibiotika in das Fruchtwasser am Ende der Schwangerschaft: 1. Teil: Ampicillin. Z Geburtshilfe Perinatal 177:330–339, 1973
19. von Voigt R, Schröder S, Meinhold P, Zenner I, Nöschel H: Klinische Untersuchungen zum Einfluss von Schwangerschaft und Geburt auf die Pharmakokinetik von Ampizillin. Zentralbl Gynaekol 100:701–705, 1978
20. Assall BM, Como ML, Miraglia M, Pardi G, Sereni F: Ampicillin kinetics in pregnancy. Br J Clin Pharmacol 8:286–288, 1979
21. Philipson A: Plasma levels of ampicillin in pregnant women following administration of ampicillin and pivampicillin. Am J Obstet Gynecol 130:674–683, 1978
22. Chatfield WR, Schramm BM, Richmond WJ: The absorption of ampicillin in late pregnancy and labour. N Z Med J 80:500–501, 1974
23. Duval J, Mora M, Chartier M, Mansour N: La Céphalexine. Son transfert placentaire. Nouv Presse Méd 1:1419–1420, 1972
24. Barr W, Graham R: Placental transmission of cephaloridine. Postgrad Med J 43 (Suppl): 101–104, 1967
25. Morrow S, Palmisano P, Cassady G: The placental transfer of cephalothin. J Pediatr 73:262–264, 1968

26. Paterson L, Henderson A, Lunan CB, McGurk, S: Transfer of cephalothin sodium to the fetus. J Obstet Gynaec Brit Comm 77:565–566, 1970

27. MacAulay MA, Charles D: Placental transfer of cephalothin. Am J Obstet Gynecol 100:940–946, 1968

28. Bastert G, Wernicke K, Müller WG, Hebauf H: Pharmakokinetische Untersuchungen zum Übertritt von Antibiotika in das Fruchtwasser am Ende der Schwangerschaft. 2. Teil: Cephalothin. Z Geburtshilfe Perinatol 178:164–173, 1974

29. Bernard B, Barton L, Abate M, Ballard CA: Maternal-fetal transfer of cefazolin in the first twenty weeks of pregnancy. J Infect Dis 136:377–382, 1977

30. Bernard B, Thielen P, Garcia-Cázares SJ, Ballard CA: Maternal-fetal pharmacology of cefatrizine in the first 20 weeks of pregnancy. Antimicr Ag Chemother 12:231–236, 1977

31. Hirsch HA, Herbst S, Lang R, Dettli L, Gablinger A: Transfer of a new cephalosporin antibiotic to the foetus and the amniotic fluid during a continuous infusion (steady state) and single repeated intravenous injections to the mother. Arch Gynaekol 216:1–14, 1974

32. Bergogne-Berezin E, Lambert-Zechovsky M, Rouvillois JL: Pharmacocinétique d'une nouvelle céphalosporine, la cephradine. Intérêt de l'étude de son passage transplacentaire. Medecine et Maladie Infectieuses 8:426–431, 1975

33. Philipson A, Stiernstedt G: Pharmacokinetics of cephradine in pregnancy. 11th Internat Congr Chemother 19th Intersc Conf Antimicrob Ag Chemother, Boston 1979

34. Bergogne-Berezin E, Lambert-Zechovsky N, Rouvillois JL: Étude du passage transplacentaire des bèta-lactamines. J Gynecol Obstet Biol Reprod 8:359–364, 1979

35. Goodwin CS, Rattery EB, Goldberg AD, Skeggs H, Till AE, Martin CM: Effects of rate of infusion and probenicid on serum levels, renal excretion, and tolerance of intravenous doses of cefoxitin in humans: Comparison with cephalothin. Antimicrob Ag Chemother 6:338–346, 1974

36. Bergogne-Berezin E, Pierre J, Rouvillois JL, Dumez Y: Placental transfer of cefuroxime. 11th Internat Congr Chemother 19th Intersc Conf Antimicr Ag Chemother, Boston 1979

37. Foord RD: Cefuroxime: Human pharmacokinetics. Antimicrob Ag Chemother 9:741–747, 1976

38. Norrby R, Foord RD, Hedlund P: Clinical and pharmacokinetic studies on cefuroxime. J Antimicrob Chemother 3:355–362, 1977

39. Philipson A, Stiernstedt G: Pharmacokinetics of cefuroxime in pregnancy and labor. 20th Intersc Conf Antimicrob Ag Chemother, New Orleans 1980

40. Weinstein AJ, Gibbs RS, Gallagher M: Placental transfer of clindamycin and gentamicin in term pregnancy. Am J Obstet Gynecol 124:688–691, 1976

41. Philipson A, Sabath LD, Charles D: Erythromycin and clindamycin absorption and elimination in pregnant women. Clin Pharmacol Ther 19:68–77, 1976

42. Daubenfeld O, Modde H, Hirsch HA: Transfer of gentamicin to the foetus and the amniotic fluid during a steady state in the mother. Arch Gynaekol 217:233–240, 1974

43. Good RG, Johnson G: The placental transfer of kanamycin during late pregnancy. Obstet Gynecol 38:60–62, 1971

44. Bernard B, Abate M, Thielen PF, Attar H, Ballard CA, Wehrle PF: Maternal-fetal pharmacological activity of amikacin. J Infect Dis 135:925–932, 1977

45. Bernard B, Garcia-Cázares SJ, Ballard CA, Thrupp LD, Mathies AW, Wehrle PF: Tobramycin: maternal-fetal pharmacology. Antimicr Ag Chemother 11:688–694, 1977

46. Plomp TA, Maes RAA, Thiery M, Yo Le Sian A: Placental transfer of thiamphenicol. Z Geburtshilfe Perinatal 180:149–156, 1976

47. Amon K, Amon I, Hüller H: Verteilung und Kinetik von Nitrofurantoin in der Frühschwangerschaft. Int J Clin Pharmacol 6:218–222, 1972

48. Ylikorkala O, Sjöstedt E, Järvinen PA, Tikkanen R, Raines T: Trimethoprim-sulfonamide combination administered orally and intravaginally in the first trimester of pregnancy: its absorption into serum and transfer to amniotic fluid. Acta Obstet Gynecol Scand 52:229–234, 1973

49. Reid DWJ, Caillé G, Kaufmann NR: Maternal and transplacental kinetics of trimethoprim and sulfamethoxazole, separately and in combination. Can Med Assoc J 112 spec issue 13:67S– 72S, 1975

60

50. Philipson A: Pharmacokinetics of antibiotics in pregnancy and labor. Clin Pharmacokinet 4:297–309, 1979
51. Wissenschaftliche Tabellen, Dokumenta Geigy. Lentner C (eds) 7th ed, Stuttgart: Georg Thieme Verlag, 1975
52. Alexanderson B: Prediction of steady-state plasma levels of nortriptyline from single oral dose kinetics: a study in twins. Eur J Clin Pharmacol 6:44–53, 1973
53. Philipson A: A protocol design for studying alterations of pharmacokinetic parameters due to pregnancy. Acta Obstet Gynecol Scand 59:311–313, 1980
54. Mirkin BL: Perinatal pharmacology: placental transfer, fetal localization, and neonatal disposition of drugs. Anestesiology 43:156–170, 1975
55. Philipson A, Sabath LD, Charles D: Transplacental passage of erythromycin and clindamycin. N Engl J Med 288:1219–1221, 1973
56. Hirsch HA, Dreher E, Perrochet A, Schmid E: Transfer of ampicillin to the fetus and amniotic fluid during continuous infusion (steady state) and by repeated single intravenous injections to the mother. Infection 2:207–212, 1974
57. Craft I, Forster TC: Materno-fetal cephradine transfer in pregnancy. Antimicrob Ag Chemother 14:924–926, 1978
58. South MA, Short DH, Knox JM: Failure of erythromycin estolate therapy in in utero syphilis. JAMA 190: 182–183, 1964
59. Mamunes P, Cave VG, Budell JW, Andersen JA, Steward RE: Early diagnosis of neonatal syphilis. Am J Dis Child 120:17–21, 1970
60. Fenton LJ, Light IJ: Congenital syphilis after maternal treatment with erythromycin. Obstet Gynecol 47:492–494, 1976
61. Gardner SE, Yow MD, Leeds LJ, Thompson PK, Mason EO, Clark DJ: Failure of penicillin to eradicate group B streptococcal colonization in the pregnant woman. Am J Obstet Gynecol 135:1062–1065, 1979
62. Yow MD, Mason EO, Leeds LJ, Thompson PK, Clark DJ, Gardner SE: Ampicillin prevents intrapartum transmission of group B streptococcus. JAMA 241:1245–1247, 1979

Author's address:
Department of Infectious Diseases
Danderyd Hospital
S-182 88 Danderyd
Sweden

3. THE TREATMENT OF URINARY TRACT INFECTIONS DURING PREGNANCY

ROBERT E. HARRIS, M.D., PhD.

INTRODUCTION

The antimicrobial therapy selected in the management of urinary tract infections during pregnancy is extremely important, not only for resolution of the infection but also for the continued well-being of mother and fetus. Therefore, the management is altered from that usually rendered for non-pregnant patients with urinary tract infections. As certain antimicrobial agents may be harmful to the fetus, drug safety is one of the most important considerations. Almost all pharmacological substances pass from the maternal to the fetal blood stream and the fetus's response to drugs is generally different from that of the mother. Usually, this response is increased toxicity due to the increase in blood-brain permeability and immature function of fetal liver enzymes.

Urinary tract infections occur frequently during pregnancy and require special attention as they produce considerable morbidity. These infections usually are not isolated events but may present as a variety of clinical situations and manifestations. Due to several altered factors during pregnancy and the postpartum period, women are at an increased risk to develop urinary tract infections. Mechanical compression of the ureters at the pelvic brim and hormonal influences result in 'physiologic hydroureters of pregnancy.' In addition to dilatation, the ureters becomes elongated, tortuous, and laterally displaced. Later in the gestation the bladder is compressed by the presenting fetal part and the ureteral orifices may be distorted or enlarged. Urinary stasis may be further complicated by vesicoureteral reflux allowing passage of infected urine from the bladder upward to the kidney. During the postpartum period, the return to the prepregnancy 'normal' status of the urinary tract is relatively slow, frequently requiring up to six weeks.

Before discussing the different rationales of therapy for pregnant patients with urinary tract infections, background information is necessary for complete understanding.

W.J. Ledger (ed.), Antibiotics in Obstetrics and Gynecology, 61–80. All rights reserved.
Copyright © 1982 by Martinus Nijhoff Publishers, The Hague/Boston/London. ISBN-13:978-94-009-7466-1

62

MICROBIOLOGY

The microorganisms which cause tract infections usually originate in the host's intestinal tract.The three principal routes for the spread of pathogens to the kidneys are hematogenous, lymphatic and ascensional [1]. The ascensional route involves a migration of microorganisms through the urinary passage, i.e. urethra, bladder, ureter to the kidneys. On the basis of clinical and experimental evidence, ascension appears to be the most common pathway.

The most frequent microorganisms causing urinary tract infections are the aerobic, gram-negative bacilli normally residing in the gastrointestinal tract. Of these, *Escherichia coli* is the most common and accounts for approximately 85% to 90% of initial urinary tract infections. Such microorganisms as *Proteus mirabilis*, *Klebsiella pneumoniae*, *Enterobacter* species, and gram-positive bacteria are those usually isolated from the remainder of patients with uncomplicated infections. Group B Beta hemolytic streptococci have also been demonstrated as potential pathogens for the urinary tract during pregnancy [2]. The presence of these microorganisms should not be considered as only a contamination, since both asymptomatic and symptomatic infections have occurred. The diagnosis of this particular microorganism as the offending etiological agent should be made only after obtaining its growth from a catheterized urine specimen.

Those patients with nosocomial urinary tract infections have a different microbiological flora. Complicated or surgical urinary tract infection is less often caused by *E. coli* but more often by such microorganisms as pseudomonas and by increasing incidences of Proteus and Klebsiella. For the usual urinary tract infections during pregnancy, these microorganisms are not as common, as most women treated are from a healthy population having their first episode of infection. Patients are seen in the childbearing years who become pregnant following urologic surgical procedures which required multiple courses of antimicrobial therapy. These patients should be carefully evaluated and followed during the pregnancy for the emergence of resistant microorganisms.

DIAGNOSTIC EVALUATIONS

Very often the clinician forgets the microscopic examination of the urine. This method is helpful in establishing the presence of infection. The presence of motile bacteria in a fresh, unspun, urine specimen, indicates possible infection. The presence of more than 50 white blood cells/high power field in a spun specimen is suggestive of urinary tract infection. If there is an intense inflammation of the bladder, erythrocytes may be present in the urine, either microscopically or gross hematuria.

Screening of all pregnant patients by means of quantitative urine cultures at the initial visit and at least once during the remainder of the pregnancy has been strongly recommended for the detection of bacteriuria. However, the detection of asymptomatic urinary tract infection within the general population by means of screening programs has not become an established preventive measure primarily because of the cost to the individual [3]. Therefore, simple economic and feasible tests, such as the Greiss test, have been developed for the detection of bacteriuria by mass screening [4, 5]. The nitrate is reduced to nitrite by the presence of urinary bacteria in significant numbers ($\geq 100\,000$/ml). One of the best and most reliable methods for the detection of significant bacteriuria is a dip stick kit, microstick, as described by Kunin and DeGroot [3].

Whenever a screening test is positive, a clean-catch midstream urine sample is obtained for culture. It is important that the urine culture be obtained properly and processed free from contamination of the lower genital tract bacteria [6]. Suprapubic and transvaginal aspiration have been accomplished in both nonpregnant and pregnant patients to obtain urine for culture [7, 8, 9]. We have not used these methods for our pregnant patients and do not recommend them as a routine. When there is a question of contamination on the culture report on a repeated urine sample, we prefer to obtain a urine sample for culture by catheterization, covering the patient with nitrofurantoin macrocrystals for three days. If $\geq 100\,000$ bacteria/ml are found in a single urine specimen by catheterization, the possibility that the patient has truly bacteriuria is greater than 95% [10]. Early onset, or low grade, infection is usually represented by the presence of 50–100 000 bacteria/ml. Appropriate antimicrobial management is dependent upon rapid identification of the offending microorganisms.

LOCALIZATION PROCEDURES

As all parts of the urinary tract are at risk of infection when the urine becomes colonized for bacteria, localization of infection has been an aim for many investigators studying urinary tract infections. By clinical evidence alone, especially in the asymptomatic patient, differentiation of renal versus bladder bacteriuria is difficult. Yet, localization studies are not clinically necessary for the immediate management of most infections, as the aim of therapy is the eradication of the microorganisms from all parts of the urinary system, both upper and lower. These methods have been reported to be of value in assessing the pathogenesis and natural history of urinary tract infections as well as with evaluations and follow up management of individual complex patients.

64

Localization studies to determine the site of infection are divided into two major groups: the direct techniques, e.g. bladder wash-out, ureteral catheterization, and indirect techniques, e.g. include fluorescent antibody-coated bacteria, or F.A. tests, [11, 12, 13, 14, 15]. In pregnant patients Harris [16] demonstrated, using the F.A. test, that renal bacteriuria occurred in 46% of asymptomatic bacteriuric patients. These data correlated well with retrograde catheterization studies of other investigators. Thus, the F.A. test appears to be valid for localization of the site of urinary tract infection for obstetric patients. However, the immunological response necessary for the F.A. test to become positive appears to be a function of the length of time of antigen exposure. Therefore, for an acutely ill patient, the result of the F.A. test *does not* alter the clinical management. Thus, the F.A. test is a beneficial, but not conclusive, aid in the management of pyelonephritis for the obstetric patient.

The positive F.A. test most often correlates with upper tract, or renal infection, whereas a negative F.A. test usually correlates with lower tract, or bladder, infection. However, physicians must be aware of the limitations in the interpretation of the results of this test, which may reflect technical aspects and/or the clinical variations of the urinary tract infection [17, 18]. (Table 1). Localization of the site of the infection is an important research endeavor but

Table 1. Utilization of the FA coated bacteria test with different clinical presentations of urinary tract infection.

Diagnosis	% Positive FA test
Chronic pyelonephritis	97
Acute pyelonephritis (pregnant)	69
Acute pyelonephritis (non-pregnant)	62
Acute pyelonephritis (children)	56
Asymptomatic bacteriuria (pregnant)	46
Asymptomatic bacteriuria (non-pregnant)	20–40
Acute cystitis	3–8

its clinical applications appear less apparent. The implications of the F.A. test in terms of the immediate management of the patient to prevent development of chronic renal complications remain to be defined [17]. For obstetric patients, antimicrobial management should not be based upon the results of F.A. tests. Under the specific antimicrobial discussions of different entities, later in this chapter, some of the implications for nonpregnant patients treated on the basis of the F.A. test results are presented. However, this is not so clear-cut, nor should it be considered so conclusive, for the pregnant patient under your care. Indeed, Mundt and Polk [18] state that the F.A. test (or antibody-coated bacteria assay – ACB assay) has *no* role in the management of patients with urinary tract infections.

Some antimicrobials are inappropriate during the gestation because of the possible adverse effects to the mother and/or the fetus. Others may be used only with considerable caution, as noted in Table 2, with possible side effects.

Tetracycline is an example of one agent that has caused problems for both mother and fetus when used during the gestation [19]. Tetracycline can be used during pregnancy in some situations but with the large number of available antibiotic formulations, its use would seem inadvisable. Whalley et al. [20] evaluated tetracycline disposition in normal pregnancy and concluded

Table 2. Antimicrobials associated with problems during pregnancy.

Antimicrobial	Problems
Tetracycline	Inhibits bone growth; discolors teeth in fetus and infant
Aminoglycosides (kanamycin sulfate, gentamicin sulfate, streptomycin	Eighth nerve damage; skeletal anomalies (streptomycin)
Trimethoprim sulfamethoxazole	Anomalies, i.e., cleft palate, in animal studies
Chloramphenicol	Gray-baby syndrome; fetal death
Sulfonamides	Hyperbilirubinemia*

* Third trimester

that it is handled similarly in pregnant and non-pregnant women. The reports showing maternal therapeutic problems, (e.g. hepatic and pancreatic dysfunction) after receiving tetracycline, were due to intravenous doses higher than necessary to provide satisfactory therapeutic blood levels. They found that satisfactory blood levels can be obtained for women with normal renal function with the intravenous administration of no more than 1 g of tetracycline daily. Both temporary and permanent discoloration of the teeth as well as inhibition of bone development in the infant has been the result of antenatal tetracycline therapy [21]. Kutscher et al. [22] pointed out that not only is the discoloration caused by antenatal administration of tetracycline, but that short-term therapy with tetracycline even after birth, especially with premature infants, results in marked discoloration of the teeth. As clinicians, we should be aware that teenage women are frequently treated for acne vulgaris with tetracycline. These patients are often overlooked as possible drug problems with pregnancy. As these patients have prolonged tetracycline therapy, frequently their physicians are not aware whenever they become pregnant, or either the patients are so accustomed to taking the antimicrobials that they fail to tell their new physicians when they enter for maternity care. Corcoran et al. [23] reported such a patient who delivered an infant with congenital abnormalities raising a teratologic question. Although the effects could have been caused by other factors, tetracycline is a general inhibitor of cell metabolism and bone changes were present suggestive of tetracycline therapy. As many women have unplanned pregnancies, all physicians treating childbearing age women with tetracycline should caution them about the drug's potential hazard should they become pregnant.

Cohlan et al. [21] demonstrated that tetracycline is deposited as a fluorescent complex in growing bone. Although of no clinical significance for the older child or the adult, tetracycline administration is suggestive of being of clinical significance with inhibition of bone growth in the fetus.

Trimethoprim Sulfamethoxazole (Septra-Bactrim), an antifolate drug, has been associated with anomalies, e.g. cleft palate in animal studies [24]. However, Brumfitt and Pursell [25] utilized this agent during pregnancy and had significantly lower incidences of side effects and no strong evidence suggesting any risk of teratogenesis. Only ten of their group were treated for bacteriuria at a critical time for teratogenesis, i.e. less than 16 weeks gestation. A total of over 200 patients had been treated with Septra-Bactrim without any evidence of fetal problems. They concluded that the potential dangers of the drug had not materialized. However, there is not enough data to conclusively state there is no increased risk for abnormalities. Of their 120 reported patients, there were four who did have variable types of congenital abnormalities.

Schiffman [26] discussed this particular problem stating that since this agent is a folate antagonist inhibiting normal development of purines, it might be expected to have a teratogenic effect. Fetal malformations commonly associated with lack of folic acid include cleft palate and abnormalities in extremities and tails: reported in several animal species when Septra-Bactrim was administered to the pregnant female. Although no abnormalities were noted by the study by Brumfitt and Pursell [25], it is known that folate levels can be marginal in many pregnant women. Thus, such a combination of antimicrobial agents is generally contraindicated or should only be used when the physician is well aware of the potential danger during the pregnancy.

Recently, Dickson [27] reported that thrombocytopenia was a serious side effect of the antimicrobial combination of trimethoprim sulphamethoxazole. Of 31 patients, two died: females being affected twice as frequently as males. Böse et al. [28] reported trimethoprim-induced interference with folate metabolism by inhibition of dihydrofolate reductase causing depression of thrombocytes. Thrombocytopenia occurred for 18% of the children treated with this agent for urinary tract infections. Folate requirements are increased by growth and may be augmented by infection. As thrombocytopenia does occur in association with toxemic patients, if this antimicrobial combination is being used during this stressful event, the resultant thrombocytopenia could be potentiated with serious consequences.

We have not used this combination agent during gestation and reserve it for postpartum patients because of the many unknown factors regarding an antifolate during the gestation and the availability of other antimicrobial agents.

The aminoglycosides are another group of antimicrobials which can cause problems, e.g. nephrotoxic and ototoxic. Streptomycin has reportedly caused skeletal anomalies. As the aminoglycosides are excreted in the urine, the clinician needs to be particularly concerned about pregnant pyelonephritis patients. Whalley et al. [29] have shown that these patients have transient renal dysfunction, with a marked lowering of the creatinine clearance which returns to normal over a period of 6 to 8 weeks following the acute episode. Because of such low clearances, if given at a regular dosage level, the amnioglycosides may indeed be not only nephrotoxic and ototoxic to the mother but also to the fetus. Therefore, these antimicrobial agents should be used with caution and serum levels should be obtained to determine the trough level of the amnioglycosides.

Chloramphenicol has been used during pregnancy but there is a danger of the Gray-baby syndrome with fetal death, particularly if given during the last part of the gestation and if the baby is born prematurely. Similarly, sulfonamides require cautious administration. Although they are safe when given during the first and second trimesters, there is a risk of hyperbilirubinemia if the mother is treated during the third trimester and the infant is delivered prematurely. The neonates, and particularly the premature, lack effective enzymes for complete and effective metabolism of antimicrobials.

ANTIMICROBIALS CONSIDERED SAFE DURING PREGNANCY

There are certain agents which are considered to be safe for urinary tract infection therapy during pregnancy (Table 3). The cost factor of these antimicrobial agents may influence the choice and may contribute to patient compliance. Patient compliance may be improved by choosing an agent which permits the fewest daily doses. For the pregnant patient, it is particularly important to control the urinary tract infection as quickly as possible, to

Table 3. Antimicrobials considered safe during pregnancy.

Methenamine mandelate
Nitrofurantoin macrocrystals
Penicillins (ampicillin, carbenicillin, ticarcillin)
Cephalosporins
Sulfonamides*

* First and second trimesters

insure microorganism eradication by the completion of therapy, and to expose mother and fetus to the minimum antimicrobial dosage that would achieve satisfactory therapeutic results.

There are other side effects to these agents which should be considered by the clinician. For example, ampicillin, erythromycin, neomycin, amnioglycosides, sulfonamides and methenamine mandelate interfere with urinary estriol determinations [30, 31]. If your department or hospital utilizes urinary estriol as a means to determine fetal well-being and you treat patients with one of these antimicrobial agents, the alteration of the urinary estriol for these particular patients can lead to false interpretations.

Furthermore, the patient may not be able to tolerate the antimicrobial agent due to allergies. Patients with penicillin allergies have cross reactions (between 15–20%) when treated with Cephalosporins. The sulfonamides, nitrofurantoin macrocrystals, and mandelamine are fairly well tolerated by patients.

Thus, although these antimicrobial agents are considered safe during the pregnancy, allergic reactions and other side effects for any antimicrobial agent must be considered.

ASYMPTOMATIC BACTERIURIA

Asymptomatic bacteriuria is one of the most commonly diagnosed urinary tract infections during pregnancy. The prevalence rate is associated with the presence of sickle cell trait, low socio-economic status, reduced availability of medical care, and increased parity. Depending upon the population studied, bacteriuria occurs for 2–10% of all pregnant women. Eradicating these infections is important as 25–30% of asymptomatic bacteriuric patients will develop symptomatic infection (i.e., pyelonephritis) during the gestational period. Almost half of the pregnant bacteriuric patients have asymptomatic upper tract (renal) infections as demonstrated by both the fluorescent antibody-coated bacteria and bladder washout techniques [16, 32].

The antimicrobial therapy for asymptomatic bacteriuria should be based upon the sensitivities of the microorganisms isolated from the urine sample. Generally, we have employed one of the regimens given in Table 4. The nitrofurantoin macrocrystals are highly concentrated by the kidneys and do not change the sensitivities for over 90% of the fecal *E. coli*. Thus, rarely do resistant bacteria emerge from the fetal *E. coli*. Urine cultures should be obtained upon completion of therapy to insure the eradication of bacteriuria. If this repeat urine culture is positive for bacterial growth, therapeutic failure has occurred. With persistence, or relapse, of infection, reevaluation of microorganism sensitivities with appropriate antimicrobial therapy should be

Table 4. Recommended therapy for asymptomatic bacteriuria during pregnancy.

Ampicillin, 250 mg q.i.d. × 10 days
        or
Cephalosporins:
  Cephalexin, 250 mg q.i.d. × 10 days
        or
  Cefadroxil, 500 mb b.i.d. × 10 days
        or
Nitrofurantoin macrocrystals, 100 mg t.i.d. × 10 days
        or
Sulfisoxazole diolamine, 500 mg q.i.d. × 10 days

---

accomplished. Recurrent infection following asymptomatic bacteriuria occurs for approximately one-quarter to one-third of patients during the same gestation. Therefore, asymptomatic bacteriuric patients should be followed closely throughout the remainder of their gestation by some type of urine screening method to detect and treat such a recurrence according to microorganism sensitivities.

The optimal duration of antimicrobial therapy for pregnant asymptomatic bacteriuric women has remained controversial over the past two decades. There is no doubt that withholding therapy from these patients results in subsequent acute pyelonephritis for at least one-quarter of them. It has been repeatedly shown that continued administration of antimicrobial agents throughout pregnancy would significantly lower the expected incidences of antepartum pyelonephritis for these women. The antimicrobial choice for short-term administration is based upon microorganism sensitivities and can include any one of the several safe agents (Table 3). Table 5 illustrates reports which have compared antimicrobial agents over varying therapy time periods

Table 5. Cure rates after treatment of bacteriuria during pregnancy for varying periods of time.

Antimicrobial	Duration of course	Number patients	% Cure rate	Author
Sulphamethoxy-Pyridazine	Until term	93	81	Savage et al. [34]
Sulphamethoxy-Pyridazine	30 days	80	60	Little [33]
Nitrofurantoin	30 days	44	82	Little [33]
Nitrofurantoin	21 days	76	92	Pathak et al. [35]
Placebo	21 days	76	13	Pathak et al. [35]
Sulfamethizole or	14 days	199	65	Whalley and Cunningham*
Nitrofurantoin	Until term	95	88	[36]

* Cure rates after first course of therapy.

with the rate of cure [33, 34, 35, 36]. The longer the duration of therapy, the more likely that the patient will be cured of her bacteriuria. However, with long-term therapy, there are certain antimicrobial agents which do have side effects. The minimum duration of time for cost and therapy effectiveness should be emphasized with antimicrobial agents. Whalley and Cunningham [36] demonstrated that patients who were carefully followed, recultured, and retreated could be effectively managed by short courses of therapy. We prefer the short-term therapy dosage, which is prescribed initially. If a patient does have a recurrence of asymptomatic bacteriuria, she is maintained on suppressive antimicrobial agents (such as Mandelamine or Macrodantin) for the remainder of the gestation.

Patient compliance has always been a problem and is a necessary consideration while treating the asymptomatic bacteriuric patient. The patient enters for a prenatal examination and is told she has bacteriuria which requires treatment. If uncertain in her mind, when she finds out the cost of the antimicrobial agent, and is not ill, she fails to see the value relative to the cost involved. In addition, many patients will forget to take their medication. Thus many investigators are discussing the possibility of using a lesser dosage and even one-dose therapy for urinary tract infections. Grüneberg and Brumfitt [37] evaluated a single dose treatment of acute urinary tract infection in their general practice and found it to be very satisfactory. However, when they extended this to pregnant patients, they found that following single dose therapy the cure rate was significantly reduced [38]. All patients took the antimicrobial agents in the clinic excluding the possibility that the patients failed to take the medication. An interesting aspect in their study was the difference between two different environments, i.e. London and Birmingham, England, where there was a marked discrepancy in the patient populations. They evaluated the sensitivities of the microorganisms at both centers and found that the Birmingham patients, who had a lesser cure rate to the antimicrobial dosage, had a higher number of resistant microorganisms. In the Birmingham population, lower socio-economic levels existed for the patient population and elevated serum antibody titers correlated with renal involvement rather than lower tract infection.

Several studies have evaluated the effectiveness of single dose antimicrobial therapy for nonpregnant patients. Fairly et al. [39] and Bailey [40] reported this regimen to be effective and suggested clinical follow-up three to five days later. The single dose therapy was considered only for certain populations: ambulatory women with symptoms of uncomplicated cystitis; those who were reliable with easy access to medical care; nonpregnant women; nondiabetic; and those free of known renal disease.

Ronald et al. [13] utilized the bladder wash-out technique for localization of bacteriuria and treated women with single dose antimicrobials, e.g. Gentamicin. The relapse rate was noted to be increased for those patients with upper tract infections. Those with lower tract infections did not have the same type of relapse. Fang et al. [41], using the fluorescent antibody-coated bacteria technique, reported that single dose or conventional dosages of amoxicillin were completely successful with patients with negative fluorescent antibody (F.A.) tests. However, for both conventional and single dose therapy only 50% of the patients with positive F.A. tests had a successful cure. Fang et al. stated that those patients who could be identified as having renal involvement would be most likely to benefit from long-term antimicrobial therapy. Turck et al. [42] had previously shown that the relapse and recurrence patterns were higher for those patients with renal involvement. Kulasinghe et al. [43] correlated relapses for those patients with positive F.A. tests but not for those patients with negative F.A. tests.

Rubin et al. [44] evaluated single dose amoxicillin therapy for urinary tract infection in a multicenter evaluation study. They reported a correlation of women with available access to medical care to the presence of lower incidences of antibody-coated bacteria, whereas those women with poor access to care had the high rates. In their population, a single three gram oral dose of amoxicillin eradicated the infecting microorganisms for 90% of patients with negative F.A. tests. These results compared favorably with ampicillin and sulfamethoxazole trimethoprim treatment regimens. However, Rumans and Vosti [17] demonstrated limitations in the F.A. test such that implications for immediate patient management remain to be defined. Mundt and Polk [18] also reported deficiencies of the test and state that there is *no* justification for basing therapy on its results.

Furthermore, we [45] have recently evaluated obstetric patients as to the predictability of clinical response following therapy of asymptomatic bacteriuria during pregnancy based on the initial F.A. test results. Our data clearly show that the F.A. test is unreliable as a predictor of therapy response for the pregnant patient. The F.A. test did have a degree of predictability as to recurrent infection rates but not to the extent that therapy should be based upon the test results. Therefore, therapy for asymptomatic bacteriuria during pregnancy should consist of a conventional regimen as outlined in Table 4. As nearly one-quarter of asymptomatic bacteriuric patients have either a relapse or recurrence during the gestation, monitoring of urine samples and retreatment are necessary components of good antenatal care.

ACUTE CYSTITIS

The incidence of acute cystitis during pregnancy is 1.3% [46]. Regardless of the detection and treatment of asymptomatic bacteriura, the incidence of cystitis remains relatively constant (Table 6). Cystitis occurs most often during the second trimester despite initially negative screening urine cultures on the first obstetric visit. Other differences have been noted between patients with cystitis and those with either asymptomatic bateriuria or pyelonephritis.

Table 6. Six year incidence of urinary tract infections in 720 obstetric patients.

Year	1974	1975	1976	1977	1978	1979	Totals
No. of deliveries	1682	1729	1676	1596	1523	1532	9738
Incidence (%) UTI							
Acute cystitis ,	1.2	1.3	1.5	1.3	1.3	0.9	1.3
Acute pyelonephritis	2.0	0.9	1.2	0.8	0.3	0.6	1.0
Asymptomatic bacteriuria	4.3	4.6	5.1	5.6	5.8	5.3	5.1
Totals	7.5	6.8	7.8	7.7	7.4	6.8	7.4

This indicates differences in the pathophysiology of these clinical manifestations of urinary tract infection [46]. Whenever the clinical diagnosis is made, therapy should be begun immediately to prevent upward extension of infection to the kidney (Table 7).

For our population, the most commonly isolated microorganisms have been equally sensitive to either of the antimicrobial regimens. As contaminated urine specimens are frequently obtained from pregnant patients, the urine sample for culture should be obtained by catheterization of the cystitis patient prior to the onset of therapy. This insures appropriate identification of microorganisms with drug sensitivities. Urine cultures should be obtained two days after the completion of therapy to insure eradication of the microorganism and to determine if resistent microorganisms or persistent infections are present. The symptomatic patient is started on empiric therapy without awaiting the return of the urine culture report. However, upon the return of the urine culture report, usually within 48 h, the resistence and sensitivity patterns of the microorganisms isolated can be determined. The patient should be contacted if she has resistant microorganisms to the antimicrobial agent prescribed. If she has an in vivo response to the antibiotic even though the microorganism is not sensitive by culture report, she should have another urine culture performed to determine if the microorganisms

Table 7. Recommended therapy for acute cystitis during pregnancy.

Ampicillin, 250 mg q.i.d. × 10 days
    or
Nitrofurantoin macrocrystals, 100 mg t.i.d. × 10 days
    or
Sulfonamides (sulfisoxazole diolamine), 500 mg q.i.d. × 10 days

have been eradicated. Only if she is not clinically responding to therapy, or has persistent infection, should she be changed to an antimicrobial agent to which the microorganism is sensitive.

Approximately 10% of cystitis patients will have recurrences of infection during the gestation. Thus, these women should be followed by urine screening tests and retreated whenever recurrences occur.

ACUTE PYELONEPHRITIS AND PREGNANCY

Acute pyelonephritis is reported to occur for approximately 1 to 2-1/2% of obstetric patients [47, 48]. As detection by screening urine samples followed by treatment of asymptomatic bacteriuria increases, the incidence of pyelonephritis for those medical centers, with such screening programs, has been markedly decreased [49] (Table 6). Early detection and elimination of bacteriuria should prevent at least two-thirds of all antenatal cases of pyelonephritis. This is more dramatically revealed by Figure 1 which shows a marked decrease in the incidence of pyelonephritis following eradication of bacteriuria. If the bacteriuric patient is not treated, subsequent symptomatic infections are very likely to occur (Table 8). Thus, there is no doubt that the bacteriuric patient should be treated to prevent subsequent pyelonephritis. Over the past seven years at Wilford Hall USAF Medical Center, there was a marked reduction in the number of pyelonephritis patients admitted to the maternity ward. In 1973 one antenatal patient was admitted every 5 days for

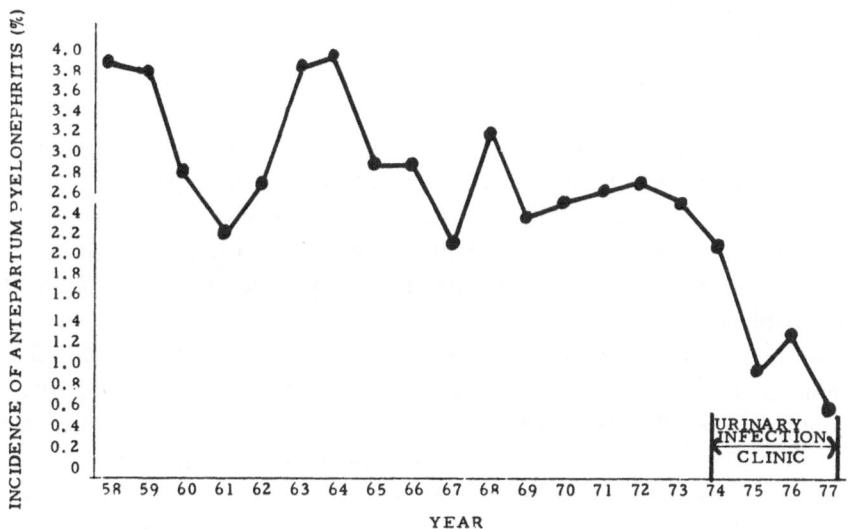

Fig. 1. The annual incidence of antepartum pyelonephritis for 35,437 women from 1 January 1958 through 31 December 1977.

Table 8. Relationship between asymptomatic bacteriuria and symptomatic urinary tract infection (literature review).

Untreated bacteriuric patients			Non bacteriuric patients		
Total #	Subsequently symptomatic #	%	Total #	Subsequently symptomatic #	%
1282	382	30	13686	241	1.8

pyelonephritis. Following the institution of routine screening and treatment of asymptomatic bacteriurics, this admission rate decreased to approximately one patient every 10 weeks in 1979 and 1980.

Pregnancy per se is one of the predisposing factors for pyelonephritis. Yet, combined urologic problems do exist during pregnancy. Urinary calculi occurring during pregnancy often present as acute infection episodes and less often with radiating pain and hematuria. Thus, patients who are seen with symptoms and signs of acute pyelonephritis during pregnancy may also have coexisting ureteral or renal calculi [50].

Hospitalization is strongly advised for the obstetric patient who has acute pyelonephritis. As this disease may lead to maternal sepsis, shock, and possible death as well as fetal wastage, immediate antimicrobial therapy is necessary prior to the return of the urine culture report [51]. The urine specimen for culture should be obtained by catheterization upon admission and prior to the institution of intravenous antimicrobial therapy. Within a few hours after initiating intravenous antimicrobials, the urine will become sterile, even though the patient remains symptomatic for longer periods. Intravenous antimicrobials are administered until the patient becomes afebrile and can tolerate oral medication, which is continued for a total of three weeks of therapy. The usual microorganisms isolated are *E coli*, which at our medical center have been sensitive (over 90% sensitivity rate) to ampicillin, our first drug of choice. However, the attending physician must be aware of the individual laboratory sensitivity patterns as well as the particular microorganisms usually isolated from the patient population presenting with pyelonephritis.

On the second day of therapy, a repeat urine sample for culture should be obtained. Following intravenous antimicrobial therapy, 85% of patients should become afebrile within 48 h, and 97% of patients within 96 h. If the patient does not respond to the initial therapy, two factors should be considered: either an underlying obstructive uropathy (i.e. stone formation) or the presence of resistant microorganisms. The initial urine culture report with sensitivity patterns should be available within 48 h. If the patient is not responding because of resistant microorganisms, switching to another antimicrobial agent should be accomplished. If the patient is responding, i.e. in vivo response, to the antimicrobial agent being used, but the in vitro laboratory testing reveals resistant microorganisms, the antimicrobial agent should not be automatically changed. Instead, the urine should be examined for the presence or absence of pyuria and bacteria. If there is persistence of bacteriuria, the antimicrobial should be changed according to sensitivity patterns. Most often the alternate antimicrobial is a Cephalosporin. Many physicians will begin the initial therapy with cephalosporins (e.g. Keflex) because of the microorganisms sensitivity patterns seen for their particular patient population. The outline for antimicrobial management of the patient with pyelonephritis is given in Table 9.

Monitoring renal function, measuring intake and output is extremely important. Transient renal dysfunction occurs in association with acute pyelonephritis during pregnancy as measured by creatinine clearances [29]. Therefore, it should be realized that certain antimicrobial agents, such as aminoglycosides, which are excreted by the kidney, must be used with caution. The dosage varies with the antimicrobial agent and the renal function status.

Table 9. Recommended therapy for acute pyelonephritis during pregnancy.

Parenteral hydration; reduce fever; monitor renal functions, intake and output.

Parenteral antimicrobials:
Ampicillin, 500–1000 mg IV q 6 h until afebrile, then oral, 250 mg. q.i.d. for 20 days total
or
Cephalosporin, 500–1000 mg IV q 6 h until afebrile, then oral 250 mg q.i.d. or 500 mg b.i.d., for 20 days total
or
Carbenicillin, 1000 mg q 4 h until afebrile, then oral 500 mg q.i.d. for 20 days
or
Aminoglycosides – varies with agent and status of renal function

Aminoglycosides should be used only if they are the only available antimicrobials either based upon the microorganism sensitivity patterns or the patient is allergic to other antimicrobial agents. Both erythromycin and nitrofurantoin macrocrystals have been used for the treatment of acute pyelonephritis but neither is our choice for the acutely ill patient.

The recurrence rates for pyelonephritis are very high for obstetric patients [48]. For this reason, careful follow-up and antimicrobial therapy are essential for continued patient well-being.

URINARY TRACT SUPPRESSION AND PROPHYLAXIS

Urinary tract prophylaxis is more often necessary due to a number of clinical situations which were formerly not as commonly seen during pregnancies. Patients who have had ureteral reimplanations or chronic renal infections frequently have recurrent infections and are on urinary suppression when they become pregnant. Antiseptic agents, e.g. nitrofurantoin macrocrystals or methenamine mandelate, are often used for this purpose. As ampicillin and cephalosporins are first line therapeutic agents, they should not be used for prophylaxis, but reserved for active infections (Table 10).

Urinary suppression and prophylaxis are closely related terms and are used interchangeably by different investigators. However, we use these terms as describing the means to prevent recurrent urinary tract infections during pregnancy. Harding and Ronald [52] and Stamey et al. [53] have shown that prophylaxis is effective when utilizing low dosage antimicrobial agents for recurrent urinary tract infections. Grüneberg et al. [54] have shown effective prophylaxis in the prevention of recurrent childhood urinary tract infections. For the adult pregnant patient, anticipation and prevention of reinfection is important. Those pregnant women who experience recurrent asymptomatic bacteriuria have a significantly higher rate of obstructive uropathy noted on postpartum pyelograms. They tend to have underlying renal disease or evidence of persistent infection. Also, if not maintained on suppressive therapy, 75% of all patients who have acute pyelonephritis can be expected to have recurrent pyelonephritis during the same pregnancy [48, 55]. This incidence can be reduced to less than 2% by the use of suppressive antimicrobial therapy.

Yet, urinary tract suppression is really necessary for only a small segment of obstetric patients. Approximately 30% of the patients with asymptomatic

Table 10. Recommended therapy for urinary tract prophylaxis and suppression.*

Complication	Therapy
For urological complications (ileal conduit, ureteral reimplantation; chronic and persistent renal infection)	Nitrofurantoin macrocrystals, 50 mg t.i.d. or 100 mg hs. or Methenamine mandelate, 500 mg t.i.d.
For recurrent asymptomatic bacteriuria or cystitis. Following initial 20 days therapy for acute pyelonephritis	Nitrofurantoin macrocrystals, 50 mg t.i.d. or 100 mg h.s. or Methenamine mandelate, 500 mg t.i.d.
For postpartum urinary retention during period of and 3 days after removal of indwelling Foley catheter	Nitrofurantoin macrocrystals, 50–100 mg t.i.d. or Trimethoprim-sulfamethoxazole, 2 tablets (80 mg trimethoprim; 400 mg sulfamethoxazol per tablet) b.i.d.

* The cephalosporins (cephalexin, 250 mg q.i.d. or cefadroxil, 500 mg b.i.d.), and ampicillin (250 mg q.i.d.) are recommended only when resistant microorganisms are encountered.

bacteriuria have recurrences. This represents only 1.5% of the total obstetric population. In addition, in our population with treatment of asymptomatic bacteriuria, fewer than 1% of patients have pyelonephritis. Therefore, approximately only 2.5% of the total obstetric population are candidates for suppressive therapy. Thus, this small group of patients at risk can be treated effectively to prevent recurrent urinary tract infections during the gestational period.

Following recurrent urinary infections, or acute pyelonephritis, suppressive therapy should be effected throughout the pregnancy and two weeks postpartum. This is continued for the two weeks postpartum because of studies of postpartum urinary tract infections. The highest incidence of postpartum pyelonephritis is during the first two weeks after delivery and only 60% of women will have resolution of the normal pregnancy physiological changes of the urinary tract within two weeks after delivery [48]. Suppressive antimicrobial therapy is begun following the initial three week course of antimicrobial therapy of acute pyelonephritis, or at the conclusion of therapeutic regimens for the recurrence of asymptomatic bacteriuria or symptomatic cystitis. An acceptable alternate to suppressive therapy is the diligent examination of the urine every two weeks for the remainder of the gestation to detect recurrent urinary infection. If patients should develop bacteriuria or pyelonephritis, they must be retreated and followed again in a similar manner. Our choice for suppressive therapy has been nitrofurantoin macrocrystals (Table 10). Those centers who perform estriol determinations late in the gestation must be aware that mandelamine can influence the urinary values obtained.

Certain postpartum patients should be considered to be at high risk to develop infections and should be treated prophylactically. The most valid time to obtain urine cultures for true bacteriuria is the third postpartum day [56]. Postpartum bacteriuria occurs for 3% of noncatheterized and for 6% of catheterized patients [57]. The incidence of positive urine cultures is significantly higher for patients catheterized for urinary retention. Approximately 40% of such patients, with retention greater than 24 h, will develop asymptomatic bacteriuria and the possibility of ensuing symptomatic infection [57, 58]. These patients should be treated prophylactically during the duration of catheterization and two days following catheter removal [59, 60, 61]. Both Septra and nitrofurantoin macrocrystals, our drugs of choice, have been used effectively.

SUMMARY

The clinician must realize that pregnant patients who present with urinary tract infections have special problems requiring precautions including the choice of antimicrobial therapy. Monitoring for and treating bacteriuria during the pregnancy is valuable in preventing symptomatic infections. Suppressive or prophylactic therapy should be given patients with recurrent infections or who are at an increased risk for recurrent infection.

Identifying infecting microorganisms and determining drug resistance and susceptibility patterns are essential in order to initiate effective therapy as rapidly as possible. The benefits must be weighed against potential hazards for any antimicrobials used during pregnancy.

REFERENCES

1. Marraro RV, Rheins MS: Consideration of the diseased human genitourinary tract: a review. J Am Med Tech 37:216, 1975
2. Mead PJ, Harris RE: Incidence of group B beta hemolytic Streptococcus in antepartum urinary tract infections. Obstet Gynecol 51:412, 1978
3. Kunin CM, DeGroot JE: Self-screening for significant bacteriuria: Evaluation of Dip-strip combination nitrate/culture test. JAMA 231:1349, 1975
4. DeShan PW, Merrill JA, Wilkerson RG, et al.: The Griess Test as a screening procedure for bacteriuria during pregnancy. Obstet Gynecol 27:202, 1966
5. Czerwinski AW, Wilkerson RG, Merrill JA, et al.: Further evaluation of the Griess Test to detect significant bacteriuria. Am J Obstet Gynecol 110:677, 1971
6. Kass EH: Role of asymptomatic bacteriuria in the pathogenesis of pyelonephritis. In: Henry Ford Hospital Symposium: Biology of pyelonephritis, p 399–412. Boston: Little Brown, 1960
7. Stamey TA, Govan DE, Palmer JM: The localization and treatment of urinary tract infection: The role of bactericidal urine levels as opposed to serum levels. Med 44:1, 1965
8. McFadyn IR, Eykyn SJ: Suprapubic aspiration of urine in pregnancy. Lancet 1:1112, 1968
9. Simpson JW, McCracken AW, Radwin HM: Transvaginal aspiration of bladder in screening for bacteriuria. Obstet Gynecol 43:215, 1974
10. Norden CW, Kass EH: Bacteriuria of Pregnancy: A Critical Appraisal. Annual Rev Med 19:431, 1968
11. Fairley KF, Bond HE, Adey FD: The site of infection in pregnancy bacteriuria. Lancet 1:939, 1966
12. Fairley KF, Whitworth JA, Radford NJ, et al.: Pregnancy bacteriuria: The significance of site of infection. Med J Aust 2:424, 1973
13. Ronald AR, Boutros P, Mourtoda H: Bacteriuria localization and response to single dose therapy in women. JAMA 235:1854, 1976
14. Thomas VL, Shelokov A, Forlund M: Antibody-coated bacteria in the urine and the site of urinary tract infection. NEJM 290:588, 1974
15. Thomas VL, Harris RE, Gilstrap LC, III, et al.: Antibody-coated bacteria in the urine of obstetrical patients with acute pyelonephritis. J Infect Dis 131 (Suppl): 57, 1975
16. Harris RE: Infections of the urinary tract during pregnancy: Use of fluorescent antibody-technique as an aid in patient evaluation. South Med J 69:1429, 1976
17. Rumans LW, Vosti KL: The relationship of antibody-coated bacteria to clinical syndromes: As found in unselected populations with bacteriuria. Arch Intern Med 138:1077, 1978
18. Mundt KA, Polk BF: Identification of urinary-tract infections by antibody-coated bacteria assay. Lancet 2:1172, 1979
19. Elder HA, Santamarina BAG, Smith S, et al.: The natural history of asymptomatic bacteriuria during pregnancy: The effect of tetracycline on the clinical course and the outcome

of pregnancy. Am J Obstet Gynecol 111:441, 1971

20. Whalley PJ, Martin FG, Adams RH, et al.: Disposition of tetracycline by pregnant women with acute pyelonephritis. Obstet Gynecol 36:821, 1970

21. Cohlan SQ, Bevelander G, Tiamsic T: Growth inhibition of prematures receiving tetracycline: A clinical and laboratory investigation of tetracycline-induced bone fluorescence. Am J Dis Child 105:453, 1963

22. Kutscher AH, Zegarelli EV, Tovell HMM, et al.: Discoloration of deciduous teeth induced by tetracycline administered antepartum. Am J Obstet Gynecol 96:291, 1966

23. Corcoran R, Castles JM: Tetracycline for acne vulgaris and possible teratogenesis. Brit Med J 2:807, 1977

24. Howard JB, Howard JE, Sr: Trimethoprim-sulfamethoxazole vs. sulfamethoxazole for acute urinary tract infections in children. Am J Dis Child 132:1085, 1978

25. Brumfitt W, Pursell R: Trimethoprim-sulfamethoxazole in the treatment of bacteria in women. J Infect Dis 128:657, 1973

26. Schiffman DO: Evaluation of an anti-infective combination: trimethoprim-sulfamethoxazole (bactrim, septra). JAMA 231:635, 1975

27. Dickson HG: Trimethoprim sulphamethoxazole thrombocytopenia. Med J Aust 2:5, 1978

28. Böse W, Karama A, Linzenmeier G, et al.: Controlled trial of co-trimoxazole in children with urinary-tract infection. Bacteriological efficacy and hematological toxicity. Lancet 2:614, 1974

29. Whalley PJ, Cunnngham FG, Martin F: Transient renal dysfunction associated with acute pyelonephritis of pregnancy. Obstet Gynecol 46:174, 1975

30. Clinical chemistry: Effects of drugs on clinical laboratory tests. J of Amer Assoc of Clinical Chemistry (CLCHAU) Vol 21 pp 294D–295D, 1975

31. Gallagher JC, Ismail MA, Aladjem S: Reduced urinary estriol levels with erythromycin therapy. Obstet Gynecol 56:381, 1980

32. Harris RE, Thomas VL, Shelokov A: Asymptomatic bacteriuria in pregnancy: Antibody-coated bacteriuria, renal function and intrauterine growth retardation. Am J Obstet Gynecol 126:20, 1976

33. Little PJ: The incidence of urinary infection in 5000 pregnant women. Lancet 2:925, 1966

34. Savage WE, Hajj SN, Kass EH: Demographic and prognostic characteristics of bacteriuria in pregnancy. Med 46:385, 1967

35. Pathak UN, Tang K, Williams LL, et al.: Bacteriuria of pregnancy: Results of treatment. J Infect Dis 120:91, 1969

36. Whalley PJ, Cunningham FG: Short-term versus continuous antimicrobial therapy for asymptomatic bacteriuria in pregnancy. Obstet Gynecol 49:262, 1977

37. Grüneberg RN, Brumfitt W: Single-dose treatment of acute urinary tract infection: A controlled trial. Brit Med J 3:649, 1967

38. Williams JD, Brumfitt W, Leigh DA, et al.: Eradication of bacteriuria in pregnancy by a short course of chemotherapy. Lancet 1:831, 1965

39. Fairley KF, Whitworth JA, Kincaid-Smith P, et al.: Single-dose therapy in the management of urinary tract infection. Med J Aust 2:75, 1978

40. Bailey RR: Single-dose antibacterial treatment for uncomplicated UTIs. Drugs 17:219, 1979

41. Fang LST, Tolkoff-Rubin NE, Rubin RH: Efficacy of single-dose and conventional amoxicillin therapy in urinary-tract infection localized by the antibody-coated bacteria technic. NEJM 298:413, 1978

42. Turck M, Anderson KN, Petersdorf RG: Relapse and reinfection in chronic bacteriuria. NEJM 275:70, 1966

43. Kulasinghe HP, Cushing AH, Reed WP: Role of antibody-coated bacteria in the management of urinary tract infections. South Med J 70:1270, 1977

44. Rubin RH, Fang LST, Jones SR, et al.: Single-dose amoxicillin therapy for urinary tract infection: Multicenter trial using antibody-coated bacteria localization technique. JAMA 244:561, 1980

45. Leveno KJ, Harris RE, Gilstrap LC, III, et al.: Bladder vs. renal bacteriuria: Recurrence after treatment. Am J Obstet Gynecol 139:403, 1981

80

46. Harris RE, Gilstrap LC, III: Cystisis during pregnancy: A distinct clinical entity. Obstet Gynecol 57:578, 1981
47. Whalley PJ: Bacteriuria of pregnancy. Am J Obstet Gynecol 97:723, 1967
48. Harris RE, Gilstrap LC, III: Prevention of recurrent pyelonephritis during pregnancy. Obstet Gynecol 44:636, 1974
49. Harris RE: The significance of eradication of asymptomatic bacteriuria. Obstet Gynecol 53:71, 1979
50. Harris RE, Dunnihoo DR: The incidence and significance of urinary calculi in pregnancy. Am J Obstet Gynecol 99:237, 1967
51. Adams RH, Pritchard JA: Bacterial shock in obstetrics and gynecology. Obstet Gynecol 16:387, 1960
52. Harding GKM, Ronald AR: A controlled study of antimicrobial prophylaxis of recurrent urinary infection in women. NEJM 291:597, 1974
53. Stamey TA, Condy M, Mihara G: Prophylactic efficacy of nitrofurantoin macrocrystals and trimethoprim-sulfamethoxazole in urinary infections: Biologic effects on the vaginal and rectal flora. NEJM 296:780, 1977
54. Grüneberg RN, Smellie JM, Leaky A, et al.: Long-term low-dose co-trimoxazole in prophylaxis of childhood urinary tract infection: Bacteriological aspects. Brit Med J 2:206, 1976
55. Harris RE: Urinary tract infection during pregnancy. Gynecology and Obstetrics Vol 3: Chaps. 38:1–8. Hagerstown, MD: Harper & Row Pub., Inc., 1979
56. Marraro RV, Harris RE: Incidence of spontaneous resolution of postpartum urinary retention. Am J Obstet Gynecol 128:722, 1977
57. Harris RE, Thomas VL, Hui GW: Postpartum surveillance of urinary tract infections: Patients at risk of developing pyelonephritis after catheterization. South Med J 70:1273, 1977
58. Brumfitt W, Davies BI, Rosser EI: Urethral catheter as a cause of urinary-tract infection in pregnancy and puerperium. Lancet 2:1059, 1961
59. Davis JH, Rosenblum JM, Quilligan EJ, et al.: An evaluation of post catheterization prophylactic chemotherapy. J Urol 82:613, 1959
60. Turck M, Petersdorf RG: A study of chemoprophylaxis of postpartum urinary-tract infection. JAMA 182:899, 1962
61. Harris RE: Postpartum urinary retention: Role of antimicrobial therapy. Am J Obstet Gynecol 133:174, 1979

Author's address:
University of Texas
San Antonio, 6402 Red Jacket
San Antonio, Texas 78238
U.S.A.

4. TREATMENT OF POST-CESAREAN SECTION
ENDOMYOMETRITIS

MARGARET LYNN YONEKURA, M.D.

Pelvic infection following cesarean section is the most common hospital-acquired infection facing the Obstetrician-Gynecologist today. The most important contributing factor is the dramatic rise in the cesarean section rate. Cesarean births in the United States have increased almost threefold, from 5.5% of all deliveries (195 000 operations) in 1970 to 15.2% (510 000) in 1978 [1]. Although the prevalence of infection following cesarean section is not uniform throughout the United States, maternal morbidity rates are generally five to ten times higher after cesarean birth than after vaginal delivery, occurring in 10% to 65% of cases [1–4]. (see Fig. 1).

The operation itself is always a contaminated procedure which results in conditions that favor the proliferation of bacteria and suppression of host defense mechanisms. These conditions include: 1) impairment of local vas-

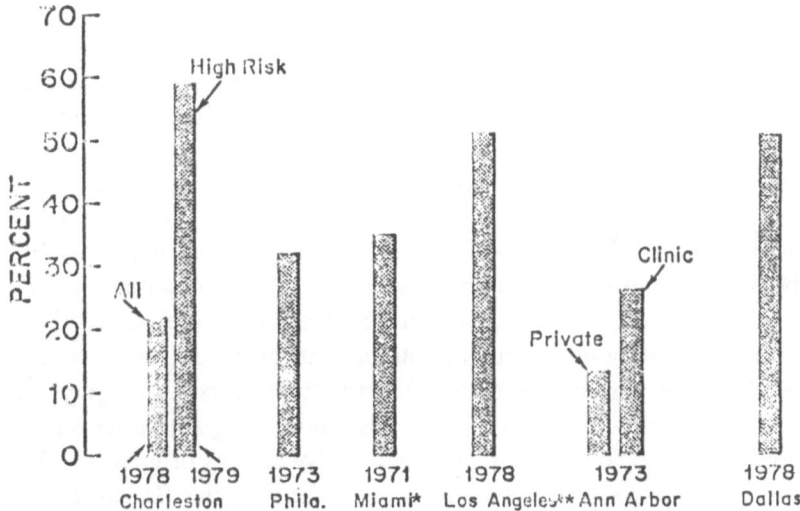

* Patients in labor, primary cesarean section.
** Patients in labor with ruptured membranes & internal fetal monitoring.

Fig. 1. Incidence of post-cesarean endomyometritis in various university hospitals (1971–1978) (Adapted from the Consensus Development Conference on Cesarean Childbirth NICHD-NIH, 1980).

W.J. Ledger (ed.), Antibiotics in Obstetrics and Gynecology, 81–98. All rights reserved.
Copyright © 1982 by Martinus Nijhoff Publishers, The Hague/Boston/London. ISBN-13:978-94-009-7466-1

cular supply resulting from vascular trauma; 2) presence of foreign bodies (i.e., sutures, talc, lint, etc.); 3) destruction of tissue by surgical manipulation (necrosis of tissue at suture line); and 4) hematoma formation [5]. The two most common causes of infectious morbidity following both cesarean and vaginal delivery are endometritis and urinary tract infection, with both complications occurring more commonly after cesarean birth [1]. Since urinary tract infections are discussed elsewhere in this volume, the scope of this chapter will focus upon post-cesarean endomyometritis.

The fact that rates of infection following cesarean section vary widely suggests that a woman's risk of developing infection postoperatively is dependent upon a variety of predisposing factors. Among these are internal fetal heart rate monitoring, prolonged rupture of the amniotic membranes, and lower socio-economic status. Although a wide variety of other clinical considerations, including frequency of pelvic exams, low hematocrit, obesity, general anesthesia, experience of the surgeon, and parity have been considered as predisposing factors to post-cesarean section febrile morbidity [6–22], insufficient data is available to permit critical evaluation. In addition, since many of these 'factors' occur concurrently, their individual assessment, in most cases, has been inconclusive.

INTERNAL FETAL HEART RATE MONITORING

The impact of internal fetal heart rate monitoring upon infectious morbidity in patients undergoing cesarean section remains one of the most important questions in operative obstetrics. When controls were used to reduce population heterogeneity, Wiechetek found no difference between the febrile morbidity in patients who were monitored during labor versus those who were not monitored [12]. Similarly, Hagen found no difference in the role of febrile morbidity in monitored and unmonitored lower socio-economic class patients who underwent cesarean section [23]. However, he observed that the infection rate among monitored private patients after cesarean section was higher than that among nonmonitored private patients. Consequently, he raised the possibility that the infection rate among indigent patients may be sufficiently high so as to obfuscate comparative studies of gross morbidity when comparing private and nonprivate patient studies. In concurrence, Gibbs et al. found no enhancement of morbidity when internal fetal heart rate monitoring was employed in a population of military dependents [10].

However, contrasting information was reported from studies utilizing a large population of indigent urban patients. Gassner and Ledger noted an increase from 20% to 40% in the incidence of endometritis when internal fetal heart rate monitoring preceded cesarean section [7] but found no statistical difference in the incidence of postpartum bacteremia (3.5% in nonmonitored patients, 4.7% in monitored patients). These data, however, may have been skewed by inclusion into the monitored group of a higher proportion of women with prolonged rupture of membranes and poor progress in labor. If internal fetal heart rate monitoring contributes to postcesarean section febrile morbidity, then the duration of monitoring should correlate positively with the number of patients manifesting infections [24]. In Gassner's study, no statistical difference was found between the duration of internal monitoring in infected and noninfected patients. Hence, any attempt to assign an arbitrary time limit for internal monitoring in order to prevent post-cesarean endometritis is not justified even in an indigent obstetric population at high risk of infectious morbidity. Thus, there is no clear evidence to suggest that internal fetal heart rate monitoring contributes, by itself, to the increased incidence of post-cesarean endomyometritis. Indeed, one of the central issues involved with invasive monitoring-related infectious morbidity is the duration of membrane rupture.

DURATION OF AMNIOTIC MEMBRANE RUPTURE

That the incidence of postpartum infection correlates with the duration of membrane rupture was described initially by Gunn and Mishell [26] and subsequently confirmed by others [6–27]. Gibbs reported that 14% of their patients developed post-cesarean infection if their membranes were intact, 28% became infected if the duration of rupture was less than 6 h, and 49% if the membranes were ruptured longer than 6 h [27]. Cunningham and co-workers demonstrated a 29% incidence of post-cesarean infection in groups of patients with intact membranes, 67% in patients with membranes ruptured less than 6 h, and 85% in patients with membranes ruptured in excess of 6 h [6]. Thus, the correlation between the incidence of post-cesarean infection and duration of membrane rupture seems assured.

When the impact of the duration of membrane rupture on the severity of post-cesarean endomyometritis was assessed prospectively in 200 patients, no statistically significant correlation was found [28]. Indeed, patients with intact membranes prior to cesarean section manifested infection-related complications distributed throughout the entire spectrum of postsurgical morbidity. Thus, it seems established that the duration of membrane rupture predisposes to an increased risk of sepsis following cesarean birth, but not necessarily to a more severe clinical course.

84

The delivery of health care to indigent patients is difficult to assess beyond the superficial consideration of general outcome. Sweet and Ledger demonstrated a statistically significant twofold increase in post-cesarean section infection when indigent patients in one hospital were compared to private patients in another [29]. In addition, significant infection-related complications of sepsis have been reported to occur more frequently in the indigent group. Anstey et al. reported on the results of infectious morbidity following primary cesarean section in a private institution [22]. Although this study was retrospective, they found no correlation between internal fetal heart rate monitoring, rupture of membranes, or the duration of membrane rupture and the incidence of intrauterine infection. However, no explanation has been put forth to account for the substantial difference in post-cesarean infectious morbidity in different socio-economic groups. Indeed, the bacteriology of the vagina in asymptomatic patients was found to be similar regardless of socio-economic background. [27, 30–34] Whether these differences relate to the quality of health care delivery, host defense response, or other factors remains unknown.

PREDISPOSING RISK FACTORS: BACTERIOLOGICAL

The optimal utilization of antibiotic therapy requires an awareness of the bacteriology of post-cesarean endomyometritis. In the pre-antibiotic era, the Group A beta-hemolytic streptococcus was thought to be the most common pathogen responsible for puerperal sepsis. [59]. With improving culture techniques, the aerobic coliforms were reported to be the most commonly isolated organisms [18]. More recently, the bacteria responsible for endomyometritis are believed to arise from the endogenous flora of the female lower genital tract [6,9,27,29,36–39] including a wide variety of aerobic and anaerobic bacteria.

Goplerud et al. obtained both aerobic and anaerobic endocervical cultures from 16 patients during the first, second, and early and late third trimesters of pregnancy as well as three days and six weeks postpartum [31]. They found a progressive decline in the isolation of *E. coli* and anaerobic organisms such as peptococci, peptostreptococci and Bacteroides species with advancing gestational age. They postulated that these changes in the cervical flora might result from either the increased vascularity of the genital tract in the third trimester resulting in better oxygenation and hence a hostile milieu for anaerobes, or to the increased steroid levels to which the endocervical cells are exposed as pregnancy progresses. In addition, important changes in the endocervical flora also occurred postpartum with a significant increase in anaerobic isolates (between 34 and 40 weeks of pregnancy, Bacteroides species were isolated from 15.8% of the cultures; whereas on the third postpartum day, they were isolated from 56.4% of the cultures). Similar trends were reported with respect to anaerobic cocci, group *D streptococci*, and *E. coli* (Table 1). One of the factors contributing to the increased prevalence of anaerobic bacterial isolates postpartum is the lochia. Composed of necrotic decidua, blood, and serous fluid, lochia provides a good medium for growth of organisms already present in the vaginal vault and endocervix.

Many of the same changes in vaginal flora were demonstrated by MacKay et al. [30] in 54 patients sequentially cultured during pregnancy and the early puerperium. This early postpartum increase in coliforms and anaerobic bacteria, all potential pathogens, suggests that puerperal sepsis is indeed a polymicrobial disease. diZerega et al. reported on the results of 53 positive blood cultures obtained from 200 patients with post-cesarean endomyometritis. They found anaerobic isolates more commonly than aerobic, with the anaerobic cocci being the most frequently recovered group of pathogens [37]. These findings are in agreement with those of Gilstrap and Cunningham who reported anaerobic isolates in 7 of 14 positive blood cultures from 100 patients with post-cesarean infection [39]. Anaerobic bacteria have also been shown to be the most common amniotic fluid isolates at the time of cesarean section [6].

Gibbs et al. also compared the flora of the endometrial cavity of two groups of puerperal patients – 47 afebrile control patients and 27 patients with post-

Table 1. Percentage of positive endocervical cultures.

Organism	Weeks Gestation				Postpartum	
Organism	8–13	14–26	27–33	34–40	3d	6 wks
Group D streptococci	37.0	30.4	35.3	23.7	43.5	31.8
E. coli	10.9	6.5	5.9	2.6	32.6	27.3
Peptococcus asaccharolyticus	52.2	47.8	47.1	42.1	63.0	63.6
Peptococcus prevotii	32.6	21.7	38.2	36.8	67.4	43.2
Peptococcus magnus	65.2	54.3	41.2	42.1	60.9	61.4
Peptostreptococcus anaerobius	30.4	15.2	11.8	15.8	41.3	25.0
Bacteroides fragilis	19.6	0.0	5.9	2.6	34.8	15.9
Bacteroides melaninogenicus	4.3	10.9	8.8	7.9	32.6	31.8
Bacteroides species	37.0	13.0	17.6	15.8	56.5	47.7

Bacterial isolates obtained from endocervical cultures during pregnancy and the puerperium. Note the dramatic increase in the prevalence of anaerobic isolates and *E. coli* in the early postpartum period. (Adapted from Goplerud et al., Am J Obstet Gynecol 126:858, 1976).

partum endometritis [27]. A transcervical intrauterine lavage technique was used to obtain specimens for aerobic and anaerobic cultures; the technique was designed to avoid vaginal and cervical contamination. The microflora of the endometrial cavity in patients with an afebrile postpartum course showed no qualitative difference from that of patients with puerperal endometritis except for peptostreptococci which were isolated less frequently from women with endometritis. In cases of endometritis, the most common pathogens isolated were peptostreptococci (37%), peptococci (33%), Bacteroides species (29%), enterococci (18%), and *E. coli* (15%). However, the fact that clinical evidence of endomyometritis was not found in the majority of patients even though bacterial colonization by known pathogens was present emphasizes that the pathogenesis of endomyometritis involves more than a source of potentially pathogenic bacteria, i.e., other host factors must be involved.

For the evaluation of puerperal sepsis, accurate microbiologic cultures are mandatory. The bacteriology of puerperal infections may seem of reduced importance in this era of broad-spectrum antibiotics but resistant strains of bacteria continue to emerge, making antibiotic susceptibility studies mandatory in the prevention of serious infection and related complications. Moreover, empirical therapy may mask the presence of a streptococcal epidemic on the postpartum ward from an outside source, such as ward personnel, which, if undetected, could persist as a reservoir of infection for other postpartum patients.

CULTURE TECHNIQUES

A frequent hindrance to the elucidation of the bacterial pathogenesis of postpartum endomyometritis is the acquisition of representative cultures. Many investigators believe that amniotic fluid obtained transabdominally at the time of cesarean section most accurately reflects the organisms potentially responsible for these infections. However, there is only a general correlation between colonization from amniotic fluid cultures obtained at the time of cesarean section and the manifestation of subsequent infection [36]. A possible explanation for this variance may result from the potential inhibition of bacterial growth by amniotic fluid. Amniotic fluid recovered from term gestations has been reported to contain a bacterial inhibitory system consisting of two components – the metal cation zinc and a peptide [40–47]. The antibacterial activity is effectively reversed by the addition of phosphate. According to Galask and co-workers, a phosphate to zinc ratio of ≤100 is usually associated with bactericidal fluid. A ratio between 100 and 200 predicts bacteriostatic fluid and a ratio of greater than 200 correlates with a noninhibitory fluid [47]. The phosphate concentration in amniotic fluid has been shown to progressively decrease from 20 weeks gestation to term such that the phosphate concentration is sufficiently low at term to allow the phosphate-sensitive inhibitory activity to be expressed. However, this bacterial growth inhibition in amniotic fluid may only be effective for *E. coli*, *Streptococcus faecalis*, and Staphylococcus aureus since anaerobes like *Peptostreptococcus anaerobius*, *Peptococcus prevotii*, and *Bacteroides fragilis* are only temporarily suppressed (8–16 h).

These data are further supported by clinical observations. Cooperman et al. demonstrated that in patients undergoing elective cesarean section at term (intact membranes, no labor), no pathogens were found in the amniotic cavity [48]. However, intact membranes offer no guarantee against contamination of the amniotic fluid once labor has begun. In patients with prolonged labor and intact membranes numerous pathogenic anaerobes and commensals were isolated. Furthermore, in patients with both prolonged labor and ruptured membranes, all three categories of organisms were present (i.e., pathogenic aerobes, pathogenic anaerobes, and commensals) [60]. Cunningham et al. have described similar results in amniotic fluid cultures obtained from 56 afebrile patients undergoing cesarean section following amniotic membrane rupture ≥ 6 h [39]. Sixty-three percent of the specimens yielded both aerobes and anaerobes. Thirty percent yielded anaerobes only, and only seven percent yielded aerobes only (Table 2). When taken together these studies suggest that at term the growth of some aerobic pathogens may be inhibited as long as the membranes remain intact; whereas anaerobic pathogens may be able to proliferate particularly after labor has begun. With rupture of the fetal mem-

Table 2. Cultures of amniotic fluid from 56 patients undergoing cesarean section with ROM ≥ 6 h.

Anaerobes	
Gram positive cocci	45%
Bacteroides species	9%
Clostridium species	3%
Other	3%
Total anaerobes	60%
Aerobes	
Gram positive cocci	28%
Staphylococcus aureus	2%
E. coli	9%
Other	1%
Total aerobes	40%

Mean number of organisms/patient = 2.5

In this series [39], 95% of the patients subsequently developed post-cesarean endometritis and required antibiotic therapy.

branes, however, amniotic fluid appears to lose its antibacterial activity, thus allowing colonization of the amniotic fluid by any of the potential pathogens in the endocervix and/or vagina.

If amniotic fluid is not available for culture, then a section of amniotic membrane excised from the area of the uterine incision may be placed in prereduced, chopped meat glucose (CMG) broth and sent for culture [48]. Alternatively, an endometrial biopsy specimen from the incision site could be cultured. Apuzzio et al. prefer a culture of the lower uterine segment at the time of cesarean section with prereduced cotton swabs if amniotic fluid is not available [35].

One of the most frequently obtained cultures in a post-cesarean section febrile patient is the transcervical endometrial swab culture. The problems with an unsheathed transcervical endometrial swab culture result from their contamination by the vaginal flora making interpretation difficult. In an attempt to avoid this problem, various sheathed transcervical endometrial culture techniques have been described [27]. Kreutner et al. utilize modified menstrual aspiration kits to obtain endometrial cultures. Gibbs recommends a transcervical endometrial lavage technique utilizing sterile Plasmolyte-148 as an irrigating solution [27]. However, most of these techniques have not achieved widespread clinical utilization, perhaps because most clinicians have not been convinced that the more accurate microbiological information gained is worth the added effort.

Ledger introduced the transabdominal intrauterine aspiration technique in an effort to obtain a culture specimen free from vaginal contamination [36]. The primary problem with this technique is knowing when the 18-gauge spinal needle is inside the endometrial cavity since many times no material is obtained for culture. Platt and associates found culdocentesis a simple, safe and reliable method of obtaining meaningful specimens for culture [5].

Blood cultures are useful in the bacteriological diagnosis of endomyometritis [35]. diZerega et al. reported that 25% of patients with endomyometritis had positive blood cultures [28, 37]. Further, they postulated that the infected soft tissue organ (uterus) functioned like an abscess in that it continually seeded the blood stream with bacteria, allowing for large bacterial inocula in the blood with resultant high recovery rates.

The necessity of utilizing culture techniques which facilitate the recovery of anaerobes must be emphasized [19,51,52]. Cotton swab cultures in an empty sterile tube expose the specimen to excessive oxygen severely limiting the recovery of anaerobic bacteria. A simple method to increase the bacterial yield is to place the cotton swab culture stick in a transport medium such as thioglycollate broth or Cary-Blair medium (Ana-port). However, transport media generally result in a lower yield of anaerobes than primary plating methods. The highest yield of anaerobes is obtained by the direct plating of the specimen at the patient's bedside followed by transport to the laboratory in an oxygen-free environment(Gas-Pak) [40].

ANIMAL MODEL

Earlier in this chapter it was stated that puerperal endomyometritis is a polymicrobial disease usually involving aerobic coliforms and anaerobic bacteria, all of which inhabit the female lower genital tract. In order to determine optimal antibiotic therapy for such infections, a useful animal model was developed to study the evolution of intra-abdominal sepsis [53–56]. Gelatin capsules containing pooled colonic contents were placed into the abdominal-pelvic cavity of rats. Thereafter, the rats developed acute peritonitis resulting in 43% mortality (See Fig. 2). All the animals that survived the acute phase went on to develop discrete intra-abdominal abscesses. This second phase was characterized by an indolent course and progressive abscess enlargement. Eventually, all the rats died from infection-related complications.

Subsequent microbiological evaluation showed that aerobic coliforms were responsible for the early mortality and that anaerobic bacteria were primarily responsible for the late complications of intra-abdominal abscess formation [56]. Recently, studies by Onderdonk et al. stressed the importance of *E. coli* in acute mortality in experimental intra-abdominal sepsis [54]. Their

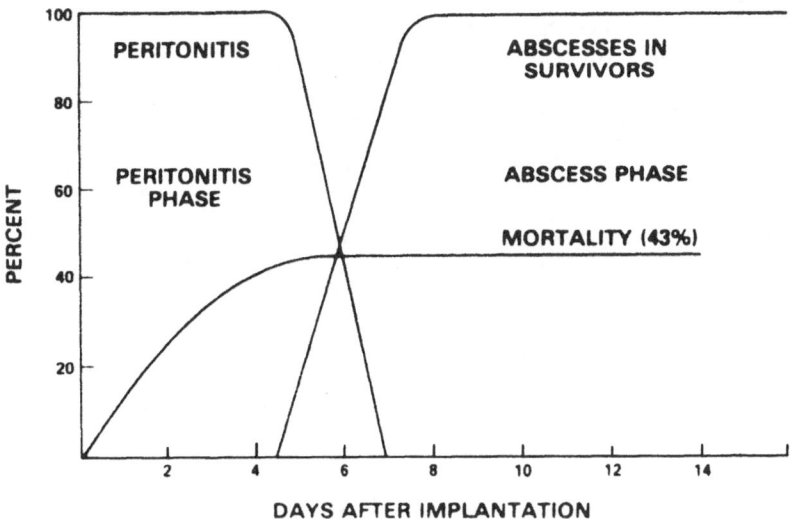

Fig. 2. A graph demonstrating the biphasic nature of intra-abdominal sepsis involving aerobic coliforms and anaerobic bacteria. (Adapted from Weinstein et al., Infect Immun 10:1250, 1979.)

results suggested that intra-abdominal abscess formation was due to a synergistic relationship between anaerobic and facultative bacteria.

Using this animal model of intra-abdominal sepsis, various antibiotics either alone or in combination, have been tested. Weinstein et al. found that gentamicin alone reduced the acute mortality from 40% to 4%, but that all of the survivors continued to develop abscesses [56]. Clindamycin alone was associated with 35% acute mortality, but the incidence of late abscess formation was reduced to 5%. However, a combination of both gentamicin and clindamycin enhanced both survival (93%) and prevention of abscess formation (94% without abscesses). (Table 3).

Louie et al. using the same experimental model, found that the use of four different cephalosporins resulted in a similar reduction in acute mortality [57]. The incidence of abscess formation after treatment with 20 mg doses of cephalosporin revealed that cefoxitin was the most effective agent, cefamandole and cephalothin were of intermediate efficacy and cefazolin was the least effective; these results may reflect the greater in vitro activity of cefoxitin against the strain of *B. fragilis* isolated from the abscesses of untreated animals. Importantly, the overall protection against abscess formation with cephalosporins was less than that with clindamycin alone – 29% vs. 6%. Nichols et al. using a similar experimental model but substituting human fecal material for rat colonic contents and employing three different inoculum sizes, found that only the combination of clindamycin and tobramycin resulted in significantly increased cure rates (survival with no abscess present at time of sacrifice) [58].

These experiments in an animal model suggest that the choice of initial antibiotic therapy is crucial in preventing late infectious complications, i.e., abscess formation. Initial therapy should be aimed at both the aerobic col-

Table 3. Treatment of intra-abdominal sepsis in animal model.

Agent	Number tested	Mortality	Abscesses in survivors
Untreated	60	37%	100%
Gentamicin	57	4%	98%
Clindamycin	60	35%	5%
Gentamicin plus Clindamycin	58	7%	6%
Cephalothin	30	3%	38%
Cefazolin	30	7%	50%
Cefamandole	30	13%	35%
Cefoxitin	30	0%	7%

Effect of antibiotic therapy upon intra-abdominal sepsis induced in rats by insertion of fecal pellets into the abdominal-pelvic cavity. Early treatment with antibiotics effective against anaerobic bacteria (clindamycin, cefoxitin) reduced the formation of abscesses in the survivors (Adapted from Weinstein et al. [56] and Louie et al. [57].

iforms and anaerobic bacteria, for a delay in initiating therapy effective against anaerobic bacteria can result in formation of intra-abdominal abscesses. A clear analogy can be drawn between this rat model of intra-abdominal sepsis and the serious pelvic infections that can occur after the initiating event of a cesarean section – early onset sepsis followed by late onset abscess formation.

TREATMENT

Post-cesarean endomyometritis is usually insidious in onset and may initially be associated with minimal localizing signs. Low-grade pyrexia ($\geq 38°$ C) associated with a slight tachycardia, malaise, and anorexia, should alert the physician to the possibility of post-cesarean endomyometritis, particularly on the third or fourth day postpartum. Other clinical manifestations which may be present include uterine subinvolution and tenderness with increased lochia, which varies from an offensive to an odorless serosanguinous discharge. More severe infections will be accompanied by chills, high fever, and clinical evidence of pelvic peritonitis with an adynamic ileus. It must be emphasized that postpartum pyrexia must be considered to result from endometritis until proven otherwise.

When post-cesarean endomyometritis is suspected, antibiotic therapy must often be instituted prior to identification of the offending organisms and assessment of their antibiotic sensitivities. It is therefore essential that the physician consider what potential pathogenic organisms may be involved and what their antibiotic susceptibility patterns are likely to be.

In order to determine which organisms were responsible for post-cesarean endomyometritis and to determine whether an antibiotic regimen which provided coverage against anaerobic organisms from the time of initiation of therapy had any clinical advantage, a prospective study was carried out by diZerega et al. on 200 patients who developed post-cesarean endomyometritis [28]. None of the patients had received prophylactic antibiotics and none were febrile prior to surgery. Patients were excluded from the study if they developed post-operative atelectasis or if a catheterized urine culture resulted in bacterial colony counts greater than 100 000 cm^3.

Patients with temperatures $\geq 38.4°$ C during the first 24 h post-op or $\geq 38°$ on two separate readings taken at least 4 h apart on any day thereafter comprised the study population. Blood cultures and transcervical endometrial swab cultures were collected from each patient prior to initiation of therapy. The patients were treated with either penicillin (5 million units i.v. every 6 h) or clindamycin (600 mg i.v. every 6 h). In addition all patients received gentamicin 80 mg i.v. every 8 h. Oral penicillin or clindamycin was begun after the patient had been afebrile for at least 36 h to complete a 10 day treatment course. The gentamicin was continued at least five days. Therapeutic decisions were made to either add other antibiotics or heparin or to perform operative procedures for patients remaining febrile ≥ 72 h after initiation of therapy.

The patients who received clindamycin-gentamicin (C-G) as their initial therapeutic regimen did better overall than those who initially received penicillin-gentamicin (P-G). Twenty-nine percent of the P-G patients required additional antibiotics for cure, whereas only 5% of the C-G patients required other antibiotics. In addition, four P-G patients developed serious, potentially life-threatening infectious complications. One patient required a TAH-BSO for a pelvic abscess, one developed a wound evisceration from a subfascial abscess, and two required heparinization for suspected septic pelvic thrombophlebitis.

A similar incidence of serious, infection-related, post-cesarean complications was reported by Gibbs et al.[9]. Following initial treatment with penicillin and kanamycin, 22% required additional antibiotics and 4% had serious complications. (Table 4). Cunningham et al. reported a 7% incidence of post-cesarean pelvic abscess formation following penicillin and tetracycline therapy and 13% after penicillin and tobramycin [6]. Therefore, a significant number (4–13%) of patients develop serious infection-related complications, including pelvic abscess, following cesarean section. To date, only the initial

Table 4. Post-cesarean endomyometritis treatment regimens.

Agent	Number tested	Therapy completed, no problems	Required additional antibiotics	Wound infection	Pelvic abscess	Septic pelvic thrombophlebitis
Clindamycin-gentamicin [28]	100	86	5 (5%)	8	0	0
Penicillin-gentamicin	100	64	29 (29%)	16	1	2
Penicillin-kanamycin [9]	160	125	35 (22%)	19	4	3
Penicillin-tetracycline [6]	61	52	9 (15%)	8	4	NS
Penicillin-tobramycin	45	32	13 (29%)	4	6	NS
Cefoxitin i.v. [65]	18	17	1	NS	NS	NS
Cefoxitin i.m.	7	6	1	NS	NS	NS
Cefamandole [66]	60	50	10 (17%)	6	1	NS
Cefamandole [67]	51	44	7 (14%)	5	10	NS
Cefotaxime	55	46	9 (16%)	NS	1	NS

NS = not specified in article

treatment regimen of clindamycin-gentamicin has been shown to prevent these sequelae.

Two indirect measures of morbidity, duration of hospital stay and fever index, also substantiate the superiority of C-G over P-G for initial treatment of post-cesarean endomyometrítis. An explanation for the difference in clinical response is provided by the blood culture results [37]. Twenty-five percent of the patients from both groups had positive blood cultures. Over 50% of the isolates were anaerobic bacteria. Those patients with anaerobic bacteremia also had significantly higher fever indices than did those with aerobic organisms isolated from their blood. (Fig. 3). Patients with *Bacteroides fragilis* bacteremia had the highest fever index overall.

The influence of antibiotic therapy on febrile morbidity as correlated with blood culture isolated is shown in Fig. 4. Only those patients who had *B. fragilis* bacteremia had a significantly different response (C-G, 71 FDH; P-G,

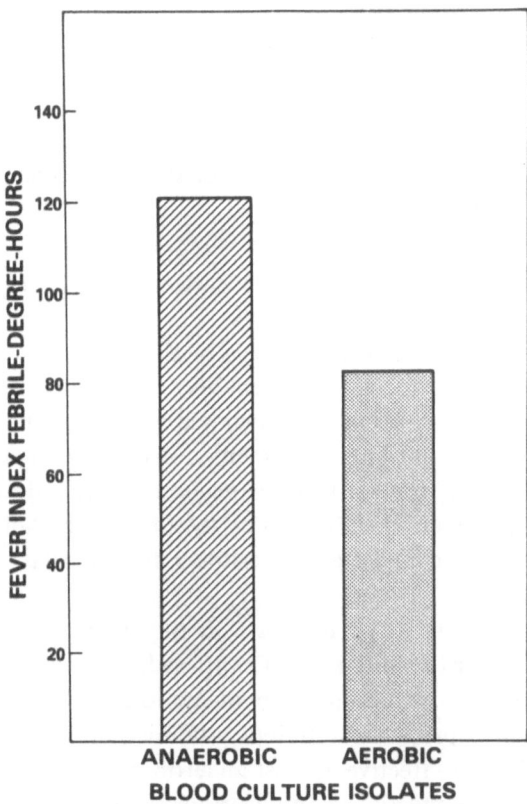

Fig. 3. Bar graphs of the blood culture isolates compiled from both treatment groups contrasting by fever index the febrile morbidity of those patients with anaerobic bacteremia (cross hatched) to those with aerobic bacteremia (stippled). (Adapted from diZerega et al., Obstet Gynecol 55:587, 1980).

94

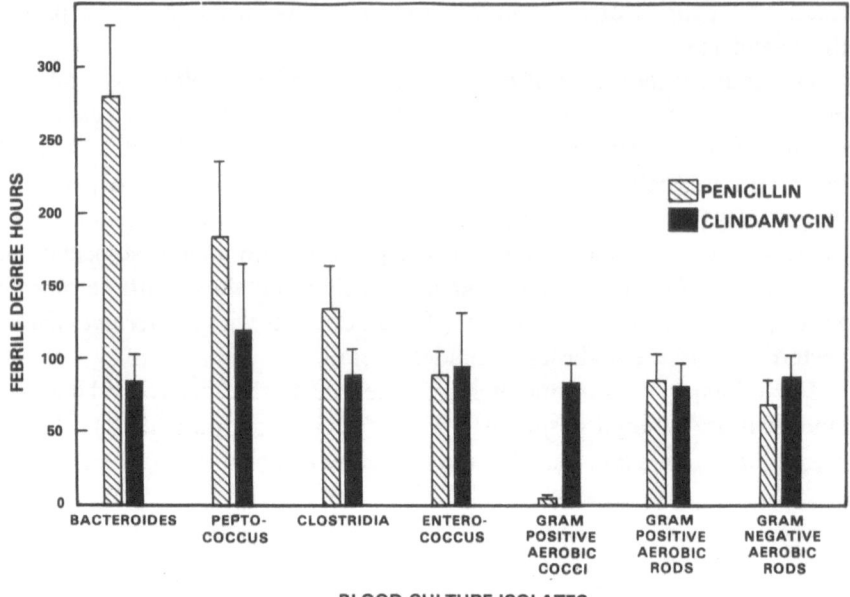

Fig. 4. Comparison of clinical response with the two treatment regimens. Shaded bars = penicillin-gentamicin; solid bars = clindamycin-gentamicin. Bacterial isolates are correlated with the compilation of the representative patients' febrile morbidity as determined by the fever index and expressed in febrile degree-hours. T bars = mean ± 1 SE. (Adapted from diZerega et al. Obstet Gynecol 55:589, 1980).

256 FDH; $p < .01$). All six of the P-G patients with *B. fragilis* bacteremia required additional antibiotics.

Because anaerobic organisms, especially *B. fragilis*, are associated with greater post-cesarean infectious morbidity, antibiotics initially effective against these organisms should be associated with a better clinical response when compared with antibiotic regimens not effective against anaerobes. Indeed, in this study, not only were the fever indices decreased and the duration of hospitalization shortened by the initial use of clindamycin-gentamicin, but even more importantly, serious infection-related complications were prevented.

Thus, there appears to be no place in the treatment of post-cesarean endomyometritis for the initial use of supposedly less toxic antibiotics, such as ampicillin alone, which do not provide good anaerobic coverage. Recall that the timing of appropriate antibiotic administration is critical. A delay in the use of antibiotics effective against anaerobes, especially *B. fragilis*, may result in serious late infectious complications such as abscess formation. By the time an abscess has formed, even the most rigorous medical therapy may not by itself be sufficient to achieve cure. At that point, surgical drainage or removal of infected pelvic organs may be required.

INITIAL TREATMENT FAILURES

For those patients who remain febrile ≥ 72 h after the initiation of C-G, one needs to carefully assess them for possible septic pelvic thrombophlebitis, a pelvic abscess, or a wound infection. Results of bacterial cultures obtained prior to the initiation of antibiotic therapy should also be available by that time and may provide important information regarding antibiotic sensitivities of the potential pathogens.

A pattern of persistent spiking fevers despite adequate antibiotic therapy may be caused by septic pelvic thrombophlebitis (SPT), particularly if there is evidence of septic pulmonary emboli [61]. Once this diagnosis is entertained, an initial bolus of 5000 units of heparin is given by IV push followed by a continuous intravenous infusion at a rate of 1000–2000 units/h. The infusion rate is adjusted to maintain the partial thromboplastin time (PTT) at $2-2\frac{1}{2}$ times control or to maintain the plasma heparin level at 0.05–0.3 iμ/ml. Heparinization is continued for 7–10 days assuming that the patient defervesces within 2 to 3 days [62–64]. However, in the absence of a significant temperature response, a reassessment of the cause of the fever is indicated. It must be emphasized, however, that failure of heparin therapy does not completely negate the diagnosis of SPT, since in some instances there may be concomitant abscesses or other septic complications.

Once a pelvic abscess is suspected, operative intervention is generally required. Occasionally, it is possible to drain the abscess via a colpotomy incision. However, a total abdominal hysterectomy and bilateral salpingo-oophorectomy may be necessary to remove all the infected tissue and achieve cure. This is indeed a high price to pay for a young woman who required a cesarean birth and then developed post-cesarean endomyometritis.

REFERENCES

1. Consensus Development Conference on Cesarean Childbirth NICHD-NIH, Bethesda, Maryland, 1980
2. Jones O: Cesarean section in present-day obstetrics. Am J Obstet Gynecol 126:521, 1976
3. Hibbard L: Changing trends in cesarean section. Am J Obstet Gynecol 125:798, 1976
4. Placek PH, Taffel SM: Demographic variation in cesarean delivery rates: United States, 1970–1978, U.S. Dept of Health, Human Services, National Center for Health Stats, 1980
5. Sweet RL: Anaerobic infections in the female genital tract. Am J Obstet Gynecol 122:891, 1975
6. Cunningham FG, Hauth JC, Strong JD, et al.: Infectious morbidity following cesarean section: comparison of two treatment regimens. Obstet Gynecol 52:656, 1978
7. Gassner CB, Ledger WJ: The relationship of hospital-acquired maternal infection to invasive intrapartum monitoring techniques. Am J Obstet Gynecol 126:33, 1976
8. Gibbs RS, DeCherney AH, Schwarz RH: Prophylactic antibiotics in cesarean section: A double blind study. Am J Obstet Gynecol 114:1048, 1972

9. Gibbs RS, Jones PM, Wilder CJ: Antibiotic therapy of endometritis following cesarean section: Treatment successes and failures. Obstet Gynecol 52:31, 1978

10. Gibbs RS, Listwa HM, Read JA: The effect of internal fetal monitoring on maternal infection following cesarean section. Obstet Gynecol 48:653, 1976

11. Tuteera G, Newman RL: Fetal monitoring: Its effect on the perinatal mortality and cesarean section rates and complications. Am J Obstet Gynecol 122:750, 1975

12. Wiechetek WJ, Horiguchi T, Dillon TF: Puerperal morbidity and internal fetal monitoring. Am J Obstet Gynecol 119:230, 1974

13. Perloe M, Curet LB: The effect of internal fetal monitoring on cesarean section morbidity. Obstet Gynecol 53:355, 1979

14. Green SL, Sarubbi FA: Risk factors associated with cesarean section febrile morbidity. Obstet Gynecol 49:686, 1977

15. Sweet RL, Ledger WJ: Puerperal infectious morbidity. Am. J. Obstet. Gynecol 117:1093, 1973

16. Middleton JR, Apuzzio S, Lange M, Sen P, Bonamo J, Louvia DB: Post-cesarean section endometritis: Causative organisms and risk factors. Am J Obstet Gynecol 137:149, 1980

17. Listwa HM, Dobeck AS, Carpenter J: The predictability of intrauterine infection by analysis of amniotic fluid. Obstet Gynecol 48:31, 1976

18. D'Angelo LJ, Sokol RJ: Determinants of postpartum morbidity in laboring monitored patients: A reassessment of the bacteriology of the amniotic fluid during labor. Obstet Gynecol 136:575, 1980

19. Rehu M, Nilsson CG: Risk factors for febrile morbidity associated with cesarean section. Obstet Gynecol 56:269, 1980

20. Weissberg SM, Edwards NL, O'Leary JA: Prophylactic antibiotics in cesarean section. Obstet Gynecol 38:290, 1971

21. Sohlberg OS, Goodlin RC: The impact of prior labor on cesarean section morbidity. Pac Med Surg 75:54, 1967

22. Anstey JT, Sheldon GW, Blythe JG: Infectious morbidity after primary cesarean sections in a private institution. Am J Obstet Gynecol 136:205, 1980

23. Hagen D: Maternal febrile morbidity associated with fetal monitoring and cesarean section. Obstet. Gynecol 46:260, 1975

24. Larson JW, Goldkrand JW, Hanson TM: Intrauterine infection on an obstetric service. Obstet Gynecol 43:838, 1974

25. Ledger WJ, Kriewall TJ: The fever index: A quantitative indirect measure of hospital-acquired infections in obstetrics and gynecology. Am J Obstet Gynecol 115:514, 1975

26. Gunn GC, Mishell DR, Norton DG: Premature rupture of the fetal membranes. Am J Obstet Gynecol 106:469, 1970

27. Gibbs RS, O'Dell TN, MacGregor RP, Schwarz RH, Morton H: Puerperal endometritis: A prospective microbiologic study. Am J Obstet Gynecol 121:919, 1975

28. diZerega GS, Yonekura ML, Roy S, et al.: A comparison of clindamycin-gentamicin and penicillin-gentamicin in the treatment of post-cesarean endomyometritis. Am J Obstet Gynecol 134:238, 1979

29. Sweet RL, Ledger WJ: Puerperal infectious morbidity. Am J Obstet Gynecol 117:1093, 1973

30. MacKay EV, Khoo SK, Baddeley A: A prospective study of the flora of the lower genital tract during pregnancy. Aust N.Z. J. Obstet Gynecol 17:133, 1977

31. Goplerud CP, Ohm MJ, Galask RP: Aerobic and anaerobic flora of the cervix during pregnancy and the puerperium. Am J Obstet Gynecol 126:858, 1976

32. Gorbach SL, Menda KB, Thadepalli H, Keith L: Anaerobic microflora of the cervix in healthy women. Am J Obstet Gynecol 117:1053, 1973

33. Ohm MJ, Galask RP: Bacterial flora of the cervix from 100 prehysterectomy patients. Am J Obstet Gynecol 122:683,1975

34. De Louvois J, Hurdley R, Standley VC, Jones JB, Foulkes JEB: Microbial ecology of the female lower genital tract during pregnancy. Postgraduate Med J 51:156, 1975

35. Ledger WJ, Norman M, Gee C, et al.: Bacteremia on an obstetric-gynecologic service. Am J Obstet Gynecol 121:205, 1975

36. Ledger WJ: Infection in the Female. Lea and Febiger, Philadelphia, 1977
37. diZerega GS, Yonekura ML, Keegan K, Roy S, Nakamura RM, Ledger WJ: Bacteremia in post-cesarean section endomyometritis: Differential response to therapy. Obstet Gynecol 55:587, 1980.
38. Gibbs RS, Hunt JE, Schwarz RJ: A follow-up study on prophylactic antibiotics in cesarean section. Am J Obstet Gynecol 117:419, 1973
39. Gilstrap LC, Gunningham FG: The bacterial pathogenesis of infection following cesarean section. Obstet Gynecol 53:545, 1979
40. Galask RP, Snyder IS: Bacterial inhibition by amniotic fluid. Am J Obstet Gynecol 102:949, 1968
41. Florman AL, Teuber D: Enhancement of bacterial growth in amniotic fluid by meconium. J Pediatr 79:111, 1969
42. Bergman N, Bercovici B, Sacks T: Antibacterial activity of human amniotic fluid. Am J Obstet Gynecol 114:520, 1972
43. Kitzmiller JL, Highby S, Lucas WE: Retarded growth of E. coli in amniotic fluid. Obstet Gynecol 41:38, 1973
44. Larsen B, Snyder IS, Galask RP: Bacterial growth inhibition by amniotic fluid. I. In vitro evidence for bacterial growth inhibiting activity. Am J Obstet Gynecol 119:492, 1974
45. Larsen B, Snyder IS, Galask RP: Bacterial growth inhibition by amniotic fluid. II. Reversal of amniotic fluid bacterial growth inhibition by addition of a chemically defined medium. Am J Obstet Gynecol 119:497, 1974
46. Thadepalli H, Appleman MD, Maidman JE, Arce JJ, Davidson EC: Antimicrobial effect of amniotic fluid against anaerobic bacteria. Am J Obstet Gynecol 127:250, 1977
47. Schlievert P, Johnson W, Galask RP: Bacterial growth inhibition by amniotic fluid. V. Phosphate to Zinc as a mediator of bacterial inhibitory activity. Am J Obstet Gynecol 125:899, 1976
48. Cooperman NR, Kasim M, Rajashekaraiah KR: Clinical significance of amniotic fluid, amniotic membranes, and endometrial biopsy cultures at the time of cesarean section. Am J Obstet Gynecol 137:536, 1980
49. Guildbeau JA, Jr, Schaub I: Uterine culture technique: A simple method for avoiding contamination by cervical and vaginal flora. Am J Obstet Gynecol 58:407, 1949
50. Platt LD,Yonekura ML, Ledger WJ: The role of anaerobic bacteria in postpartum endomyometritis. Am J. Obstet Gynecol 135:814, 1979
51. Ledger WJ: Anaerobic infections. Am J Obstet Gynecol 123:111, 1975
52. Sweet RL: Anaerobic infections of the female genital tract. Am J Obstet Gynecol 122:891, 1975
53. Onderdonk AB, Weinstein WM, Sullivan-Siegler NM, et al.: Experimental intra-abdominal abscess in rats: Qualitative bacteriology of infected animals. Infect Immun 10:1256, 1975
54. Onderdonk AB, Bartlett JG, Louie TJ, et al.: Microbial synergy in experimental intra-abdominal sepsis. Infect Immun 13:22, 1976
55. Weinstein WM, Onderdonk AB, Bartlett JG, et al.: Experimental intra-abdominal abscesses in rats: Development of an experimental model. Infect Immun 10:1250, 1974
56. Weinstein WM, Onderdonk AB, Bartlett JG, Louie TJ, Gorbach SL: Antimicrobial therapy of experimental intra-abdominal sepsis. J Infect Dis 132:282, 1975
57. Louie TJ, Onderdonk AB, Gorbach SL, Bartlett JG: Therapy for experimental intra-abdominal sepsis: Comparison of four cephalosporins with clindamycin plus gentamicin. J Inf Dis Suppl 518, 1977
58. Nichols RL, Smith JW, Fossedal EN, Condon RE: Efficacy of parenteral antibiotics in the treatment of experimentally induced intra-abdominal sepsis. Review of Inf Dis 1:302, 1979
59. Gibbs RS, Weinstein AJ: Puerperal infection in the antibiotic era. Am J Obstet Gynecol 124:769, 1976
60. Lewis JF, Johnson P, Miller P: Evaluation of amniotic fluid for aerobic and anaerobic bacteria. Am J Obstet Gynecol 65:58, 1976
61. Dunn LJ, VanVoorhis LW: Enigmatic fever and pelvic thrombophlebitis: Response to anticoagulants. NEJM 276:265, 1967

98

62. Josey WE, Cook CC: Septic pelvic thrombophlebitis: Report of 17 patients treated with heparin. Obstet Gynecol 35:891, 1970
63. Josey WE, Staggers SR: Heparin therapy in septic pelvic thrombophlebitis: A study of 46 cases. Am J Obstet Gynecol 120:228, 1974
64. Ledger WJ, Peterson EP: The use of heparin in the management of pelvic thrombophlebitis. Surg Gynecol Obstet 131:1115, 1970
65. Sweet RL, Ledger WJ: Cefoxitin: Single-agent treatment of mixed aerobic-anaerobic pelvic infections. Obstet Gynecol 54:93, 1979
66. Gibbs RS, Huff RW: Cefamandole therapy of endomyometritis following cesarean section. Am J Obstet Gynecol 136:32, 1980
67. Cunningham FG, Gilstrap LC, Kappus SS: Treatment of obstetric and gynecologic infections with cefamandole. Am J Obstet Gynecol 133:602, 1979

Author's address:
George Washington University Medical Center
Department of Obstetrics and Gynecology
The H.B. Burns Memorial Building
2150 Pennsylvania Avenue, N.W.
Washington, D.C. 20037
U.S.A.

PART II

ANTIBIOTIC THERAPY IN GYNECOLOGY

5. DIAGNOSIS AND TREATMENT OF SALPINGO-OOPHORITIS

DAVID ESCHENBACH, M.D.

Acute salpingitis is a spontaneous infection which occurs among sexually active, menstruating, nonpregnant women. The majority of infections are caused by bacteria and a polymicrobial bacterial infection is common. *Neisseria gonorrhoeae, Chlamydia trachomatis* and a wide variety of aerobic and anaerobic bacteria are most frequently isolated from women with acute salpingitis. Genital mycoplasmas also have been recovered from a small number of infections. A tuberculous, parasitic or fungal salpingitis is rare among women in industrialized countries.

Salpingitis is a common infection [1] which is most likely to occur in young women. The rate of salpingitis is highest for women between the ages of 15 and 25 [2]. From 5–10% of all gynecologic admissions occur because of salpingitis.

Approximately 15% of women who develop salpingitis have had a predisposing event [3] which introduces bacterial flora from the normally colonized cervix and vagina into the normally sterile uterine and fallopian tube portion of the upper genital tract. Predisposing events include dilatation and curettage, intrauterine device (IUD) insertion or hysterosalpingography. The remaining 85% of women develop salpingitis spontaneously without prior genital tract instrumentation.

Among the women who spontaneously develop salpingitis, the ascent of bacteria from a cervical location to the uterus and fallopian tubes probably occurs most commonly during menses. The association between infection and menses is most striking among women who develop acute salpingitis in the presence of cervical *N. gonorrhoeae* in whom the onset of abdominal pain occurs within seven days of menses in 1/2 to 2/3 of patients [4, 5]. This circumstantial evidence suggests that gonococci are disseminated from their cervical location during menses. The cervical mucus barrier which possesses mechanical and antibacterial properties to prevent bacterial ascent into the uterus at other times of the menstrual cycle, is lost with menses [5]. Gonococcal growth, particularly of more virulent strains of gonococci may be stimulated during menses. These events during the menstrual period make the patient susceptible to the development of salpingitis.

Obviously salpingitis occurs only during an occasional menstrual period. In addition to menses, the presence of certain virulent bacteria within the

W.J. Ledger (ed.), Antibiotics in Obstetrics and Gynecology, 101–117. All rights reserved.
*Copyright © 1982 by Martinus Nijhoff Publishers, The Hague/Boston/London.*ISBN-13:978-94-009-7466-1

cervix are more likely than others to cause salpingitis. *Neisseria gonorrhoeae*, especially type I gonococci and those which produce endotoxin [6] and *Chlamydia trachomatis* are two virulent organisms capable of causing salpingitis. Genital mycoplasmas may also occasionally manifest virulence.

The virulence of the organism can be countered if the patient develops specific antibodies. It is generally believed that from 10 to 17% of women who are identified to have gonorrhea develop clinically recognized salpingitis [2, 7]. Probably most of these women develop salpingitis within the first one or two menstrual periods following gonococcal acquisition before they have developed gonococcal bactericidal antibodies [8]. The development of specific bactericidal antibodies against the antigens of gonococci appears to protect women from salpingitis [8, 9]. The failure of a patient to develop antibodies may be associated with an increased risk of salpingitis. For instance, up to 50% of women who present to an emergency room with gonorrhea have salpingitis [10]. Because most of the women in this study had symptoms it is likely that these women only recently acquired gonorrhea and perhaps a high proportion developed salpingitis because they did not have time to develop antibodies prior to the onset of infection. The increased rate of salpingitis among younger, rather than older, women may be due to a large proportion of young patients who lack bactericidal antibodies because they had not been previously exposed to gonorrhea. *C. trachomatis* infection may be inhibited by similar specific humoral or local immunity systems.

Normal cervico-vaginal flora has also been associated with salpingitis. These organisms are less virulent than the organisms previously mentioned. Frequently they secondarily invade the fallopian tube following a primary gonococcal [11] or chlamydial infection. These organisms also are frequently associated with infection which develops because of previous tubal damage [5] or with an IUD.

The presence of an IUD is an independent factor in the development of salpingitis [12]. It is most likely that the IUD tail wicks normal cervical and vaginal flora into the otherwise sterile uterus [13]. This mechanism of IUD-associated salpingitis is supported by the finding of intrauterine bacteria at the time of hysterectomy only among tailed IUD users, but not among tailless IUD users or women without an IUD in place [13]. It is also possible that anaerobic bacterial growth is enhanced by the IUD's presence. *Actinomyces israelii* [14] and anaerobic vaginitis [15] are both present more frequently among IUD and non-IUD users. In addition, the IUD may increase salpingitis rates by producing micro-ulcers or by producing a chronic inflammatory reaction.

The usual route of infection is a continuous spread of organisms ascending from the cervix into the endometrial cavity and the fallopian tubes. Lymphatic or hematogenous spread of organisms from the uterus to the tubes and ovaries is uncommon in nonpregnant women except perhaps those with mycoplasma [16] or IUD infection [17]. Once bacteria reach the uterus, organisms most commonly reach the fallopian tube by contiguous spread along the mucosa, although it is possible that organisms may be transported through the fallopian tubes by cilia, or even carried by their attachment to spermatoza. Infectious organisms attach to the fallopian tube mucosa and initiate an endosalpingitis.

Studies of gonococcal infection within human fallopian tube culture serves as a model for salpingitis infection [18]. Following gonococcal attachment to the epithelial cells of the fallopian tube mucosa, gonococci are phagocytized into the cell. The cell then becomes markedly distorted and it loses its ciliary motility. Because the tubal lumen remains open during the early stage of infection, infected material can be exuded through the fimbriated end which produces a peritonitis and contamination of the ovarian surface. If organisms reach the tubal subepithelial connective tissue, muscular and serosal surfaces become involved in the inflammatory process and subsequent scarring is likely. It is probable that aerobic and anaerobic bacteria of the normal flora are more likely to reach the subepithelial connective tissue than gonococci and hence these organisms are more likely than gonococci to produce infertility [19]. Obstruction of the fallopian tube produces distention of the tubal lumen. Intraabdominal abscess formation occurs in 7–16% of patients with acute salpingitis [20,21] as a result of a mixed aerobic and anaerobic peritoneal infection within the tube, within the ovary or between genital and gastrointestinal structures.

Damage of the epithelial cell cilia or surface and even connective tissue damage from an initial infection undoubtedly causes an increased susceptibility of the fallopian tube for further infection. Approximately 20% of women with acute salpingitis develop further episodes of salpingitis [19]. Repeated tubal infection markedly increases infertility. The infertility rate increases from 13% with one episode to 35% with two episodes and to 75% with three episodes of salpingitis [19].

BACTERIOLOGY

Four groups of organisms have been associated with acute salpingitis (Table 1). The proportion of these organisms which cause infection is dependent largely upon the population studied. Previously, patients with salpingitis had been categorized to have either gonococcal or nongonococcal salpingitis. The term gonococcal salpingitis was used when cervical *N. gonorrhoeae* was recovered and the term nongonococcal salpingitis was used among the remaining patients without cervical gonorrhea. There are at least 14 epide-

104

Table 1. Microorganisms isolated from women with acute salpingitis.

Neisseria gonorrhoeae
Chlamydia trachomatis
Genital mycoplasmas
  Mycoplasma hominis
  Ureaplasma urealyticum
Nongonococcal bacteria
  Aerobic bacteria
  Anaerobic bacteria

---

miologic, microbiologic and clinical characteristics which are different between the two groups [22]. However, it has become apparent that while the categorization of salpingitis into gonococcal and nongonococcal forms is clinically useful, it has limited use when discussing the bacteriology because of the wide variety of organisms associated with both types of infection. Women with gonococcal salpingitis can have fallopian tube infection with *N. gonorrhoeae* only, with a combined infection of *N. gonorrhoeae* and the other organism or with the other organisms, *C. trachomatis*, genital mycoplasmas and nongonococcal bacteria. Women with nongonococcal salpingitis can have fallopian tube infection caused by *C. trachomatis*, genital mycoplasma or nongonococcal aerobic and anaerobic bacteria individually or in combination. Although there is a large number of possible combinations of organisms, we will try to simplify the microbiology by discussing each group separately.

Many physicians have mistakenly believed that virtually all salpingitis was caused by *N. gonorrhoeae*. Most investigators have recovered cervical *N. gonorrhoeae* from only 40 to 50% of women with acute salpingitis [23, 24]. However, the proportion of women with salpingitis who have gonorrhea varies widely. Cervical *N. gonorrhoeae* can be recovered from 70 to 80% of interurban U.S. populations [7, 25], but from less than 20% of Swedish women with salpingitis [12]. However, gonorrhea does not cause the majority of salpingitis among women of most populations.

N. gonorrhoeae is the most common intraabdominal isolate from women with acute salpingitis and cervical *N. gonorrhoeae* [11, 23]. The recovery of *N. gonorrhoeae* from the abdomen is greatest during the early stage of the infection [24]. The decrease of *N. gonorrhoeae* recovery rates during the later stage of infection probably occurs because of gonococcal inhibition by leukocytes and because as the inflammatory response progresses more organisms may remain totally intracellular. At a later stage of infection, a tissue sample and not a simple swab sample may be required for the recovery of *N. gonorrhoeae*. It is a common misconception that only *N. gonorrhoeae* is recovered from the tubes of women with gonococcal salpingitis. Although the exact proportion differs among studies, a significant number of patients with salpingitis and cervical gonorrhea have *N. gonorrhoeae* with other aerobic and anaerobic bacteria (5–30%) or other bacteria alone isolated from the abdomen (20–50%) [11, 23–28] (Table 2).

Table 2. Bacterial isolates from the cul-de-sac in patients with salpingitis and cervical *N. gonorrhoeae.*

Author (ref.)	No. of patients	Cul-de-sac isolates			
		N. gonorrhoeae			Aerobic and anaerobic bacteria
		Isolated	Alone	With other bacteria	
Chow et al. [27]	25	4 (16%)	Not stated		
Thompson et al. [28]	30	10 (33%)	Not Stated		
Eschenbach et al. [23]	21	7 (33%)	6 (28%)	1 (5%)	4 (19%)
Monif et al. [11]	28	11 (39%)	5 (18%)	6 (21%)	6 (21%)
Cunningham et al. [25]	56	30 (54%)	12 (31%)	18 (32%)	26 (46%)
Sweet et al. [24]	13	8 (61%)	4 (31%)	4 (31%)	4 (31%)

At present it is believed that gonococci also have the ability to produce infection in a manner that allows subsequent infection by other bacteria. It has been proposed that an orderly progression of a gonococcal and then an increasingly anaerobic infection occurs [11]. However it is not clear whether infection by other bacteria, including anaerobes, occur at the same time and by the same mechanism as gonococcal infection or whether these bacteria enter the infectious process subsequent to an initial gonococcal infection. It is important to recognize mixed infections because women with a polymicrobial, particularly an anaerobic infection, either may respond slowly to antibiotic therapy or may require alternative antibiotic therapy.

C. trachomatis is the second most frequent sexually-transmitted organism which causes acute salpingitis. Cervical *C. trachomatis* can be isolated from 20 to 36% [23, 29] of women with salpingitis. In Sweden, 30% of women with salpingitis have *C. trachomatis* isolated from the fallopian tube. *C. trachomatis* was isolated from the fallopian tube of six or seven women with salpingitis who had cervical *C. trachomatis* [29]. An additional group of patients with salpingitis have significant chlamydial antibody changes which suggest acute chlamydial infection. Recovery of Chlamydia from fallopian tube infection and the initiation of salpingitis in primates infected with Chlamydia clearly demonstrates the ability of Chlamydia to produce salpingitis [30, 31]. As with gonorrhea the rates of Chlamydial recovery from women with salpingitis vary widely [24]. Symptomatic perihepatitis associated with salpingitis (Fitz-Hugh-Curtis syndrome) occurs in from 4% to 9% of women with salpingitis [32, 33]. An additional 5% of women may have asymptomatic

106

perihepatitis [32]. This common cause of pleuritic upper quadrant pain was formerly attributed solely to *N. gonorrhoeae* but recently it has become evident that *C. trachomatis* can also cause perihepatitis [31]. It is also of interest that Chlamydia can be recovered from fallopian tubes and intra-abdominal adhesions of women undergoing tuboplasty because of infertility months to years following an episode of recognized salpingitis [34]. The ability of this organism to remain latent within the abdomen will require a closer scrutiny of antibiotic therapy for patients with salpingitis. Poly-microbial infections with other organisms among women with Chlamydial salpingitis requires further study.

Genital mycoplasma comprises the third group of sexually-transmitted organisms associated with salpingitis. Intraabdominal genital mycoplasma can be recovered from 2 to 16% of patients with acute salpingitis [23, 24, 35]. *Mycoplasma hominis* but not *Ureaplasma urealyticum* produces salpingitis in the Grivet monkey [16]. However, the ubiquity of mycoplasmas in the normal lower genital tract flora and their infrequent isolation from intraabdominal samples suggests that they possess little virulence and that they may only have a minor role in salpingitis.

The fourth group of organisms which have been associated with acute salpingitis are the nongonococcal aerobic and anaerobic bacteria. These organisms are isolated from culdocentesis samples of the abdomen in 30 to 60% of women with salpingitis who do not have cervical gonorrhea (non-gonococcal salpingitis) [23, 24] (Table 3) and from 20 to 50% of women who have salpingitis with cervical gonorrhea (gonococcal salpingitis) (Table 2). Although the frequency of these organisms may be overestimated by con-tamination of the culdocentesis samples by normal vaginal flora, they clearly are important acute salpingitis pathogens. As previously mentioned, among women with cervical gonorrhea and salpingitis, it is currently believed that nongonococcal bacteria secondarily invade the fallopian tube and infect the peritoneum following the initial gonococcal infection. An analogous situa-tion undoubtedly could occur following a primary *C. trachomatis* infection. These organisms are usually the primary pathogens among women who have

Table 3. Bacteria isolated from the cul-de-sac of patients with salpingitis and without cervical *N. gonorrhoeae.*

Author (ref.)	No. of patients	Cul-de-sac isolates		
		Aerobic bacteria alone	Anaerobic bacteria alone	Aerobic and an-aerobic bacteria
Eschenbach et al. [23]	33	7 (21%)	4 (12%)	11 (33%)
Sweet et al. [24]	13	2 (15%)	0 –	2 (15%)

an IUD in place and perhaps among the women with recurrent salpingitis who have had previous tubal epithelial damage. Other unidentified factors, however, must still be present to allow infection with these normal cervicovaginal aerobic and anaerobic bacteria among the women with none of these factors.

The most common isolates from women with nongonococcal salpingitis include aerobic nonhemolytic streptococci, *E. coli* and *H. influenzae* and anaerobic peptococci, peptostreptococci and Bacteriodes [11, 23, 24, 26, 28]. Anaerobic bacteria alone or, more commonly, a polymicrobial mixture of anaerobic and aerobic bacteria have been isolated from 15 to 33% of women with nongonococcal salpingitis. As expected, anaerobic bacteria are virtually always isolated from intraabdominal abscesses caused by salpingitis. Although the absence of *B. fragilis* recovery by some investigators has lead to a doubt of the importance of this organism in salpingitis, we found that not only was it the most common Bacteroides isolated [23], but the demonstration of a specific *B. fragilis ss. fragilis* antibody response among those patients in whom the organism was recovered [36] supports the concept that an infection and not simple colonization of *B. fragilis* occurred. The importance of anaerobic bacteria is further illustrated by the finding of a poor clinical response or early recurrence among 6 of 15 women with anaerobes recovered and 3 of 51 women without anaerobes recovered (p <0.005) [37].

RISK FACTORS

Because many of the organisms which cause salpingitis are sexually-transmitted, it is logical to assume that a further factor in the development of salpingitis would be the number of sexual partners of the women. Women with multiple partners were 4.6 times more likely to have pelvic inflammatory disease (PID) than women with one partner [12]. Another risk factor is the untreated male with gonorrhea; over 80% of male contacts of women with gonococcal salpingitis were not examined or treated before the female presented with salpingitis. One half of the males with gonorrhea was symptomatic but untreated and one half was asymptomatic. The asymptomatic male contact of the women with gonococcal salpingitis had a 40% rate of urethral *N. gonorrhoeae* [38].

As previously discussed, damage to the fallopian tube from prior salpingitis is a risk factor for subsequent salpingitis. A patient who has had salpingitis is over twice as likely as the patient who has not previously had salpingitis to develop subsequent salpingitis [12]. Patients who have had gonorrhea are also at an increased risk of the development of subsequent salpingitis either because of subclinical fallopian tube damage which may occur among asymptomatic women with gonorrhea or because of the increased likelihood of subsequent gonorrhea in this population [38].

Women who have an intrauterine device (IUD) are two to four times more likely to develop salpingitis than women not using an IUD [5, 12, 39, 40]. To date, at least 16 studies have reported a higher IUD usage rate among patients with salpingitis than controls without salpingitis [41]. The intrauterine device may be more commonly associated with the development of salpingitis among nulligravid females (7–9-fold increase in risk) than among multigravid patients (2–3 fold increase in risk) [5, 39], although recent studies found the same increased salpingitis risk for both groups [42]. The relatively high risk of salpingitis among IUD users was not related to a higher rate of salpingitis co-risk factors among IUD than non-IUD users such as the presence of gonorrhea, age, race, marital status, gravidity or the number of sexual partners. Some or all of these factors were matched in these studies. The IUD is more of a relative risk for the development of nongonococcal (2.8%) than for gonococcal salpingitis (6.8%) [5]. There is probably no difference in the severity between IUD-associated salpingitis and the severity of salpingitis among non-IUD users.

Recently the presence of cervical *Actinomyces israelii* has been identified among up to 8% of IUD users [14]. Most of the women were using the IUD for more than 24 months. The organism was not identified in non-IUD users. In an attempt to reduce the rate of *Actinomyces israelli* caused salpingitis, women with this organism should either have the IUD removed, undergo treatment with ampicillin or perhaps both [43]. However, this anaerobic organism has been infrequently isolated from women with IUD-associated salpingitis and the identification of Actinomyces and removal of the IUD in these women would be expected to have little effect on the overall salpingitis rate among IUD users.

DIAGNOSIS

A series of determinations should be made when a patient has acute lower abdominal pain so that either salpingitis can be promptly treated or other pelvic conditions can be distinguished from salpingitis. In patients who have overt salpingitis, it is possible to establish the diagnosis with reasonable certainty by a combination of methods which include history, physical examination, gram stain of the cervix, culdocentesis and examination of the male sexual partner [38]. However, when the diagnosis is uncertain and these methods fail to provide a positive diagnosis, particularly if there is a possibility of surgical disease, laparoscopy should by performed. Physicians should approach the rate of accuracy provided by laparoscopy if they use other diagnostic methods. Laparoscopy remains the standard for the diagnosis of salpingitis; it is a relatively safe procedure and there is no evidence that laparoscopy exacerbates the infection [3, 46].

Clinical Diagnosis

There is a tremendously broad spectrum of clinical manifestations that can result from salpingitis which ranges from mild manifestations leading to a false negative clinical diagnosis, to severe manifestations. The insistence upon rigid criteria such as fever, severe tenderness, leukocytosis and an elevaed sedimentation rate leads to a failure of diagnosis in non-overt cases. The diagnosis of acute salpingitis in the United States is usually made on clinical criteria, which relies almost totally upon the history and the physical examination. This method had been plagued by both false positive and false negative rates. The largest study to address the difficulties of accurately establishing a clinical diagnosis of salpingitis is reported by Jacobson and Westrom [3] who studied 814 consecutive patients with a clinical diagnosis of acute salpingitis. Salpingitis was confirmed by laparoscopy in only 65%. Surprisingly, 12% of patients had other clinical diagnoses established and 23% of patients had no pathology demonstrated. Other investigations have reported similar results [24, 44], although the clinical diagnosis was 89% accurate among the patients with more overt salpingitis studied by Sweet et al. [24].

History

Lower abdominal pain is the most frequent symptom in patients with laparoscopically visualized acute salpingitis, although the pain may be mild or even absent in 6% of patients [3]. The abdominal pain is usually continuous, bilateral and more severe in the lower quadrants. It frequently increases with movement, Valsalva maneuver and intercourse. Pain resulting from salpingitis is usually present for a short time. Pain was present less than 15 days in 83% of patients with visually confirmed salpingitis [45]. Chronic pain of longer than three weeks duration, particularly intermittent pain that does not increase in severity is unlikely to be caused by PID.

The presence or absence of other symptoms may be of only limited use in establishing the diagnosis. Jacobson and Westrom [3] found that patients with visually confirmed salpingitis and patients without salpingitis had the same rate of increased vaginal discharge, irregular vaginal bleeding, urinary symptoms and vomiting. Only a history of fever or chills and proctitis was found more frequently among patients with salpingitis than in patients without the infection.

Table 4. Laparoscopic observation in patients with a clinical diagnosis of PID.

Diagnosis	Jacobson and Westrom	Chaparro et al.	Sweet et al.	Total (%)
Salpingitis	532	103	24	661 (62)
Normal findings	184	51	0	235 (22)
Ovarian cysts	12	39	0	51 (5)
Ectopic pregnancy	11	27	1	39 (4)
Appendicitis	24	2	1	27 (3)
Endometriosis	16	0	0	16 (1)
Other	35	1	1	37 (3)

PID = Pelvic inflammatory disease
From: *Obstet Gynecol* 55:142S, 1980

Salpingitis may be particularly common among women who have recently had the infection and among sexual contacts of men with gonococcal or chlamydial urethritis.

Physical Examination

Patients with salpingitis commonly have lower abdominal, cervical, uterine and bilateral adnexal tenderness. Unilateral salpingitis was demonstrated in 8% of laparoscoped patients [46]. It is of interest that 21 of 26 women believed to have unilateral disease by clinical criteria had bilateral salpingitis by laparoscopy [46]. Few physical findings among women with salpingitis are specific and patients with other disease or no visible disease may have these physical findings. A visually abnormal vaginal discharge was present in less than half of the patients [3], although vaginal leukocytosis is common. A temperature $\geq 38°$ C was present more often among patients with salpingitis than among controls [3] but only 33% of patients with visually confirmed salpingitis had a temperatue greater than 38° C. Physicians who diagnose the infection only among febrile patients clearly diagnose only the most overt disease.

Laboratory Examination

Many physicians place undue emphasis upon laboratory testing for assistance in establishing the diagnosis of salpingitis. The hematocrit level, white blood count and sedimentation rate are of benefit only when abnormal. For example, only 47% of patients with laparoscopically confirmed salpingitis had an elevated white count of 7900 or greater [46]. The sedimentation rate was elevated above 15mm/h in only 76% of women with visually confirmed salpingitis [3].

A cervical gram stain is a helpful laboratory procedure when positive, but unfortunately, it is the least used. Although it is not useful in establishing the diagnosis of gonorrhea among asymptomatic women who are at low risk for gonorrhea, it can be beneficial for diagnosing complicated gonorrhea. Because the gram stain is only 67% sensitive in identifying women who have *N. gonorrhoeae* recovered from the cervix [23], a negative gram stain does not exclude gonococcal disease. The gram stain, however, is 98% specific if performed by experienced physicians and a positive result would allow a presumptive diagnosis of gonococcal salpingitis.

Culdocentesis

Culdocentesis can be used to establish the diagnosis of salpingitis and to obtain culture data. Culdocentesis is beneficial when the abdominal fluid contains white blood cells or non-clotting blood. One would have to exclude appendicitis or other causes of peritonitis that could also be associated with intraabdominal white blood cells. Culdocentesis, of course, is of no diagnostic benefit when no fluid or fluid devoid of white blood cells is obtained.

Examination of the Male

An opportunity to help establish a diagnosis occurs when the male sexual partner is accompanying a patient with suspected salpingitis. Even male partners without an overt discharge should have urethral material obtained by a calcium alginate swab or wire loop. Urethral material should be cultured for gonorrhea and gram stained. Gonococci within the urethral gram stain is strong evidence that a symptomatic female sexual contact has salpingitis.

CULTURES

A cervical culture for *N. gonorrhoeae* is mandatory and a cervical culture for *C. trachomatis* will probably also be required when more is learned about its prevalence in salpingitis. However with rare exception, there is no evidence that the recovery of other bacteria from the cervix will identify the organism in the fallopian tube [26]. The normal cervical flora contains all of the other aerobic and anaerobic bacteria which have been recovered from intraabdominal infections. However, patients with acute salpingitis do not have an increased prevalence of these bacteria in the cervix compared to normal patients. Because the identification of all of these bacteria is not only costly but is of no proven clinical significance, routine culture of the cervix for these organisms is not advocated.

Culdocentesis fluid within a syringe should be made free of air and either immediately injected with anaerobic transport media or placed on anaerobic media. The culture media for aerobic bacteria should include both solid Thayer-Martin and chocolate media for the recovery of *N. gonorrhoeae* because liquid media usually fails to recover this organism [26].

During laparoscopy or laparotomy, purulent material can be obtained by a needle and syringe. The tube can be cannulated with a small catheter or a calcium alginate swab. However tissue is the most ideal abdominal material to culture. *N. gonorrhoeae*, anaerobic bacteria and *C. trachomatis* are more likely to be recovered from infected tissue than from pus.

Ultrasonography

Grey-scale ultrasound scans have been advocated to diagnose the presence of a pelvic abscess because of the high degree (87%) of accuracy [47]. Recent information suggests that an adnexal mass which represents an abscess can be differentiated by ultrasonography from an inflammatory adnexal mass which consists of swollen tube, ovary and bowel. At the present time, ultrasonography is recommended for any large adnexal mass to distinguish an inflammatory mass from an abscess. However ultrasonography should not be used to replace an adequate pelvic examination or to routinely search for an adnexal mass when none is suspected.

TREATMENT

The adequate treatment of salpingitis includes: 1) an assessment of the severity of infection, 2) antibiotic administration, 3) adjacent health measures administration, 4) close patient follow-up and 5) treatment of the male sexual partner.

Because of the cost, most of the patients with salpingitis have not been hospitalized in the United States, although hospitalization of all patients has been advocated and is the standard in many European countries. However, if the recently reported higher treatment failure rate among women receiving oral antibiotics on an outpatient basis is confirmed [48], most women with salpingitis may require hospitalization.

At the present time patients with the following criteria should be admitted: patients with severe clinical manifestations (severe peritonitis, severe nausea, or a temperature >38°), patients with a suspected pelvic abscess, patients who fail to respond to outpatient antibiotics and patients in whom the diagnosis of salpingitis is unclear.

Ideally antibiotic therapy should be directed towards the organism recovered from the fallopian tube but unfortunately, the fallopian tube is not easily cultured. In addition, antibiotics must be empirically administered prior to identification of the organisms so the physician must be aware of the most prevalent organisms isolated from patients with salpingitis. Several recent reports of various antibiotic regimens have been published and are outlined in Table 5. The clinical response to the administration of each of the various antibiotic regimens was usually favorable and, to date, no particular regimen has been shown to be superior over another. Although other antibiotic combinations are possible, until better comparative antibiotic therapy data is available, it seems logical to initiate treatment with antibiotic regimens which have a known response rate.

Patients selected for outpatient therapy usually respond to a loading dose of 1.5 g of tetracycline hydrochloride followed by 500 mg of tetracycline every 6 h for 10 days [48]. An alternative treatment is a loading dose of either 4.8 million units of intramuscular aqueous procaine penicillin G or 3.5 g of oral ampicillin together with 1.0 g of oral probenacid followed by 500 mg of ampicillin every 6 h for 10 days [48]. Both regimens are effective for gonococcal PID. Nongonococcal PID appears to respond best to tetracycline although patients with nongonococcal PID respond more slowly to both regimens than patients with gonococcal PID. Regimens of doxycycline 100 mg twice daily and cephalexin 500 mg four times daily are more expensive and no more effective than the first two regimens.

Hospitalized patients with severe peritonitis but without an adnexal mass usually respond to intravenous administration of aqueous crystalline penicillin G 20 million units daily, 1.0 to 2.0 g of ampicillin every 4 to 6 h or doxycycline 100 mg every 8 h. The combination of penicillin and an aminoglycoside and penicillin and doxycycline has also been used. In contrast, hospita-

Table 5. Antibiotic regimens for salpingitis.

---

1) *Outpatient regimens*
    Tetracycline hydrochloride [49]
        Loading dose 1.5 g, 2 g daily for 10 days
    Ampicillin [49]
        Loading dose 3.5 g plus probenecid, 2 g daily for 10 days
    Doxycycline
        200 mg daily for 10 days
2) *Inpatient regimens*
    Peritonitis
        Aqueous crystalline penicillin G
        Aqueous crystalline penicillin G and an aminoglycoside [28]
        Doxycycline [51]
    Adnexal mass or suspected abscess
        Aminoglycoside and clindamycin
    Penicillin G and chloramphenicol
    Aminoglycoside and metronidazole

114

lized patients with large adnexal masses even without extensive peritonitis should receive an antibiotic that inhibits *B. fragilis* because this organism is recovered from more than 80% of the adnexal abscesses [50]. A combination of either gentamycin 3 to 5 mg/kg in three divided doses combined with clindamycin 600 mg every 6 h or a combination of penicillin 20 million units daily and cloramphenicol 500 mg every 6 h is indicated.

IUD users should have the IUD removed. Although no control data is available at the present time, most investigators recommend removal after 1–2 days of antibiotic therapy.

All patients should be reexamined at 2–3, 7 and 21 days from the beginning of therapy to document a satisfactory clinical response and to obtain repeat cervical specimens from gonorrhea cultures. This represents the minimum number of outpatient visits. Patients who are having a slow response should be seen more frequently.

All recent male sexual contacts of women with acute salpingitis including those who are asymptomatic should be examined and have cultures obtained for *N. gonorrhoeae*, and if possible, *C. trachomatis*. Males with intracellular gram negative diplococci or more than four polymorphonuclear leukocytes per high powered field should be treated for either gonorrhea or nongonococcal urethritis.

With the use of antibiotics which inhibit anaerobic bacteria, particularly *B. fragilis*, therapeutic surgery has become less common. Clearly, the best result in the treatment of a ruptured pelvic abscess is immediate exploration. Early operative transvaginal drainage is also the preferred method of treating a fluctuant pelvic abscess which becomes attached to the vagina in the midline of the cul-de-sac. More difficulty arises in the treatment of an inflammatory mass which does not attach to the vagina, making only a transperitoneal approach possible. Not all of these masses, even large masses, represent abscess formation [3, 46]. Our current recommendation remains the institution of antibiotic therapy which is continued if the mass size declines. Surgical exploration is delayed unless a definite abscess is identified or the mass size remains unchanged. The operative rate with this method is low. If abdominal exploration is necessary, the least extensive amount of surgery which is likely to be effective should be performed, particularly among women who wish to retain their fertility. For instance, the removal of a unilateral abscess without removal of the opposite tube and ovary and the uterus is usually successful when the patient is operated upon under an adequate antibiotic regimen, which would include antibiotics that inhibit *B. fragilis*.

A limited number of patients with salpingitis will have persistent abdominal pain without evidence of an abscess or adnexal pathology except for mild tenderness. If the pain continues for several weeks, laparoscopy should be performed to exclude other pelvic pathology or pelvic adhesions which can then by lysed. In many instances, however, no discernable pelvic pathology is present among patients with persistent pain.

REFERENCES

1. Westrom L: Incidence, prevalence, and trends of acute pelvic inflammatory disease and its consequences in industrialized countries. Am J Obstet Gynecol 138:880, 1980
2. Forslin L, Falk V, Danielsson D: Changes in the incidence of acute gonococcal and nongonococcal salpingitis. Br J Vener Dis 54:247, 1978
3. Jacobson L, Westrom L: Objectionalized diagnosis of acute pelvic inflammatory disease. Am J Obstet Gynecol 105:1088, 1969
4. Falk V, Krook G: Do results of culture for gonococci vary with sampling phase of menstrual cycle? Acta Dermatol Venereol 47:190, 1967
5. Eschenbach DA, Harnisch JP, Holmes KK: Pathogenesis of acute pelvic inflammatory disease: Role of contraception and other risk factors. Am J Obstet Gynecol 128:838, 1977
6. McGee ZA, Melly MA, Gregg CR, et al.: Virulence factors of gonococci: Studies using human fallopian tube organ culture, Immunobiology of N. gonorrhoeae. (Ed. GF Brooks, EL Gotschlich, KK Holmes, et al.) Washington DC: Am Soc Microbiol 1978, p. 258
7. Rendtorff RC, Curran JW, Chandler RW, et al.: Economic consequences of gonorrhea in women. J Am Vener Dis Assoc 1:40, 1974
8. Kasper DL, Rice PA: Antigenic specificity of lipopolysaccharides to the bactericidal antibody response in gonococcal infection, Immunobiology of N. gonorrhoeae. (Ed. GF Brooks, EL Gotschlich, KK Holmes, et al.) Washington DC: Am Soc Microbiol, 1978, p 187
9. Buchanan TM, Eschenbach DA, Knapp JS, Holmes KK: Gonococcal salpingitis is less likely to recur with Neisseria gonorrhoeae of the same principal outer membrane protein (POMP) antigenic type. Am J Obstet Gynecol 138:978, 1980
10. McCormack WM, Stumacher RJ, Johnson K, et al.: A clinical spectrum of gonococcal infection in women. Lancet 1:1182, 1977
11. Monif GRG, Welkos SI, Baer H, et al.: Cul-de-sac isolates from patients with endometritis-salpingitis-peritonitis and gonococcal endocervicitis. Am J Obstet Gynecol 126:158, 1976
12. Flesh G, Weiner JM, Corlett RC, et al.: The intrauterine contraceptive device and acute salpingitis. Am J Obstet gynecol 135:402, 1979
13. Sparks RA, Purrier BGA, Watt PJ, et al.: The bacteriology of the cervical canal in relation to the use of an intrauterine contraceptive device, The Uterine Cervix in Reproduction. (Ed. V Insler, G Bettendorf) Stuttgart: Thieme, 1977, p. 271
14. Hagar WD, Douglas B, Majmudar B, et al.: Pelvic colonization with Actinomyces in women using intrauterine contraceptive devices. Am J Obstet Gynecol 135:680, 1979
15. Amsell R, Eschenbach DA, Spiegel C, et al.: Intrauterine contraceptive devices and nonspecific vaginitis. JAMA, in press
16. Møller BR, Freundt EA, Block FT, et al.: Experimental infection of the genital tract of female Grivet monkeys by Mycoplasma hominis. Infect Immunol 20:258, 1978
17. Taylor ES, McMillan JH, Greer BE et al.: The intrauterine device and tuboovarian abscess. Am J Obstet Gynecol 123:338, 1975
18. Ward ME, Watt PJ, Robertson JN: The human fallopian tube: A laboratory model for gonococcal infection. J Infect Dis 129:650, 1974
19. Westrom L: Effect of acute pelvic inflammatory disease on fertility. Am J Obstet Gynecol 121:707, 1975
20. Lardaro HH: Spontaneous rupture of tuboovarian abscess within the free peritoneal cavity. JAMA 156:699, 1954
21. Pedowitz P, Bloomfield RD: Ruptured adnexal abscess (tuboovarian) with generalized peritonitis. Am J Obstet Gynecol 88:721, 1964
22. Eschenbach DA, Holmes KK: The etiology of acute pelvic inflammatory disease. Sex Trans Dis 6:224, 1979

116

23. Eschenbach DA, Buchanan TM, Pollock HM, et al.: Polymicrobial etiology of acute pelvic inflammatory disease. N Engl J Med 293:166, 1975
24. Sweet RL, Mills J, Hadley KW, et al.: Use of laparoscopy to determine the microbiologic etiology of acute salpingitis. Am J Obstet Gynecol 134:68, 1979
25. Cunningham FG, Hauth JC, Gilstrap LC, et al.: The bacterial pathogenesis of acute pelvic inflammatory disease. Obstet Gynecol 52:161, 1978
26. Chow AW, Patten V, Marshall JR: Bacteriology of acute pelvic inflammatory disease. Am J Obstet Gynecol 133:362, 1979
27. Chow AW, Malkasian KL, Marshall JRL: The bacteriology of acute pelvic inflammatory disease. Am J Obstet Gynecol 122:876, 1975
28. Thompson SE, Hagar WD, Wong KH, et al.: The microbiology and therapy of acute pelvic inflammatory disease on hospitalized patients. Am J Obstet Gynecol 136:179, 1980
29. Märdh PA, Ripa T, Svensson L, et al.: Role of *Chlamydia trachomatis* infection in acute salpingitis. N Engl J Med 296:1377, 1977
30. Ripa KT, Møller BR, Märdh PA, et al.: Experimental acute salpingitis in Grivet monkeys provoked by *Chlamydia trachomatis*. Acta Pathol Microbiol Scan Sect B Microbiol Immunol 87:65, 1979
31. Møller BR, Märdh PA: Experimental salpingitis in Grivet monkeys by *Chlamydia trachomatis*. Acta Path Microbiol Scand 88:107, 1980
32. Onsrud M: Perihepatitis in pelvic inflammatory disease – association with intrauterine contraception. Acta Obstet Gynecol Scand 59:69, 1980
33. Wang S-P, Eschenbach DA, Holmes KK, et al.: *Chlamydia trachomatis* infection in Fitz-Hugh-Curtis syndrome. Am J Obstet Gynecol 138:1034, 1980
34. Henry-Suchet J, Loffredo V: Chlamydia and mycoplasma genital infection in salpingitis and tubal sterility. Lancet 1:539, 1980
35. Märdh PA, Westrom L: Tubal and cervical cultures in acute salpingitis with special reference to *Mycoplasma hominis* and T-strain mycoplasmas. Br J Vener Dis 46:179, 1970
36. Kasper DL, Eschenbach DA, Hayes ME et al.: Quantitative determination of the serum antibody response to the capsular polysaccharide of *Bacteroides fragilis* subspecies *fragilis* in women with pelvic inflammatory disease. J Infect Dis 138:74, 1978
37. Eschenbach DA: Acute pelvic inflammatory disease. Presented at the 13th Interscience Conference on Antimicrobial Agents and Chemotherapy, Washington DC, September 19–21, 1973
38. Eschenbach DA: Epidemiology and diagnosis of acute pelvic inflammatory disease. Obstet Gynecol 55:142S, 1980
39. Westrom L, Bengtsson LP, Märdh PA: The risk of pelvic inflammatory disease in women using intrauterine contraceptive devices as compared to non-users. Lancet 2:221, 1976
40. Vessey M, Doll R, Peto R, et al.: A long term follow-up study of women using different methods of contraception – an interim report. J Biosoc Sci 8:373, 1976
41. Senanayake P, Kramer DG: Contraception and the etiology of pelvic inflammatory disease: New perspectives. Am J Obstet Gynecol 138:852, 1980
42. Osser S, Liedholm P, Gullberg B, Sjoberg NO: Risk of pelvic inflammatory disease among intrauterine devise users irrespective of previous pregnancy. Lancet 1:386, 1980
43. Spence MR, Gupta PK, Frost JK, et al.: Cytologic detection and clinical significance of *Actinomyces israelii* in women using intrauterine contraceptive devices. Am J Obstet Gynecol 131:295, 1978
44. Chaparro MV, Ghosh S, Nashed A, et al.: Laparoscopy for the confirmation and prognostic evaluation of pelvic inflammatory disease. Int J Gynecol Obstet 15:307, 1978
45. Westrom L, Märdh PA: Epidemiology, etiology and prognosis of acute salpingitis: a study of 1457 laparoscopically verified cases in nongonococcal urethritis and related diseases. (Ed by D Hobson, KK Holmes) Washington DC: Am Soc Microbiol, 1977, p. 84
46. Falk V: Treatment of acute non-tuberculous salpingitis with antibiotics alone and in combination with glucocorticoids. Acta Obstet Gynecol Scand 44 (Suppl 6), 1965
47. Taylor KSW, Wassen JF, deGraaff C, et al.: Accuracy of grey-scale ultrasound diagnosis of abdominal and pelvic abscesses in 220 patients. Lancet 1:83, 1978

48. Thompson S, Holcomb G, Cheng S, et al.: Antibiotic therapy of outpatient pelvic in-flammatory disease. Presented at the 20th Interscience Conference on Antimicrobial Agents and Chemotherapy, New Orleans, La, 22–24 September 1980
49. Cunningham FG, Hauth JC, Strong JD, et al.: Evaluation of tetracycline or penicillin and ampicillin for treatment of acute pelvic inflammatory disease. N Engl J Med 296:1380, 1977
50. Thadepalli H, Gorbach SC, Keith L: Anaerobic infections of the female genital tract: bacte-riology and therapeutic aspects. Am J Obstet Gynecol 117:1034, 1973
51. Monif GRG, Welkos SC, Baer H: Clinical response of patients with gonococcal endocer-vicitis and endometritis-salpingitis-peritonitis to doxycycline. Am J Obstet Gynecol 129:614, 1977

Author's address:
Department of Obstetrics and Gynecology RH-20
University of Washington School of Medicine
Seattle, Washington 98195
U.S.A.

6. DIAGNOSIS AND TREATMENT OF
THE PATIENT WITH AN INFECTED ABORTION

RICHARD SCHWARZ

Despite the fact that revised attitudes and laws concerning abortion have led to a concomitant increase in medically performed abortions and a decrease in non-medical procedures, the serious problems of the patient with an infected abortion persist [1]. The frequency of non-medical abortion and its sequelae vary geographically throughout the world, in a fashion which is generally inversely related to the sanction of medical abortion. The high rank of septic abortion in the maternal mortality and morbidity statistics in the United States has been greatly reduced in the past two decades [2]. Nonetheless, because of the persistence of non-medical abortion in some areas as well as the result of complications of medical abortions, the practioner must still deal with the clinical entity.

PATHOPHYSIOLOGY

In most instances non-medical abortion attempts are initiated by the introduction through the cervix of a foreign body such as a urethral catheter. The result is a degree of separation of the products of conception from the implantation site along with the introduction of bacteria from the normal cervical and vaginal flora. If the uterus is not emptied promptly and completely the combination of blood and necrotic products of conception provide an ideal culture medium for the growth of both the aerobic and anaerobic microflora. The process is initially confined to the products and the superficial decidua but untreated may spread to the deeper layers of the myometrium and also probably by lymphatic spread to the adnexae resulting in abscesses which may at times be microscopic in size. Septic thrombophlebitis in the contiguous pelvic veins is often seen in advanced cases presumably because of the proximity of anaerobic infections with heparinase producing organisms (*B. fragilis*). Bacteremia may occur and with the predominant gram negatives (*E. coli*), endotoxin may lead to shock, disseminated intravascular clotting, shock lung and death. Renal failure is also a common end-stage problem in the form of acute tubular necrosis or in some cases bilateral cortical necrosis. Renal failure is especially a problem with clostridial sepsis which is accompanied by hemolysis.

W.J. Ledger (ed.), Antibiotics in Obstetrics and Gynecology, 119–135. All rights reserved.
Copyright © 1982 by Martinus Nijhoff Publishers, The Hague/Boston/London. ISBN-13:978-94-009-7466-1

There is a number of variations in this clinical sequence which may result from the nature of the abortion attempt or immediate complications thereof. Uterine perforation at the time of the attempt may lead to intraperitoneal bleeding and hypovolemia. However, more often there is no continuing bleeding at the perforation site and the impact is simply to seed the myometrium and the peritoneum with blood and bacteria. In some cases caustic and/or toxic substances are instilled through the catheter. These may produce chemical burns and even absorption which is prone to occur because of the vascularity. The latter may lead to systemic toxicity. Soap and detergent solutions have been employed commonly and besides producing extensive necrosis, cause hemolysis on gaining access to the intravascular space. Potassium permanganate tablets may be placed in the vagina instead of the cervical canal causing severe burns.

Intrauterine devices are associated with a unique syndrome of septic abortion in that the process begins with migration of organisms along the tail of the device into the extraovular space, producing chorioamnionitis [3]. This infection then leads to spontaneous abortion in contrast to the usual process in which the abortion is initiated and becomes secondarily infected. Also peculiar to this process in which a patient becomes pregnant with an I.U.D. in place, is the initial clinical presentation which often does not focus attention on the pregnancy. Endotoxin shock or shock lung may actually precede gross signs of uterine infection or abortion [4]. Because of the insidious nature of the problems it is generally advised that patients who conceive with IUD's in place have them removed as soon as possible if the pregnancy is desired. If the string is not available for removal, termination should probably be urged since the potential for serious infection is significant and the ability to monitor for its onset limited.

MICROBIOLOGY

In most cases the bacteria involved in septic abortions are representatives of the normal cervical and vaginal flora acting opportunistically in the presence of altered host defenses [5, 6, 7]. Microbiologically, then, there is no difference between this and other polymicrobial soft tissue pelvic infections. Patients in the reproductive age groups commonly have several facultative as well as anaerobic species present in the genital tract. Among the facultatives, *E. coli* predominates and classically is the dominant organism in the early stages of the process and often the source of endotoxin shock. Anaerobes which are also inoculated at the start of the process tend to flourish as the facultative organisms consume oxygen and the oxidation reduction potential diminishes. Anaerobes dominate late in the process with abscess formation and although most of the species are susceptible to penicillin as well as other common antibiotics, Bacteroides especially *B. fragilis*, is a problem because of its penicillin resistance. The selection of antibiotics to cover *B. fragilis* is a special problem in management. However antibiotics are frequently a secondary consideration since penetration of abscesses and necrotic tissue reduces effectiveness and necessitates surgical drainage.

A few organisms merit special mention. *Clostridium welchii* is present in the normal vaginal flora in 8–10% of women [8, 9]. Although this organism is capable of producing often fatal gas gangrene, its recovery from the cervix of a patient with an infected abortion does not necessarily imply causality. The full-blown clinical syndrome includes extensive myonecrosis with gas formation and hemolysis [10]. If not treated aggressively, particularly with extensive surgical debridement, shock, renal failure and death are almost inevitable.

Neisseria gonorrheae is exogenous to the genital flora but can be recovered from the cervix of asymptomatic women in some populations with a frequency which may exceed 5%. Any abortion attempt in the presence of cervical gonorrhea may result in endometritis, and if unchecked, adnexal involvement as well [11]. Some workers have suggested the administration of prophylactic tetracycline at the time of curettage for abortion which would theoretically control this problem. Because of the relatively low frequency of infectious morbidity with early therapeutic abortion, a more logical approach would be pre-operative screening with treatment of culture proved carriers.

Listeria monocytogenes is also associated with reproductive failures including late pregnancy stillbirths as well as spontaneous abortion [12]. Little is known about the epidemiology of this organism and the matter is further complicated by the fact that the organism is difficult to grow and often not identified. It is not likely that *Listeria* will be found as a common pathogen in septic abortion but it requires special attention to detect when present.

DIAGNOSIS

By definition a septic abortion is a threatened, inevitable or incomplete abortion upon which the infectious element is superimposed and consequently both parts of the diagnosis must be established. The confirmation of a diagnosis of pregnancy may range from simple in a patient in whom this has been done previously to exceedingly difficult in a seriously ill patient who has had a clandestine attempt at abortion and is frightened about divulging the facts. The history is extremely important if the patient will comply. Knowing the precise nature of the attempt at induction of abortion is critical especially when toxic substances are involved. The timing is also important.

The longer the delay between intervention and presentation for medical care, the more likely the infectious process is to be widespread and microbiologically the more likely there will be abscess formation with anaerobic bacteria. It should be noted that since many of these cases become legal matters, careful recording of the history and indeed of all medical information is critical. The history should be as complete as possible and obviously preexisting diseases are also important.

The general physical examination should begin with an overall assessment of the severity of the problem. Recognizing that both blood loss and sepsis may produce shock in these patients it should include recording of the vital signs as well as such other parameters as the state of consciousness, skin color and temperature and especially in the more seriously ill some rapid assessment of urinary output by measuring the quantity of bladder urine. In the seriously ill patient this should be accomplished simultaneously with establishing intravenous and other necessary lines and collecting appropriate samples for laboratory evaluation.

Specifically, the physical examination should address the status of the lungs (pulmonary emboli and congestive heart failure), the heart (rate and arrhythmia) and the abdomen. The latter examination provides evidence of the extent of the process and thereby a guide to therapy. When the process is limited to the endometrial cavity, abdominal signs will be absent except for direct tenderness over the uterine fundus if it is palpable suprapubically. If the process has spread laterally with parametritis, adnexitis or abscess formation, lower abdominal signs will become more prominent. Uterine perforation with bleeding or abscess rupture will lead to four quadrant signs with evidence of peritonitis and ileus. In advanced and incompletely treated cases, upper abdominal and chest signs may indicate subhepatic or subphrenic collections.

The pelvic examination is critical and should be accomplished promptly and by the most experienced person available. The vulva is inspected and then the vagina, looking especially for evidence of trauma or chemical burns. All tissue and foreign material in the vagina should be saved. If there is a catheter or other foreign object protruding from the cervix it is best left in place until X-rays can be done to localize the tip. The cervix should also be inspected for trauma and its status with regard to dilatation be determined since this may be the only way to differentiate a threatened from an inevitable abortion. Microbiologic samples are obtained at this point as subsequently outlined. Bimanual palpation is then directed toward the determination of uterine size. The presence of tenderness and the extent of tenderness and induration or adnexal masses is critical to management. However when abscesses are present the tenderness is often such that accurate definition of the masses is difficult [13]. The cul de sac should be evaluated by both bimanual and rectovaginal palpation for the presence of a collection. Ultrasound may be useful in clarifying these points.

LABORATORY ASSESSMENT

A. Microbiology

The general principles of clinical microbiology which apply to all mixed pelvic infections apply as well to the patient with a septic abortion and include:
1. There is usually not a single pathogenic bacteria isolated.
2. Recovery from the cervix or vagina of aerobic or anaerobic organisms which are part of the 'normal' flora does not imply causality and does not assist appreciably in determining therapy.
3. Blood cultures are helpful if positive but are not regularly so.
4. Sensitivity studies are not particularly helpful because of the polymicrobial etiology and also because anaerobes grow slowly making such testing impractical, and often inaccurate.
5. The presence of an exogenous pathogen such as *Neisseria gonorrheae* in the cervix or vagina is significant but does not indicate its role in the upper tract.
6. Antibiotic selection must be based upon knowledge of the usual organisms involved and their antibiotic sensitivities.

Sources of cultures:

1) *Blood* – blood cultures are advisable in all but the most mildly ill patient with an infected abortion. If positive they rather clearly indicate a pathogenic role for the organism and of additional importance is the fact that in many hospitals these are the most anaerobically obtained and handled cultures. The number of blood cultures and their timing is a much discussed matter. In the septic abortion patient, it is not likely that a blood culture will be obtained with the chill prior to the fever spike and the best compromise is to obtain it at the initiation of therapy. As to the number, two samples obtained from separate sites with careful skin preparation should suffice.

2) *Genital tract* – cervical cultures are of importance *only* for the recovery of exogenous organisms and in this case the major one of consequence is *Neisseria gonorrheae*. Although it is difficult if not impossible to obtain uncontaminated samples from the endometrial cavity, it is worth an attempt if the cervix is widely dilated. Such a sample should be evaluated both by culture and gram stain to check for the predominant organism. A reasonable alternative is to send a fragment of placental tissue for culture. An anaerobic transport system may be used to handle these samples. However, even with the best techniques of obtaining or handling samples, the information gained will be of limited clinical value.

3) *Peritoneal – upper genital* – samples obtained from the peritoneal cavity or the tubes which would normally be sterile are obviously of great value in the patients with more advanced pathology. In the patient with peritonitis, if the cul de sac is free, culdocentesis is a reasonable approach to obtaining a useful sample for microbiologic study. There is always some fluid present in the peritoneal cavity and with peritonitis the quantity increases. Although some have raised the question of contamination as the needle penetrates the posterior vagina, such contamination is of relatively minor import if a significant volume of fluid is obtained. The fluid should be evaluated by gram stain as well as by aerobic and anaerobic culture. It is best transported to the laboratory in the syringe which has been capped after the air is evacuated. Presumptive identification of bacteria may be possible by the combination of odor and gram stain characteristics if pus is obtained. Fecal odor indicates anaerobes and if the morphology is gram positive cocci the organism is likely peptostreptococcus (anaerobic streptococcus), while if gram negative rods *B. fragilis* is likely. In the absence of a fecal odor gram negative rods are most probably *E. coli*. In the case of *C. welchii* the rather typical dumbbell-shaped gram positive rods are quite suggestive especially if they predominate in the smear. In addition to culdocentesis, fluid collected at laparotomy or by abscess drainage is appropriate for detailed microbiologic study and should be handled as already detailed.

4) Urine sediment examination and cultures may be done if there is any concern or if the source of the fever is not clear.

B. Other Laboratory Studies

1) *Hemoglobin – hematocrit* – these may reflect the degree of blood loss or preexisting anemia while in other cases, particularly if blood loss is acute, dilution may not have occurred and they may not reflect the true problem.

2) *White count and differential* – although elevation of the white count with a shift in the differential toward immature forms is classical for severe infection, the variation may be from a transient leukopenia to a leukemoid reaction.

3) *BUN creatinine* – these values are not likely to be abnormal except in the most severe cases but should be determined as a base line even in the moderately ill patient.

4) *Glucose* – blood sugar values are expected to be normal in the absence of diabetes. However, the release of catecholamines with stress can bring about glycogen mobilization with increase in blood sugars followed in a more advanced and exhaustive phase by hypoglycemia.

5) *Electrolytes and blood gasses* – these may not be necessary in mild infections but in severe cases and certainly if there is any evidence of shock they are essential. Anticipated changes in the critically ill patient include progressive metabolic lactoacidosis with hypoxemia. Serial evaluations are necessary.

C. Radiographic Studies

1) *Chest* – an upright chest film in addition to scanning the lungs and cardiac configuration is the best approach to detecting air under the diaphragm, a finding which may be present with uterine perforation or in gas forming infections.

2) *Abdominal film* – this is important for the detection of foreign bodies as well as gas formation in pelvic tissues in the case of clostridial infections.

3) Other studies including contrast studies of bowel and urinary tract may be indicated in specific cases.

D. Physiologic Monitoring

In the critically ill patient it may be necessary to monitor all these functions while in the mild case nothing more than the routine vital signs may be needed. Although all of these measures may be of value in the immediate assessment of the critically ill patient it is intermittent or continuous recording that provides the most useful information about prognosis and treatment response.

1) *Urinary output* – although this can be monitored by measuring voided urine, catheter placement is necessary in more seriously ill patients with hourly recording of urine formation. Output is a good index of effective central perfusion and should exceed 20 ml/h.

2) Blood pressure may be recorded intermittently in the standard fashion or with Doppler instruments but in the seriously ill patient an arterial line can afford continuous recording as well as a ready source for intermittent blood gas determinations. The response of the blood pressure to postural change is a useful technique for rapidly assessing blood volume.

3) *Central venous pressure* – this can be measured by placing a catheter into the right atrium most commonly by way of the subclavian vein although it can also be placed through the antecubital or the jugular veins. Catheter place-

126

ment can be checked radiographically or by appropriate fluctuations with respirations. Measurements of 5–12 cm of water are normal with lower values generally indicating decreased blood volume. Although this technique has some pitfalls when applied to patients with heart disease or significant shunts, it is in the young, otherwise healthy individual a guide to blood volume and a good means to monitor volume replacement.

4) Pulmonary wedge pressure can be monitored by placement of a Swan Ganz catheter. This is a more sophisticated approach of choice in the critically ill patient.

5) ECG and heart rate should also be continuously recorded in the seriously ill patient.

TREATMENT

The general principles of management of the patient with an infected abortion are not different from those involved in the treatment of any surgical infection. The establishment of adequate drainage and debridement of necrotic tissue although accomplished somewhat differently (by dilatation and curettage) are the primary concerns while antibiotic therapy is important but secondary to the surgical approach. Supportive measures are also a concern and especially so in seriously ill patients with complications such as septic shock.

SURGICAL MANAGEMENT

In the majority of patients with infected abortions, cure is accomplished by evacuating the infected products of conception from the uterus. This is indicated in all patients with infected abortions although the patient with a septic threatened abortion may be a rare exception. When a patient presents with an apparently intact pregnancy and uterine infection, a short carefully monitored trial of conservative therapy with parenteral antibiotics may be justified. The likelihood of success is small with the process usually progressing in the face of infection to an inevitable or incomplete status. Even if this does not occur the integrity of the pregnancy should be closely monitored by HCG levels or if far enough along by real time ultrasound. At the opposite end of the spectrum it is unwise to consider any septic abortion complete until a curettage has been carried out. Although this is sometimes done in the non-infected patient, leaving placental fragments with infection simply delays the recovery and increases the risk of complications.

Uterine size is the main constraint in the approach to evacuation. Conventional or suction curettage is usually considered to be safe with uteri up to 12 weeks in size and perhaps slightly larger. When the uterus is larger the risk of perforation increases. The use of oxytocin for a short period may bring about sufficient uterine contraction and evacuation of some contents so as to make curettage safer. In rare cases hysterotomy or hysterectomy may be necessary. The technique for curettage is a matter of preference of the surgeon. However, the danger of perforation is lessened by using the largest instruments which can be readily passed through the cervix and some feel that the large suction curet is even safer than the blunt or sharp curet.

Timing of uterine evacuation is also an important matter. In the past there was reluctance to proceed with curettage in the infected patient. However, experience has lead to an awareness that this was not an effective approach. Without evacuation patients continued a febrile course in spite of antibiotics. For most patients the ideal approach is to evacuate the uterus promptly after the establishment of an antibiotic level. With intravenous administration, the delay should be no longer than one or two hours, time which is commonly consumed by other preparations unless the situation is emergent. Bleeding at the time of admission can usually be controlled by removal of placental fragments from the cervical canal with ring forceps and the administration of oxytocin by infusion. Since in most cases the cervix is already dilated the procedure can be accomplished readily, often with sedation and local anesthesia, obviating the delays inherent in the use of general anesthesia for the patient who has recently eaten. Some have suggested that the presence of significant parametritis might be a reason to delay the manipulation of curettage. However, even under those circumstances evacuation of the infected products from the cavity will in the long run most probably hasten rather than delay resolution.

The role of more extensive surgery in infected abortion is extremely limited. As already suggested, the uterus which is too large for safe curettage can often be dealt with by delay and the use of oxytocin. Hysterotomy is a procedure which is associated with a significant infectious morbidity even when applied primarily as a means of mid-trimester pregnancy termination. Consequently it is not a desirable approach to emptying an infected uterus. There is perhaps a rare case of an advanced gestation septic abortion in a young low parity patient in whom hysterotomy might be tried if oxytocin is unsuccessful. It would of necessity be coupled with intensive antibiotic therapy and with the recognition that further surgery might be necessary at a later time to adequately deal with the problem. Nonetheless the calculated risk could be worth taking in these special circumstances. Hysterectomy is not often needed but if the same contingencies occur in an older multiparous woman or if there is

128

evidence of spread of infection to the adnexal structures or if there is a failure to respond to more conservative measures it may become necessary. In most instances if this occurs removal of the tubes and ovaries should probably be carried out as well. Even if there is no obvious adnexal involvement, micro-abscesses may be present and consequently the risk exists of doing non-curative surgery. Although it is not often necessary to treat it surgically, pelvic thrombophlebitis is a complication of anaerobic pelvic infection. At times because of the extent and failure to respond to anticoagulant therapy high ovarian vein and vena canal ligation may be indicated.

MEDICAL MANAGEMENT

The role of antibiotics in the management of an infected abortion is significant but clearly secondary to the role of surgery. The situation is analogous to all surgical infections. In the infected abortion drainage and debridement generally mean uterine evacuation. Antibiotic selection should be guided by the following principles:
1) A single drug whenever possible.
2) The narrowest spectrum of activity which will cover the pathogens and consequently impact least upon the flora.
3) Low toxicity.
4) Bactericidal.
5) Lowest cost.
Because there is not a single identifiable pathogen in these mixed infections it is not possible to select an antibiotic with a narrow area of action, but rather there must be wide coverage for the many possible pathogens, a fact which often leads to the use of combinations of drugs. Although there is a theoretic advantage to bactericidal antibiotics, it is probably of real importance only when dealing with infections such as subacute bacterial endocarditis and not in most mixed infections of this type. Toxicity is likely to be the major determinant of antibiotic selection as well as development in the future. Some of the most potent of the currently available agents such as the aminogly-cosides and chloramphenicol provide the greatest concerns about toxicity. Although in many instances the septic abortion patient is seriously ill and consequently the exposure to a toxic drug justified, it would be an obvious advantage to have an antibiotic or combination of agents of low toxicity even under these circumstances. Because of the method of action of the penicillin-cephalosporin family (*Beta lactam*) antibiotics, they tend to have the lowest level of serious toxicity. This is because they inhibit cell wall synthesis and while bacteria have cell walls human cells do not. Also critical in the selection of antibiotics is the severity of the patient's illness. Often in a patient with a

septic incomplete abortion who is only mildly or moderately ill, recovery is prompt after uterine evacuation, irrespective of the drug selected and regardless of its spectrum of activity. In contrast, the proper selection may be critical in a patient who is desperately ill with impending septic shock. It is also apparent that there are a number of agents or combinations which may be appropriate [6, 14] and therefore they will be discussed individually with respect to the spectrum of activity as well as potential for toxicity.

Penicillin

When administered parenterally in high doses (20 million units/24h) there is reasonably broad activity with two important exceptions for the septic abortion patient. First among the gram negative aerobes there will be a number of resistant strains of *E. coli* as well as some other enterobacteriacae of lesser importance. Among the anaerobes most will be sensitive with the very important exception of *Bacteroides fragilis*. Since this is a significant organism in mixed infections penicillin alone is not appropriate for patients with infection associated with abortion. Toxic reactions are for the most part not serious or life threatening.

Ampicillin

Ampicillin has a similar spectrum of activity to penicillin when given in equivalent doses (approximately 8.0 g/24 h). *E. coli* resistance is common (< 30–40% in many institutions) and *B. fragilis* is not covered. Ampicillin is the most effective agent against enterococcus. However, this is not a common pathogen in these patients. Toxicity is frequent in the form of skin rashes but not often serious. The skin eruptions with ampicillin do not necessarily indicate true penicillin allergy. Because of the deficits in coverage ampicillin alone is insufficient for a patient with an infected abortion who is more than mildly ill.

Carbenicillin

Carbenicillin has expanded coverage in the gram negative area as well as among the anaerobes. The coverage for *B. fragilis* requires high doses (30–40 g/24 h) and can only be achieved by the intravenous route. Thus the selection of carbenicillin implies a commitment to a full course of parenteral therapy. Toxicity is similar to that of other penicillins, but in addition the high parenteral doses present a large sodium load which may be a concern for older patients or those with hypertension or cardiac disease. Because of those constraints carbenicillin is not a first line selection for patients with infected abortions.

Ticarcillin and Piperacillin

Ticarcillin and piperacillin are also new synthetic penicillins with expanded coverage, but there is insufficient experience at this time for suggesting their use for septic abortion.

Cephalosporins

The first generation of cephalosporins is currently represented by cephalothin and cefazolin in the parenteral form and cephalexin orally. These agents have significant gaps in coverage amongst gram negative aerobes as well as anaerobes and fail to cover enterococcus. Toxicity is local for the most part, in the form of phlebitis, pain on IM injection or gastrointestinal disturbances with the oral form and there is an approximately 8% risk of cross reaction in penicillin allergic patients. Because of the spotty coverage these antibiotics are inadequate in this clinical situation.

Aminoglycosides

As a group these antibiotics provide the best coverage for the gram negative aerobes, but no anaerobic coverage and consequently must only be used in combination in the case of mixed infections. Oto- and nephrotoxicity are major concerns as is the development of R factor resistance by bacteria. Currently the aminoglycosides of choice are tobramycin, gentamicin and kanamycin in the combinations as subsequently outlined.

Clindamycin

Clindamycin provides excellent coverage for anaerobes as well as gram positive aerobes. Consequently, as with many other drugs, it cannot be used along in mixed infections. There is the potential of pseudomembranous enterocolitis especially with the oral form but this complication is not limited to clindamycin. Clindamycin is at present the standard against which other antibiotics are judged for activity against *B. fragilis*.

Chloramphenicol

Chloramphenicol is an extremely potent albeit bacteriostatic antibiotic which is infrequently used because of its potential bone marrow toxicity. The latter is rare (1:20 000–1:50 000) and most often seen with oral use but it is nearly always fatal. The coverage is excellent including *B. fragilis* and therefore chloramphenicol alone or in combination is a reasonable selection for a patient with an infected abortion especially if the patient is seriously ill.

Combinations

1) Penicillin (ampicillin) and aminoglycoside – the addition of the amino-glycoside broadens the gram negative aerobic coverage especially against resistant *E. coli*. This is useful but still leaves *B. fragilis* uncovered. Consequently this combination is inadequate for the seriously ill patient with a mixed infection.

2) Cephalosporin (first generation) and aminoglycoside – these two agents leave two significant gaps, *B. fragilis* and enterococcus and therefore offer little to support their selection.

3) Clindamycin and aminoglycoside – this combination is currently the standard for the treatment of seriously ill patients with mixed soft tissue pelvic infections against which new agents must be judged. The coverage is quite broad with enterococcus being the only organism of potential clinical importance that is not covered. Toxicity of course is additive.

4) Triple therapy with the addition of ampicillin to clindamycin and gentamicin fills in the gap for enterococcus and is often selected as the approach in seriously ill patients. The decision to add the third drug must be based upon balancing the added toxicity against the likeliood of enterococcus playing a major role in the mixed infections.

Newer Agents

1) Cefoxitin – this relatively new product is a cephamycin with expanded coverage especially for anaerobes and specifically for *B. fragilis* of which roughly 85% are sensitive. Because of this coverage and its low order of toxicity, this agent has considerable appeal as a single agent for serious mixed infections. The only reservation at this time is that the clinical studies have involved a mixture of patients, many of whom were not seriously ill and consequently there is no extensive experience with cefoxitin in critically ill patients.

2) Cefamandole is also a new cephalosporin with expanded gram negative aerobic coverage. Unlike cefoxitin it does not cover the majority of *B. fragilis* (40–60% in most reports). It has proved efficacious in a number of studies of mild to moderate mixed infections, presumably because of its expanded coverage of enterobacteriacae. There is insufficient evidence to recommend this agent in a critically ill patient with a septic abortion.

3) Metronidazole has very recently been marketed in a parenteral form and provides excellent anaerobic coverage. Because of its lack of aerobic coverage it will have to be used in combination. The oral form does provide excellent serum levels so that follow-up therapy may be oral. The major concerns with metronidazole are related to a suggestion of carcinogenesis in animals.

132

4) The future certainly holds many new agents with even more expanded coverage coupled with reduced toxicity. For reasons already stated it is likely that much of this development will be in the beta lactam group of antibiotics. In addition, there is on-going research with beta lactamase inhibitors which, if effective, might resurrect a number of drugs which have been set aside because of inactivation by the bacteria produced enzyme.

As of this time, then, the choice of antibiotics for moderately or seriously ill patients with an infected abortion involves a combination of drugs with significant toxic potential. Clindamycin with an aminoglycoside, most likely gentamicin or tobramycin, is the most common recommendation. Many add ampicillin to provide coverage for enterococcus, a relatively uncommon pathogen. Chloramphenicol alone in combination is preferred by others. Of the new 'cepha' products, cefoxitin would seem to have the greatest potential for single agent treatment of patients with infected abortions because of its activity against *B. fragilis*. Metronidazole also has great promise but must be used in combination.

MAJOR COMPLICATIONS OF INFECTED ABORTIONS

Although it is beyond the scope of this writing to discuss in great detail the management of the major complications, they are of such importance that it is essential to understand and anticipate their occurrence in order to properly manage any patient with an infected abortion.

A) *Septic Shock* – This is the most dramatic complication and a potentially lethal one. It arises because of the release of endotoxin upon the disintegration of gram negative bacteria [14]. Occasionally it is precipitated by the administration of bactericidal antibiotics. The pathophysiology of septic shock is extremely complex involving the interaction of endotoxin and a variety of vasoactive intermediaries. The net result is reduced organ perfusion or a so-called 'low flow state'. The characteristics of this state vary from time to time and patient to patient but include myocardial depression, varying combinations of vasoconstriction and vasodilatation, disseminated intravascular clotting and adult respiratory distress syndrome or shock lung. The cause of shock in the septic abortion patient may not always be obvious since blood loss and hypovolemia are common concurrent events. The management can be conveniently discussed from two perspectives [15]. Primary therapy is directed toward the control of the focus of infection and therefore the source of endotoxin. As has already been pointed out the surgical approach is the key and antibiotics somewhat secondary. Most patients can be managed with curettage alone although occasionally more extensive surgery is needed to clear the source of endotoxin. The other aspect of management is supportive, i.e., an attempt to support life functions until the endotoxin is cleared. The modalities in this category include fluid therapy, corticosteroids, heparin, correction of lactoacidosis, inotropic agents and a variety of vaso-active agents. Application of specific approaches is dependent upon the careful assessment of the physiologic derangements in the individual patient and cannot be done empirically. The prognosis for the patient with septic shock secondary to an infected abortion is considerably better than for patients with septic shock generally. The reasons for this are the early age and good health of the patients at the onset and the fact that the site of infection is surgically accessible. An important exception to the generally good prognosis occurs as a result of failure of the patient to seek medical care in a timely manner. Sophisticated modern management of patients with septic shock has also contributed to survival and when deaths occur they are more likely to result from shock lung and its sequelae than from the cardiovascular collapse. The management of severe shock lung is often frustrating with limited therapeutic tools available to provide respiratory support in the presence of non-functioning lungs.

B) *Renal failure* – This is a second major complication of septic abortion which must be anticipated in order to deal with it in an appropriate fashion. Several etiologic mechanisms are operative. The most common is acute tubular necrosis related to shock and reduced renal perfusion. This may be aggravated in the case of clostridial sepsis by the hemolysis produced by the exotoxins. When disseminated intravascular clotting occurs, the renal lesion may be bilateral corical necrosis, a lesion with a poor prognosis if other than patchy in its distribution. A third mechanism of renal failure relates to toxic substances which might have been utilized in the abortion attempt. Diagnosis is not especially difficult as long as the suspicion exists since the monitoring of urinary output should be a part of the normal approach to these patients. When oliguria occurs it must be assessed in relation to circulatory volume and perfusion pressure. A fluid volume challenge may be employed in an effort to clarify the problem provided the central venous or pulmonary wedge pressure is not elevated. This may be done with 500–1000 ml of a balanced salt solution or with an osmotic diuretic such as mannitol. The latter may also be used during the low flow period to preserve renal tubular flow and thereby act as prophylaxis against acute tubular necrosis (ATN). Management of acute renal failure is dependent to some extent on the etiology, but regardless of the cause, the early phases of treatment are similar, i.e., restriction of fluid intake to cover the output and insensible loss. In some cases of ATN a spontaneous diuresis will occur before dialysis becomes necessary and then the problem is to keep up with the losses during the diuretic phase. In all other cases

134

regardless of the cause, hemodialysis must be instituted before serious complications such as hyperkalemia ensue and be maintained until function returns. Obviously when function does not return as in the case of bilateral necrosis, the options are limited to chronic dialysis or transplantation. The prognosis with renal failure and septic abortion is dependent upon the pathology. In most cases patients with acute tubular necrosis recover completely provided support is adequate during the acute phase of the illness. As in the case of septic shock this good outlook is related to the youth and antecedent good health of most women in this population.

SUMMARY

Septic abortion was a far more common problem in the United States before the reform in abortion laws took place. It has, not however, disappeared completely and in some parts of the world remains a very frequent problem for the obstetrician/gynecologist. Infection generally results from the entry of opportunistic vaginal flora into the uterus, which contains an excellent culture medium in the form of blood and necrotic products of conception. Most often the process is confined to the cavity and consequently uterine evacuation is the crucial management step. More serious problems arise when infection spreads deeply into the myometrium or to the adnexal structures or if the uterus has been perforated and the peritoneum seeded. Antibiotic therapy is of secondary importance to surgical evacuation but should provide broad coverage for both aerobes and anaerobes and may require a combination of antibiotics in the seriously ill patient. The prognosis is generally good unless major complications such as septic shock or renal failure occur.

REFERENCES

1. Seward PN, Ballard CA, Ulene AL: The effect of legal abortion on the rate of septic abortion at a large county hospital. Am J Obstet Gynecol 115:335, 1973
2. Schwarz RH: Septic Abortion, p 7–15. Philadelphia: Lippincott, 1968
3. Eisenger SH: Second trimester spontaneous abortion, the I.U.D. and infection. Am J Obstet Gynecol 119:441, 1974
4. Christian CD: Maternal deaths associated with an intrauterine device. Am J Obstet Gynecol 119:441, 1974
5. Rotheram ED, Schick SG: Nonclostridial anaerobic bacteria in septic abortion. Am J Med 46:80, 1969
6. Chow AW, Marshall JR, Guze LB: A double-blind comparison of clindamycin with penicillin plus choramphenicol in treatment of septic abortion. J Infect Dis 135 (Suppl.): 35, 1977
7. Sweet RL: Anaerobic infections of the female genital tract. Am J Obstet Gynecol 122:891, 1975
8. O'Neill RT, Schwarz RH: Clostridial organisms in septic abortion. Obstet Gynecol 35:458, 1970

9. Ledger WJ, Hackett KA: Significance of clostridia in female reproductive tract. Obstet Gynecol 41:525, 1973

10. Kadner JL, Anderson GV: Septic abortion with hemoglobinaria and renal insufficiency with special reference to Clostridium welchii infection. Obstet Gynecol 21:886, 1963

11. Burkman RT, Tonascia JA, Atienza MG, King TM: Untreated endocervical gonorrhea and endometritis following elective abortion. Am J Obstet Gynecol 126:648, 1976

12. Ansbacher R, et al.: Clinical investigation of Listeria monocytogenes as a possible cause of human fetal wastage. Am J Obstet Gynecol 94:386, 1966

13. Neuwirth RJ, Friedman EA: Septic abortion. Am J Obstet Gynecol 85:24, 1963

14. Ostergard DR: Comparison of two antibiotic regimens in the treatment of septic abortion. Obstet Gynecol 36:473, 1970

15. Schwarz RH, Polin JJ: Septic Shock. In: Davis gynecology and obstetrics (Ed. JJ Rovinsky), Vol. I, Chapter 46, p. 1–16. Hagerstown, MD: Harper and Row, 1971

Author's address:
Department of Obstetrics and Gynecology
Downstate Medical Center
450 Clarkson Avenue
Brooklyn, New York 11203
U.S.A.

PART III

REVIEW OF ANTIBIOTICS EFFECTIVE IN THE TREATMENT OF SOFT TISSUE PELVIC INFECTION

7. TETRACYCLINES AND PENICILLINS

WILLIAM J. LEDGER

INTRODUCTION

The tetracyclines are useful drugs for the obstetrician-gynecologist. They are broad spectrum antibiotics with a wide range of activity against many gram positive and gram negative organisms, both aerobes and anaerobes. In view of the multibacterial etiology of many soft tissue pelvic infections, this family of antibiotics has great theoretical appeal, and clinical studies have indicated effectiveness. Tetracyclines are bacteriostatic in their antimicrobial activity against bacterial pathogens. They act by inhibiting protein synthesis in susceptible bacteria at the 30 S ribosomal level within the cell.

A number of clinical modifications has been made in the tetracycline structure with pharmacologic and microbiologic changes in activity. The parent compound was derived from actinomycetes, and the chemical structure is shown in Fig. 1. This figure depicts the basic chemical structure of four

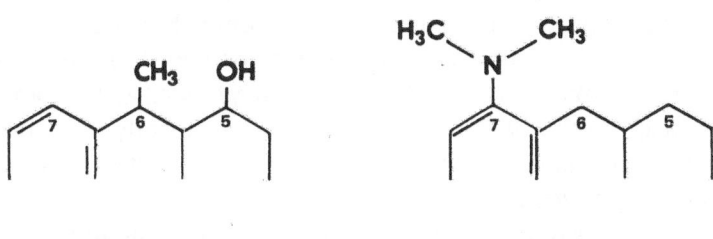

Fig. 1. The chemical structure of the tetracyclines.

W.J. Ledger (ed.), Antibiotics in Obstetrics and Gynecology, 139–158. All rights reserved.
Copyright © 1982 by Martinus Nijhoff Publishers, The Hague/Boston/London. ISBN-13:978-94-009-7466-1

benzene rings. With chemical alterations of the one and six positions, scientists developed the newer tetracyclines, minocycline and doxycycline (Fig. 1). These compounds are primarily eliminated in the gut and have a wider range of activity against anaerobic organisms than the parent tetracycline compound.

CLINICAL USE – HISTORICAL PERSPECTIVE

There have been wide swings in the popularity of the tetracyclines among Obstetrician-Gynecologists. Better understanding of the trends in the employment of antibiotics should give us more insight into the role of tetracyclines in medical practice in the 1980's.

During the 1950's, tetracyclines were frequently prescribed by the obstetrician-gynecologist. There was a number of factors for this popularity. The tetracyclines had a broad spectrum of antibacterial coverage, with good activity against organisms considered pathogens by clinicians in the 1950's. These included gram negative aerobes, especially *Escherichiae coli* and *Neisseria gonorrhea*. The enthusiasm by physicians for the tetracyclines in this decade must be analyzed within the perspective of the antibiotics then available for prescription. Penicillins such as ampicillin, with a wider spectrum against gram negative aerobes, were not yet in use and the only available aminoglycoside was streptomycin with known eighth nerve and renal toxicity plus the rapid development of bacteral resistance when the drug was used. Another factor in the acceptance of tetracyclines was the lack of appreciation by most clinicians of the role of anaerobic bacteria in pelvic infection. Tetracyclines were effective against most aerobic pathogens. Within this framework of microbiologic understanding of pelvic infection it is understandable that tetracyclines were frequently prescribed. On a practical level, tetracyclines were versatile. They could be employed intravenously for hospitalized patients. In fact, a popular combination of antibiotics for seriously ill patients was intravenous penicillin and intravenous tetracycline. The oral form of the drug was also available. This meant that a prolonged course of the antibiotics could be employed in patients treated in the hospital because of infection, so that their treatment could be completed as an outpatient. Milder infections, not requiring hospitalization could be adequately treated with an oral form as an outpatient. In the 1950's, tetracyclines were frequently prescribed as an adjunct to treatment in seriously ill patients as well as being standard therapy for less sick outpatients.

The 1960's saw a tremendous drop in the overall usage of the tetracyclies by the obstetrician-gynecologist. A number of diverse factors contributed to this nationwide drop in popularity.

The most important blow to the widespread popularity of the tetracyclines was the discovery of its toxicity during pregnancy, to both the mother and the fetus. In 1963, the New England Journal of Medicine article documented a number of cases of maternal mortality in which high dosage intravenous tetracycline had been used for the treatment of pyelonephritis during pregnancy [1]. All of these women died of liver failure and at postmortem examination were found to have extensive fatty infiltration of the liver. On theoretical grounds, it was presumed that the liver during pregnancy was more susceptible to this toxic action of the tetracyclines, particularly in view of the more usual pharmacokinetics of antibiotics during pregnancy, documented by Phillipsen in her chapter in which lower serum levels of antibiotics were frequently found.This reasoning was probably incorrect. These patients with pyelonephritis may have represented a special situation, Whalley et al. have shown a marked diminution in renal functions, particularly renal blood flow and glomerular filtration rate (GFR) in some women with acute pyelonephritis in pregnancy [2]. The mechanisms are not known, but dehydration preceding admission to the hospital as well as inflammation of the kidneys in the acute stage of infection may be factors. These early observations on diminished renal function in pyelonephritis were followed by measures of tetracyclines in the serum in pregnant women with pyelonephritis [3]. Much higher than expected levels were found in some women. The impact of this finding of serious maternal results led to a marked decrease in the employment of these agents during pregnancy and the puerperium. The ill effects of tetracyclines during pregnancy were not limited to the mother. If these drugs are administered during pregnancy, they will cross the placenta and expose the fetus to the drug. If given after the middle of pregnancy when the crowns of deciduous teeth have begun to form, a chelated metabolite of the drug will be incorporated into the developing tooth and this will appear as a brown band on the tooth and cause hypoplasia of the tooth when it becomes visible as the newborn matures [4]. There are other causes for concern for the fetus. Animal studies demonstrated the deposition of chelated forms of tetracyclines in the epiphyses of the long bones of the fetus of mothers receiving this drug [5]. More important, there was diminishment of long bone growth while the mother was receiving the drug. All of these maternal and fetal observations led to the virtual abandonment of the use of this family of drugs during pregnancy.

Another big factor in the diminished use of the tetracyclines in the 1960's was the emergence of newer aminoglycosides, particularly kanamycin. This bactericidal antibiotic did not have the rapid emergence of resistance by gram negative aerobic bacteria, that had been noted with streptomycin. Of more importance, was the acute awareness of clinicians in the 1960's of the increasing importance of gram negative aerobic organisms in pelvic infections, particularly infected abortions, and the emerging significance of septic endotoxic shock [6]. Because of this, there was much interest in new bactericidal antibiotics for the treatment of these gram negative aerobic infections, replacing the bacteriostatic agent, tetracycline. Penicillin in combination with kanamycin, largely replaced the combination of penicillin and tetracycline.

Another factor in the reduced employment of tetracyclines by obstetrician-gynecologists in the 1960's was the sudden emergence of *Bacteroides fragilis* resistant to tetracycline [7]. The decade of the 1960's saw this antibiotic agent go from the drug of choice in *Bacteroides fragilis* infections, that were infrequently recognized to a situation in which clinicians were more aware of this anaerobe and a large number of the isolates was resistant. All of these developments contributed to a lessened prescription of this family of antibiotics in hospitalized patients.

The 1970's saw a rebirth of interest in the tetracyclines by obstetrician-gynecologists. This renewed prescription zeal was stimulated by a number of independent developments. All of these resulted in greater use of these agents in women with pelvic infections.

The most important ingredient in the renewed interest in tetracyclines was the development of new analogues, minocycline and doxycycline. These agents had many attributes to stimulate clinician interest. They were versatile and easy to use. Both an intravenous and oral form were available, and the pharmacokinetics of these drugs was such that only twice a day dosage was needed instead of the more frequent four times a day administration of the standard tetracyclines. These agents had different pharmacologic routes of elimination, for they were largely cleared by the bowel and thus there was no problem of the buildup of serum levels in the face of renal failure or diminution of renal function [8]. This stimulated hope that these new analogues would have less toxicity for humans than the standard form of tetracycline. The major factor for increased physician enthusiasm for the prescription of these newer tetracyclines was the discovery in microbiologic laboratories of their broadened activity against anaerobic bacteria, particularly *Bacteroides fragilis* [7]. This discovery occurred at the same time there was a re-awakening of awareness of the importance of anaerobic bacteria in soft tissue pelvic infections in the female [9,10]. All of these developments increased the interest of clinicians in prescribing tetracyclines for obstetric-gynecologic patients.

Another significant development in the 1970's, leading to wider use of the tetracyclines, was the possibility that other organisms might be involved in pelvic infections. There have been many studies attempting to pinpoint the significance of mycoplasma in pelvic infections in women. Although evidence for widespread involvement does not exist, there are isolated cases in which mycoplasmas seem to be significant pathogens [11]. This occasionally may be of importance for the clinician for these organisms are exquisitely susceptible to the tetracyclines. Of much more clinical significance is chlamydia. A number of studies have suggested involvement in nongonococcal salpingitis [12] and post-partum endomyometritis [13]. The most convincing case for their involvement in non-gonococcal salpingitis was the laparoscopy evaluation of patients with non-gonococcal salpingitis done by Märdh et al. [12]. In this study, these organisms were recovered from 6 of 20 (30%) fimbrial biopsies in women with untreated acute salpingitis. Of special interest to the clinician dealing with patients with either postpartum endometritis or salpingitis in a non-pregnant population is the susceptibility of this group of organisms to tetracycline. Again, this has sparked an increased utilization of these broad spectrum antibiotics in obstetric-gynecologic patients.

CURRENT USE

The tetracyclines have been recommended by the Center for Disease Control in the United States as second line agents for the treatment of infections due to *Neisseria gonorrhea* and *Treponema pallidum*. The drug of choice in each instance is penicillin and the tetracyclines are not recommended for the penicillin allergic pregnant woman. For the non-pregnant patient who is allergic to penicillin, this is an effective alternative antibiotic. The recommended treatment regimen for the various clinical manifestations of gonococcal disease are listed in Table 1. There is no evidence that the newer analogues of tetracycline (i.e. minocycline and doxycycline) are any more effective than standard tetracyclines in the treatment of these clinical entities. There is a number of studies to indicate the effectiveness of tetracycline. A large compilation of treatment data from the Center for Disease Control indicates that this drug resulted in a microbiologic cure in 4.3% of women with uncomplicated gonococcal disease, as compared to a failure rate of 4.7% with spectinomycin, 8.0% with ampicillin, and 4.2% with aqueous procain penicillin G. [14]. One outpatient study comparing ampicillin with tetracycline in the treatment of gonococcal salpingitis had similar results [15]. Tetracycline is the drug of choice for the treatment of syphilis in the nonpregnant woman. In the spirit of a more rational method of classification, infectious syphilis is judged to be either less than one year in duration or the alternative group of either more than one year or unknown duration or the alternative group of either more than one year or unknown duration. Table 2 lists the treatment regimens for these entities. Since the effectiveness of tetracycline in asymptomatic central nervous system syphilis is not known, a spinal fluid analysis should be done prior to therapy in those women who have had syphilis for more than a year or unknown duration.

144

Table 1. Tetracycline treatment of gonorrhea in women.

Clinical diagnosis	Treatment regimen
1. Asymptomatic gonorrhea – i.e. culture positive women or sexual partners of culture positive males.	1. Tetracylcine hydrochloride 0.5 g orally four times a day for five days. Doxycycline or minocycline 100 mg twice a day can be used as an alternative.
2. Rectal and oral pharyngeal gonorrhea.	2. Tetracycline hydrochloride 0.5 g orally four times a day for 10 days. Doxycycline or minocycline 100 mg twice a day can be used as an alternative.
3. Gonococcal salpingitis.	3. Outpatient treatment – Tetracycline hydrochloride 0.5 g orally four times a day for 10 days. Doxycycline or minocycline 100 mg twice a day can be used as an alternative. Inpatient treatment – Inpatient therapy. Tetracycline 0.25 g intravenously four times a day until afebrile for at least 24 h. Then tetracycline HCl 0.5 grams orally four times a day to complete 10 days of therapy. As an alternative, 100 mg doxycycline or minocycline intravenously every 12 h until afebrile for at least 24 h. Then 100 mg orally every 12 h to complete 10 days of therapy.
4. Gonococcal arthritis.	4. Tetracycline hydrochloride 0.5 g orally four times a day for 7 days. Doxycycline or minocycline 100 mg twice a day can be used as an alternative.

Table 2. Treatment of syphilis with tetracycline in the non-pregnant woman.

Type of infection	Recommended treatment
1. Syphilis of less than one years' duration.	1. Tetracycline 0.5 g qud for 15 days. A total of 30 g.
2. Syphilis of more than one year or unknown duration.	2. Tetracycline 0.5 g qud for 30 days. A total of 60 g.

Recently, there has been much enthusiasm for the tetracycline therapy of women with acute salpingitis. A number of reports have documented short-term successful treatment, i.e. the women have been identified as clinical cures, although long-term evaluation of future fertility has not been done. One study from California focused upon the significance of *Neisseria gonorrhea* in salpingitis, but demonstrated good clinical results with doxycycline [16]. In a series of studies from the University of Florida, Monif et al. have championed the classification of salpingitis or pelvic inflammatory disease as *Endometri-tis-Salpingitis-Peritonitis*, [17, 18] (ESP). In the evaluation of tetracycline treatment of these patients, the authors have found the combination of penicillin-tetracycline to be superior to the use of a tetracycline alone, and attributed the treatment failures in the tetracycline alone group to the recovery of anaerobic bacteria from peritoneal fluid obtained by culdocentesis to be resistant to the tetracyclines and susceptible to the penicillins. My own experience with the tetracyclines, both minocycline and doxycycline has been that it is highly effective in the treatment of patients with acute salpingitis without pelvic masses, and I was unable to correlate treatment failures with the isolation of tetracycline resistant organisms from culdocentesis samples [19]. In addition, I found the temperature response to be more rapid in patients with salpingitis treated with a tetracycline as compared to ampicillin alone. Until long-term studies are made to determine the impact of this therapy upon future fertility, it is impossible to be dogmatic about the exact place of tetracycline in the treatment of salpingitis. These preliminary findings are encouraging indeed. Prospective studies evaluating the frequency of recovery of mycoplasma or chlamydia from the fallopian tube of patients with salpingitis should help to better delineate the role of tetracyclines in these disease entities. Based upon the clinical observations to date, it is likely that these will be a frequently employed family of antibiotics.

The tetracyclines have been used in patients with hospital acquired infections, but there has not been the widespread reporting as noted with other families of antibiotics. One great source of reluctance for the prescription of these agents is the already mentioned concern about maternal toxicity with these agents. This may be less of a factor in the future. Doxycycline, which is almost totally eliminated by the gastro-intestinal route, does not reach toxic levels in the presence of renal impairment, and has been employed in post-partum women. If more data is found to implicate mycoplasma or chlamydia in post-partum infections, there will be more interest in the agents. One evaluation recovered mycoplasma from genital sites and the blood stream in patients with a post-partum endomyometritis and found tetracycline effective [20]. A recent evaluation from the University of Washington recovered chlamydia from patients with a postpartum endomyometritis, particularly those with a late developing infection, i.e. patients who became symptomatic after discharge from the hospital [13]. If this is reconfirmed by future studies, it will lend great impetus to the use of tetracycline in post-partum women, particularly those with late developing infections. There has not been widely reported experience with tetracyclines in post-operative pelvic infection in gynecology, but tissue levels would suggest this to be an effective form of therapy [21].

Tetracyclines have been employed as prophylactic agents in obstetric-gynecologic patients. To date, reports have documented the use of these agents in women undergoing pregnancy termination [22] and in women undergoing hysterectomy [23]. A more detailed description of these studies is contained in Dr Mead's chapter on prophylactic antibiotics in gynecology.

There are side effects that can be noted with the administration of tetracyc-

146

line to women. In addition to the problems with the mother and fetus during pregnancy, other difficulties have been noted. Reactions in the form of a skin rash or sensitivity to sunlight have been associated with tetracyclines. Minocycline has been plagued in particular by a high incidence of central nervous system symptomatology. These symptoms are primarily vestibular in origin, manifested by dizziness, loss of balance, light-headedness, and tinnitus, as well as the associated problem of nausea. Since women have these troubling side effects more often than men, 53.5% vs. 27.8%, one theory has been that the smaller body size of most women produced higher serum levels than in the male when standard doses were used [24]. The hypothesis that the higher serum levels accounted for the symptomatology was evaluated in a study in Vermont and refuted [24]. Using a lower dosage regimen in women, that produced lower serum levels, all central nervous system symptomatology remained unchanged except for nausea which was reduced. The reasons for the increased frequency of symptoms in women remain unclear for it occurs when similar serum levels of doxycycline are seen in male and female study subjects. The frequency of these problems and the debility associated with this symptomatology seriously restrict the clinical use of this antibiotic by obstetrician-gynecologists.

PENICILLINS

Introduction

The family of penicillin antibiotics was originally isolated from the mold, *Penicillium notatum*. The core chemical structure of all penicillins consists of a thiazolidine ring, a beta lactam ring, and a side chain. Since the elucidation of the chemical structure of the parent compound, modifications have been made in the various side chains that have influenced the antibacterial activity of the resulting compounds. The wide variety of these chemical variants is noted in Fig. 2. These chemical innovations have resulted in the introduction into clinical practice of a wide variety of penicillins with an expanded spectrum of activity.

The penicillins have many favorable attributes that have helped to account for their popularity. They have little direct toxicity in the human. This means that huge doses can be used with almost complete impunity. In elderly patients with reduced renal function, massive penicillin doses of 40–80 million units/day, have resulted in increased central nervous system irritability and even convulsions [25]. This is a rare event on an obstetric-gynecologic service for this high dosage level is rarely used and most of our patients are young women with good renal function. There is widespread usage of from 20–40

TYPE OF PENICILLIN   SIDE CHAIN

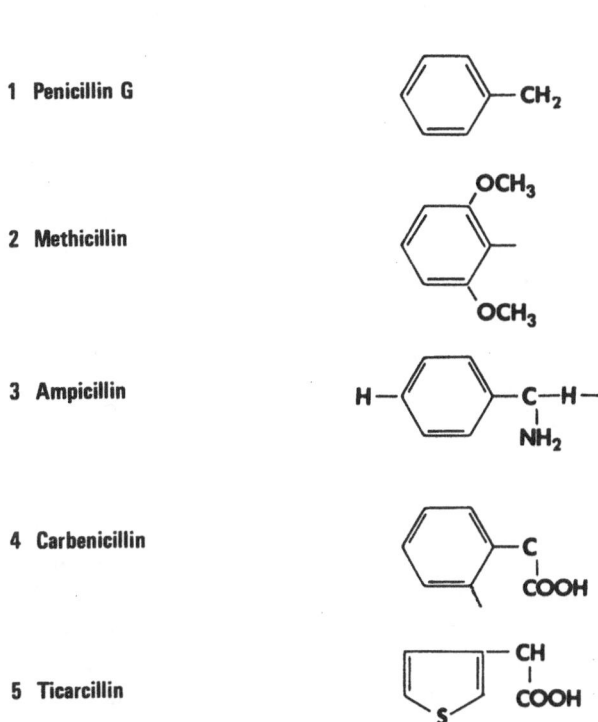

1 Penicillin G

2 Methicillin

3 Ampicillin

4 Carbenicillin

5 Ticarcillin

Fig. 2. Side chain variations among various penicillins.

million units of penicillin/day in patients with serious infections, and this dosage produces serum levels that exceed the MIC's of many susceptible organisms by a factor of hundreds. In addition, the penicillins are versatile for they offer the prescribing physician a wide variety of routes of administration. Various types of penicillin can be given by the intravenous route, intramuscularly, or in an oral form. The versatility of the penicillins applies in another characteristic of this family of antibiotics. The varied chemical forms make it possible to treat a wide spectrum of both gram negative and gram positive bacteria. The continued development of newer penicillins is a good sign for future widespread use of this family of antibiotics. A wide variety of adverse responses can be seen with all forms of penicillins employed. These may be related to toxic reactions to the drugs or an allergic response. The allergic side effect may range from a mild skin eruption to anaphylaxis and death. Fortunately, the latter outcome is rare. To reduce the possibility of any allergic response, a careful history of a prior penicillin allergy should be obtained before these drugs are administered. Toxicity to penicillin takes many forms.

It may be related to electrolyte changes, effects upon platelet function, or the results of alterations in the bacterial flora of the bowel. Prescription of this family of antibiotics implies knowledge and recognition of these toxic effects. The varied types of agents in the penicillin family provide the framework for the discussion of the antibacterials.

Benzathine Penicillin

Benzathine penicillin has a unique place in therapeutic armamentarium of the obstetrician-gynecologist. The chemical formulation of this penicillin results in its slow release from the intramuscular site repository. This low release extends over a period of two to four weeks with low serum levels, much less than 1.0 μg/ml. These pharmacologic characteristics define a penicillin with a limited and specific role in the therapy of sexually acquired diseases. The serum levels achieved are far too low for the treatment of an infection in women due to *Neisseria gonorrhea*, because they do not exceed the MIC's of this organism. In contrast, the spirochete *Treponema pallidum* is uniquely amenable to treatment with this penicillin. *Treponema pallidum* is exquisitely susceptible to penicillin with MIC's of less than 0.1 μg/ml. In addition, the slow replication rate of this spirochete, requiring from 24–28 h, means that elimination of the organism from the site of infection will require the presence of an effective antibiotic for long periods of time. Benzathine penicillin meets both of these requirements, a serum level above the MIC of *Treponema pallidum* and maintenance in the serum for many days. Syphilis in women has been characterized as being less than one year's duration or more than one year's duration. Those women with a disease of less than one year's duration either have a chancre (primary syphilis) or a diffuse skin eruption (secondary syphilis), or a serology that has converted during the past year. For these patients with a reagin serologic test that has become positive, a specific treponemal test, such as a Fluorescent Treponemal Antibody ABSorption test, (FTA-ABS) should be done and be positive to confirm the diagnosis. For patients with syphilis of less than one year's duration, the recommended treatment is 2.4 million units of benzathine penicillin administered intramuscularly. For the woman with syphilis for more than a year or of unknown duration, the recommended treatment is 2.4 million units of benzathine penicillin given intramuscularly at weekly intervals for three doses for a total of 7.2 million units. For the patient with a positive serology, the test of cure is a fourfold or greater drop in the titer of non-treponemal quantitative antibody tests over a period of six months. Because of the low serum levels achieved with this penicillin, it should be considered adequate antibacterial therapy for only the spirochete, *Treponema pallidum*, and not for other sexually acquired infections such as *Neisseria gonorrhea*.

Penicillin G

Penicillin G has been the mainstay of therapy for patients who are candidates for the parenteral form of penicillin. This potassium salt is soluble in water and thus can be administered by the intravenous route. For seriously ill female patients with soft tissue pelvic infections, penicillin G has been administered intravenously with dosage ranges of 20 000 000 to 60 000 000 units/day. The drug can be administered at 4 to 6 h intervals and has been given by continuous infusion or by bolus administration. The advantage of continuous perfusion is that serum levels of penicillin are maintained at a nearly constant rate. With bolus infusion, much higher peak levels are obtained, with a rapid drop-off as penicillin is cleared by the kidney. If 6 h intervals are used with bolus administration in a patient with normal renal function, there will be no detectable level of penicillin for 3–4 h, every 6 h time frame. The advantage of the bolus dosage strategy is that higher levels of penicillin have been achieved in the poorly perfused animal model simulation of an abscess [26]. Theoretically, this would be of some advantage in the woman with a serious pelvic infection and a suspected abscess.

Penicillin G has been widely employed in the treatment of serious pelvic infections in hospitalized patients. In general, this antibiotic has been used in combination with an aminoglycoside. The aminoglycoside provides better coverage of gram negative aerobes and in combination with penicillin is effective against the enterococcus. Support for this treatment regimen comes from the comparative study of the combinations of penicillin-kanamycin and clindamycin-kanamycin [27]. In that treatment evaluation, no differences were noted in the therapeutic results. This was the basis for the commonly used antibiotic strategy of beginning therapy with penicillin and an aminoglycoside and then adding either clindamycin or chlorampenicol to cover *Bacteroides fragilis* in the occasional patient who remained febrile. The physician prescribing intravenous penicillin G should be aware that each one million units contains 1.7 meq of potassium, or sodium depending upon the type of penicillin G used. This is rarely a problem in the usually young obstetric-gynecologic patient with good renal function, but could cause problems in a woman with diminished renal clearances. Recently, this penicillin-aminoglycoside combination as initial therapy has been questioned in women with a post-partum endomyometritis following cesarean section. Unlike the previous study comparing clindamycin and penicillin, all of these women were treated early in the course of the infection. Better clinical results were obtained in the group receiving clindamycin-gentamicin, as compared to penicillin-gentamicin [28]. Four per cent of this population had serious problems with the penicillin-gentamicin combination, exactly the same percentage found by Gibbs et al. when penicillin-kanamycin was employed initially [29].

150

The decision to use one or the other of these combinations of antibiotics must weigh the desire to avoid these serious complications of infection in a small percentage of the treated population, against the toxicity of clindamycin when employed routinely. Since there is a wide variation in the number of women developing gastrointestinal symptomatology with clindamycin, this decision may vary from hospital to hospital. As an alternative, many services employ a combination of penicillin and tetracycline, usually with success in these patients.

Penicillin G is the drug of choice for the woman with a gonococcal infection, except for an oropharyngeal site. In the asymptomatic woman who is cervical culture positive for *Neisseria gonorrhea* or who has been a sexual contact of a culture positive male, the treatment is aqueous procaine penicillin G 4.8 million units given in two divided intramuscular doses with 1 g of oral probenecid. This dosage is also effective for the patient with incubating syphilis who is still serology negative. For the patient with gonococcal salpingitis who is to be treated as an outpatient, aqueous procaine penicillin G 4.8 million units can be given intramuscularly in two divided doses with one gram of oral probenecid to be followed by an oral form of penicillin to complete ten days of therapy. The patient with gonococcal salpingitis, treated as an inpatient, is given 20 million units of intravenous penicillin G daily until clinical improvement occurs with a switch then to an oral form of penicillin to complete ten days of therapy. All of these treatment regimens will be ineffective if the strain of *Neisseria gonorrhea* is penicillinase producing. Alternative agents, either spectinomycin or cefoxitin should be employed in such cases.

Penicillin G is one of the alternative forms of treatment for the patient with syphilis. For the woman with syphilis of more than one year's duration, an alternative therapy to benzathine penicillin is to employ procaine penicillin G, 600 000 units IM daily for eight consecutive days. The need to rely upon the patient to return for eight consecutive daily visits and the difficulty in maintaining an outpatient clinic open seven days per week has lessened physician enthusiasm for this treatment. For the patient with documented central nervous system syphilis, based upon a positive reagin test in a cerebrospinal fluid sample, one popular form of therapy has been to admit the patient to the hospital and employ intravenous penicillin G, 12–14 million units a day for ten days. This maintains higher serum levels of penicillin, which in time ensures higher levels in the cerebrospinal fluid and the central nervous system. These higher levels theoretically should result in a higher percentage of cures.

Antibiotic prophylaxis, a widespread practice pattern in obstetrics and gynecology, has included penicillin G with success. Most of the effective regimens in hysterectomy and cesarean section have employed cephalosporins, in part due to the fact that cephalosporins have been less frequently used than the penicillins in the treatment of infections and also because funding for the evaluation of cephalosporins was more available than for the penicillins. The evidence seems to be that penicillins are equally effective. In a careful study of antibiotic prophylaxis in hysterectomy at Yale, intravenous penicillin G 1 000 000 units given every 6 h for 48 h with the first dose given before the operation was equally effective as cefazolin 500 mg, used in a similar manner [30]. For the patient not allergic to penicillin, this drug is an alternative for use in prophylaxis.

Semi-Synthetic Penicillins

The semi-synthetic penicillins, methicillin, nafcillin, cloxacillin and dicloxacillin have a limited therapeutic role for the obstetrician-gynecologist. They were developed to resist the beta lactamase activity of the coagulase positive staphylococcus, so that infections due to this organism could be effectively treated. For this indication alone, they have been helpful additions to the therapeutic armamentarium of practicing physicians. These are not convenient penicillins for the practitioner to employ. They are expensive and each form can be administered by only one route. For example, methicillin is only given intravenously, while dicloxacillin is administered by the oral route. Of much more importance is the extreme protein binding by some of these penicillins that are administered orally. Table 3 documents the protein binding of the various penicillins. Since free unbound antibiotic is that portion of the administered dose which has antibacterial activity and is available for passage from the intravascular compartment into soft tissue sites of infection, it is easy to see that only very susceptible organisms would be effectively treated by the oral forms of these semi-synthetic penicillins. Because of this lack of flexibility in dosage forms, the only indication for the use of these agents is a documented infection with a penicillin G resistant coagulase positive staphylococcus. Even these specific infections are less frequently

Table 3. Protein binding of commonly employed penicillins.

Type of penicillin	Percentage bound to protein
Ampicillin	17%
Amoxicillin	17%
Methicillin	35%
Carbenicillin	50%
Ticarcillin	50%
Penicillin G	55%
Nafcillin	87%
Oxacillin	93%
Cloxacillin	94%
Dicloxacillin	97%

152

treated by these penicillins. In some hospital centers, particularly in urban centers in Europe, widespread resistance of the coagulase positive staphylococcus to methicillin has developed. In addition, alternative antibiotics such as the cephalosporins and clindamycin have been developed. These are effective against the coagulase positive staphylococcus and the free serum levels of these antibiotics are higher than most of the semi-synthetic penicillins. These semi-synthetic penicillins may have problems related to their use. In addition to the standard allergic responses seen with the penicillins, the employment of methicillin has resulted in interstitial nephritis in some patients. This can be recognized by the appearance of hematuria with proteinuria, skin rash, fever, and mild to moderate renal insufficiency. It is best treated by discontinuing the antibiotics, and generally this results in complete recovery.

AMPICILLIN

The introduction of ampicillin into clinical practice in the 1960's was accompanied by a great enthusiasm for the drug by physicians. Ampicillin had a broader spectrum of activity than the parent compound penicillin G, with excellent coverage of the common gram negative aerobes found in pelvic infections. It was an easily administered antibiotic with both an intravenous and an oral form available. The oral form was particularly appealing for it achieved the best serum levels of any of the then available penicillins. A new derivative of ampicillin, amoxicillin, achieves even higher serum levels. The frequent clinical successes with oral ampicillin caused many doctors to develop the habit of rapidly switching to the oral form of this agent with the first evidence of a clinical response to parental ampicillin. The major drawback to this agent was the frequent development of a skin rash often late in the course of therapy or after treatment has ended with this form of penicillin. A less frequent, but more serious problem is the development of diarrhea during therapy and the rare discovery of pseudomembranous enterocolitis in some of these women. The diagnosis depends upon proctosigmoidoscopic examination with the discovery of friable bowel that bleeds easily and the presence of raised plaques. Stool culture is usually positive for *Clostridium difficili*. The treatment is discontinuation of the ampicillin therapy and the use of oral vancomycin [32].

Ampicillin has been widely used in the treatment of women with sexually acquired infections. One alternate therapy for the asymptomatic woman who is culture positive for the gonococcus or who is a sexual contact of a culture positive male is 3.5 g of ampicillin or 3.0 g of amoxicillin given orally plus 1 g of probenecid at the same time. The rate of success with this therapy is not as great as with the injection of aqueous procaine penicillin G. Ampicillin is not recommended for the treatment of oropharyngeal gonorrhea, instead tetracycline should be prescribed. For the patient with gonococcal salpingitis, ampicillin can be employed. For the outpatient, the initial therapy is either intramuscular aquemous procaine penicillin G, 4.8 million units or 3.5 g of oral ampicillin or 3.0 g of oral amoxicillin plus one gram of oral probenecid. Following any of these initial therapies, the patient should receive either 0.5 g of ampicillin or 0.5 g of amoxicillin orally, four times a day for ten days. For the inpatient, the patient is given intravenous penicillin G 20 000 000 units/day or ampicillin 8.0 g/day until improvement occurs and then ampicillin or amoxicillin 0.5 g orally four times a day to complete ten days of therapy. Since the successful treatment of *Neisseria gonorrhea* infections is dependent upon high serum levels of penicillin, ampicillin and amoxicillin are the only acceptable oral forms of penicillin to be used. Similar treatment regimens have been employed in the therapy of women with non-gonococcal salpingitis. I have not been impressed that the immediate therapeutic response has been as effective as that seen with the tetracycline regimen. Certainly, ampicillin and amoxicillin did not provide as effective antimicrobial coverage of either Chlamydia or *Bacteroides fragilis* as do the tetracyclines.

Ampicillin has been a popular antibiotic for the treatment of soft tissue pelvic infections in hospitalized patients. It is frequently used alone in the therapy of low risk infections, such as the patient with a post-partum endomyometritis following vaginal delivery. For more serious infections in patients with an infected abortion, a post-partum endomyometritis following cesarean section, or a post-operative pelvic infection, ampicillin is frequently used in combination with an aminoglycoside to provide better antimicrobial coverage of gram negative aerobes. In many hospitals, a disproportional percentage of gram negative aerobes recovered from patients with hospital acquired infections are resistant to ampicillin, necessitating this addition. This combination has generally been quite effective, with either clindamycin or chloramphenicol added to provide coverage of *Bacteroides fragilis*, when there has been no response to this combination after 48 h of treatment. The widespread development of resistance of gram negative aerobes to ampicillin and the increased awareness of the lack of coverage of *Bacteroides fragilis* has resulted in a diminished popularity for the prescription of this drug for the treatment of soft tissue infection in hospitalized patients.

Ampicillin remains a popular form of therapy for patients with urinary tract infections. There are a number of obvious reasons for this preference. The availability of an intravenous and an oral form of the drug means that hospitalized patients can be sent home on oral therapy to complete a prescribed treatment course with the same drug that was employed during hospital therapy. In addition, ampicillin is concentrated in the urine, yielding even higher levels than attained in serum. This is an added help in the therapy of urinary tract infections, for over 90% of the organisms in these infections are gram negative aerobes, and the concentration effect makes most of them susceptible. This concentration phenomenon is often the source of confusion for the clinician in the interpretation of laboratory tests. In the woman with a urinary tract infection with an organism resistant in the laboratory to ampicillin, who is responding clinically to ampicillin therapy, there are two possible explanations. Either the organism is susceptible to the higher levels of ampicillin achieved in the urine or the bacterial growth in the urine has been suppressed and eliminated symptomatology, but the organisms have not been eradicated. This differential diagnosis is quickly resolved by a urine culture. No growth suggests the first possibility while bacterial growth of the same organism originally cultured should result in a change of antibiotics to one effective against this isolate. Another factor in the popularity of ampicillin for the treatment of urinary tract infection is its apparent safety in pregnancy. For this reason, it is widely employed for the treatment of pyelonephritis in pregnancy. The major drawback in microbiologic coverage of ampicillin in urinary tract infections is the lack of susceptibility of most strains of Klebsiella. If Klebsiella is a frequent isolate from the urine of women with urinary tract infections on your service, ampicillin would not be a wise routine choice for initial therapy. In this event one of the cephalosporins would be a more appropriate initial choice.

Ampicillin has been frequently employed as a prophylactic agent in obstetrics and gynecology. It has been successfully used in hysterectomy [33] and in cesarean section [34]. In addition, it had been one of the long-term agents used to suppress urinary tract bacterial growth in patients following treatment of pyelonephritis in pregnancy [35].

CARBENICILLIN AND TICARCILLIN

Carbenicillin is the prototype for a highly appealing form of penicillin for the clinician. It was introduced originally into clinical practice because of its extended antibacterial coverage of gram negative aerobic organisms. The emergence of these organisms, particularly *Pseudomonas aeruginosa*, in serious hospital acquired infections was the major source of interest in this form of penicillin. High dosages of carbenicillin were effective against many of these resistant strains. This drug had a synergetic activity with gentamicin and other aminoglycosides, against pseudomonas [36], if certain precautions in administration were followed. Since the beta lactam ring of carbenicillin has the capacity to link with the amino groups of aminoglycosides in vitro and inactivate both drugs [37], it is important that these two drugs not be mixed and administered in the same intravenous solution. If these precautions were followed, carbenicillin could be frequently employed in the treatment of the patient who was seriously ill, with a hospital acquired infection in which gram negative aerobic organisms were suspected. This linkage of carbanicillin and an aminoglycoside in vivo seems only important in the patient with renal failure [37]. Since relatively few women on an obstetric-gynecologic service had serious infections due to these resistant gram negative organisms, carbenicillin was infrequently employed outside of the oncology service.

In addition to the allergic responses that carbenicillin and ticarcillin share with the penicillins, these two drugs have a number of unique side effects. If clinicians are aware of these toxic possibilities, appropriate clinical and laboratory observations can be made to avoid continued difficulties. The administration of these drugs may be accompanied by serum electrolyte imbalances. Carbenicillin is a disodium salt and each gram contains 4.7 meq of sodium. Since seriously ill patients receive 30–40 g of carbenicillin/day, this sodium load may be excessive, particularly in patients with abnormal cardiac or renal disease. The sodium load per gram of ticarcillin is also large, 5.2 meq/g, but the advantage of this agent is that only 18–21 g/day are used as a therapeutic dose. In addition to the difficulties of administration of both drugs related to the sodium load, hypokalemia can be a problem. Both carbenicillin and ticarcillin act as a nonreabsorbable anion in the distal renal tubule and increase passive potassium excretion [38]. In patients receiving massive doses of these drugs, frequent evaluations of the serum potassium should be done and some authors have advocated the use of supplemental potassium treatment [39]. Both drugs also have the potential of causing bleeding problems. They bind to the ADP of platelets and may induce abnormalities of platelet aggregation. Any bleeding diathesis should be investigated, and alternative antibiotics employed if another cause of the bleeding is not apparent on testing.

The increasing clinical recognition of the importance of anaerobic organisms, particularly *Bacteroides fragilis*, in soft tissue pelvic infections led to wider employment of carbenicillin and ticarcillin in obstetric-gynecologic patients. The major concern of clinicians has been *Bacteroides fragilis*, particularly subspecies [40] fragilis, and there is some evidence that this virulence is related to the presence of a capsule [41]. The drugs of choice for the treatment of infections in which these organisms have been involved have been either clindamycin or chloramphenicol. A recurring concern for clinicians has been the toxicity of these two antibiotics, the pseudomembraneous enterocolitis with clindamycin and the aplastic anemia associated with chloramphenicol. There was interest in carbenicillin, because the toxicity associated with this antibiotic seemed less severe. This interest was further spurred by the laboratory discovery that high doses of carbenicillin were effective against *Bacteroides fragilis*. Sutter and Finegold reported that carbe-

156

nicillin inhibited 96% of strains of *Bacteroides fragilis* at a concentration of 100 μg/ml. These levels are easily achieved by megadose intravenous therapy with carbenicillin. These laboratory findings were followed by clinical trials in which the drug proved efficacious [43]. Indeed, one comparative study found ticarcillin as effective as either clindamycin or chloramphenicol in the therapy of serious soft tissue infections [39]. Despite this rate of favorable reports, there is a number of concerns voiced by many experts in infectious disease. The most common one is related to the high dosage levels of carbenicillin needed to be effective against *Bacteroides fragilis*. For the physician treating the patient with a suspected or proven *Bacteroides fragilis* infection, this means that the large doses of intravenous antibiotic must be maintained for the total duration of therapy. There is no alternative oral therapy. In addition, not everyone is convinced of the effectiveness of carbenicillin and ticarcillin against *Bacteroides fragilis*. Tally et al. found only 60% of strains of *Bacteroides fragilis* were inhibited by 128 μg/ml [44], and Maki et al. have suggested that high doses of penicillin G would be equivalent to carbenicillin for the treatment of *Bacteroides fragilis* infections and showed equivalent activity in the laboratory [45]. At the present time, these drugs are approved for use in anaerobic infections by the Food and Drug Administration. Because of disadvantages of prolonged megadose intravenous therapy, these drugs have not been widely used by most obstetrician-gynecologists as primary therapy. For the patient in whom neither clindamycin nor chloramphenicol is indicated, it remains an effective alternative.

There is one report of carbenicillin as effective prophylaxis in women undergoing hysterectomy [46]. Although effective, it seems no better than the cephalosporins or ampicillin in this regard. Because this drug is so effective in uncommon, but serious gram negative aerobic infections, most clinicians have preferred not to use it as a prophylactic, but instead reserve it for therapy of seriously ill patients. It is hoped this strategy will delay the emergence of resistant gram negative organisms.

1. Schultz JC, Adamson TS, Jr, Workman WW, et al.: Fatal liver disease after intravenous administration of tetracycline in high dosage. N Engl J Med 269:999, 1963
2. Whalley PJ, Cunningham FG, Martin FG: Transient renal dysfunction associated with acute pyelonephritis of pregnancy. Obstet Gynecol 46:174, 1975
3. Whalley PJ, Adams RH, Combes B: Tetracycline toxicity in pregnancy. JAMA 189:357, 1964
4. Kutscher AH, Zeqarelli EV, Tovell HMM, et al.: Dislocation of teeth induced by tetracycline administered antepartum. JAMA 184:586, 1963
5. Cohlan SO, Bevelander G, Tiomsic T: Growth inhibition of the developing skeleton due to

tetracycline deposition in bone: Clinical and laboratory investigation. Am J Dis Child 104:480, 1962

6. Neuwirth RS, Friedman FA: Septic abortion. Am J Obstet Gynecol 85:24, 1963
7. Sutter VL, Tally FP, Kwok Y, et al.: Activity of doxycycline and tetracycline versus anaerobic bacteria. Clin Med 80:31, 1973
8. Whelton, A.: Tetracyclines in renal insufficiency: Resolution of a therapeutic dilemma. Bull NY Acad Med 54:223, 1978
9. Swenson RM, Michaelson TC, Daly MJ, et al.: Anaerobic bacterial infections of the female genital tract. Obstet Gynecol 42:538, 1973
10. Thadepalli H, Gorbach SL, Keith L: Anaerobic infections of the female genital tract: Bacteriologic and therapeutic aspects. Am J Obstet Gynecol 117:1034, 1973
11. Sweet RL, Mills J, Hadley KW, et al.: Use of laparoscopy to determine the microbiologic etiology of acute salpingitis. Am J Obstet Gynecol 134:68, 1979
12. Mårdh PA, Ripa T, Jensson I, et al.: Chlamydiatrachomatis infection in patients with acute salpingitis. N Engl J Med 296:1377, 1977
13. Wager GP: Postpartum endometritis in women with antepartum chlamydia birth infections. Am J Obstet Gynecol. In press
14. Kaufman RE, Johnson RE, Jaffe HW, et al.: National gonorrhea therapy monitoring study. N Engl J Med 294:1, 1976
15. Cunningham FG, Hauth JC, Strong JD, et al.: Evaluation of tetracycline or penicillin and ampicillin for treatment of acute pelvic inflammatory disease. N Engl J Med 296:1380, 1977
16. Chow AW, Patten V, Marshall JR: The etiology of acute pelvic inflammatory disease: Value of cul de sac culture and relative importance of gonococci and the aerobic and anaerobic bacteria. Am J Obstet Gynecol 122:876, 1975
17. Monif GRG, Welkos SL, Baer H, et al.: Cul de sac isolates from patients with endometritis-salpingitis-peritonitis and gonococcal endocervicitis. Am J Obstet Gynecol 124:838, 1976
18. Monif GRG, Welkos SL, Baer H: Clinical response of patients with gonococcal endocervicitis and endometritis-salpingitis-peritonitis doxycycline. Am J Obstet Gynecol 129:614, 1977
19. Ledger WJ: Personal observation.
20. Tully JG, Smith LG: Postpartum septicemia with Mycoplasma hominis. JAMA 204:827, 1968
21. Whelton A, Blanco LJ, Carter GG, et al.: Therapeutic implications of doxycycline-cephatothin concentrations in the female genital tract. Obstet Gynecol 55:28, 1980
22. Hodgson JE, Major B, Portman K, Quattlebaum FW: Prophylactic use of tetracycline for first trimester abortion. Obstet Gynecol 45:574, 1975.
23. Wheeless CR, Jr, Porsey JH, Wharton LR, Jr: An evaluation of prophylactic doxycycline in hysterectomy patients. J Reprod Med 21:146, 1978
24. Gump DW, Ashikoqa T, Fink TJ, et al.: Side effects of minocycline: Different dosage regimens. Antiagents & Chemo 12:642, 1977
25. Weinstein L, Lerner PI, Chew WH: Clinical and bacteriologic studies of the effect of 'massive' doses of penicillin G on infections caused by gram negative bacilli. N Engl J Med 271:525, 1964
26. Barza M, Samuelson T, Weinstein L: Penetration of antibiotic into fibrin loci in vitro. J Infect Dis 129:73, 1974.
27. Ledger WJ, Kriewall T, Sweet R, et al.: A comparison of penicillin-kanamycin and clindamycin-kanamycin in the treatment of severe obstetric-gynecologic infections. Obstet Gynecol 43:490, 1974
28. DiZerega G, Yonekura L, Rey S, et al.: A comparison of clindamycin-gentamicin and penicillin-gentamicin in the treatment of post cesarean section endomyometritis. Am J Obstet Gynecol 134:238, 1979
29. Gibbs RS, Jones PM, Wilder CJ: Antibiotic therapy of endometritis following cesarean section, treatment successes and failures. Obstet Gynecol 52:31, 1973
30. Grossman JH, Creco TP, Minkin MJ, et al.: Prophylactic antibiotics in gynecologic surgery. Obstet Gynecol 53:537, 1979

158

31. Kagan BM: Antimicrobial therapy – Third Edition, Saunders, Philadelphia, 1980. Neu AC, Chapter 3, Penicillins: microbiology, pharmacology, and clinical usage.
32. Tedesco FR, et al.: Oral vancomycin for antibiotic associated pseudomembraneous colitis. Lancet II:226, 1978
33. Glover MW, Nagell JR: The effect of prophylactic ampicillin on pelvic infection following vaginal hysterectomy. Am J Obstet Gynecol 126:385, 1976
34. Miller RD, Crichton D: Ampicillin prophylaxis in cesarean section. S Afr J Obstet Gynecol 6:69, 1968
35. Harris RE, Gilstrap LC, III: Prevention of recurrent pyelonephritis during pregnancy. Obstet Gynecol 44:637, 1974
36. Ryes MP, El-Khabib MR, Brown WY, et al.: Synergy between carbenicillin and an amino-glycoside (gentamicin or tobramycin) against *Pseudomonas aeruginosa* isolated from patients with endocarditis and sensitivity to isolates to normal human serum. J Inf Dis 140:192, 1979
37. Riff LJ, Jackson GG: Laboratory and clinical conditions for gentamicin inactivation by carbenicillin. Arch Int Med 130:887, 1972
38. Chesney RW: Drug induced hypokalemia. Am J Dis Child 130:1055, 1976
39. Harding GKM, Buckwaldi FJ, Ronald AR, et al.: Prospective randomized comparative study of clindamycin, chloramphenicol, and ticarcillin, each in combination with genta-micin, in therapy for intra abdominal and female genital tract sepsis. J Inf Dis 142:384, 1980
40. Polk BF, Kasper DL: *Bacteroides fragilis* subspecies in clinical isolates. Ann Inter Med 86:469, 1977
41. Onderdonk AB, Kasper DL, Cisneios RL, et al.: The capsular polysaccharide of *Bacteroides fragilis* as a virulence factor: comparison of the pathogenic potential of encapsulated and unencapsulated strains. J Inf Dis 136:82, 1977
42. Sutter VL, Finegold SM: Susceptibility of anaerobic bacteria to carbenicillin, cefoxitin, and related drugs. J Inf Dis 131:417, 1975
43. Swenson RM, Lorber B: Clindamycin and carbenicillin in treatment of patients with intra-abdominal and female genital tract infections. J Inf Dis 135:S40, 1977
44. Tally FP, Jacobus NV, Bartlett JG, et al.: In vitro activity of penicillin against anaerobes. Antimicrob Agents Chemother 7:413, 1975
45. Maki DG, Kurzynski TH, Agger WA: Carbenicillin for treatment of *Bacteroides fragilis* infections: Why not penicilln G. J Inf Dis 138:859, 1978

Author's address:
Department of Obstetrics and Gynecology
The New York Hospital – Cornell Medical Center
New York, NY 10021
525 East 68th Street
U.S.A.

8. CHLORAMPHENICOL, CLINDAMYCIN AND METRONIDAZOLE

DAVID CHARLES, M.D.

INTRODUCTION

In recent years, the significance of anaerobic bacteria as part of the normal commensal flora of the lower genital tract, and of their role in a variety of obstetric and gynecologic infections, has become widely appreciated. One of the consequences of the increasing awareness of anaerobic non-sporing organisms in infectious processes has been the increasing interest in the assessment of the antimicrobial susceptibility of these organisms. Clinically, the most important species is the *Bacteroides fragilis* group, and because of their resistance to penicillins, cephalosporins and tetracyclines, other antimicrobial agents must be used in order to contain the infectious process at the primary site and treat life-threatening *Bacteroides fragilis* bacteremia.

In this chapter, three of the antimicrobial agents which are available and effective for the treatment of serious polymicrobial infections involving *Bacteroides fragilis* are discussed. It is, however, essential not to forget that surgical aspects of therapy are extremely important.

CHLORAMPHENICOL

This antibiotic was the first of the synthetically prepared broad spectrum bacteriostatic antimicrobial agents introduced into medical practice. As large quantities of this antibiotic can be produced relatively inexpensively, it is cheaper than other available antibiotics. It has been extensively used in many parts of the globe and in some countries is even sold without a prescription. In the United States its use has been drastically curtailed because of its potential to cause aplastic anemia with the result that this antimicrobial agent is only prescribed for a few relatively specific infections.

This antibiotic owes its bacteriostatic effect to its ability to inhibit protein synthesis. Pongs et al. [33] demonstrated that chloramphenicol binds to the 50S subunit of the ribosomes at the site where the enzyme peptidyltransferase is located. By suppression of this enzyme, peptide-bond formation is prevented so that protein synthesis is impeded. Chloramphenicol is a relatively specific inhibitor of mitochondrial biosynthesis and in pharmacologic doses sup-

160

presses the biosynthesis of cytochrome oxidase. Its ability to inhibit the biosynthesis of mitochondrial enzymes may be the basis for the aplastic anemia which is encountered in some patients.

Chloramphenicol is rapidly absorbed from the gastrointestinal tract and peak serum levels occur within 2 h following oral administration. Dupont et al. [14] showed that it is one of the few antibiotics which achieves equally efficacious serum levels after oral or parenteral administration. This drug is mainly converted by hepatic glucuronyltransferase to an inactive metabolite which is eliminated from the body by renal tubular secretion. About 10% of any dose of chloramphenicol is excreted unchanged in the urine by glomerular filtration. Konin et al. [21] reported that chloramphenicol has the ability to bind to an intracellular soluble hepatic protein, and this may account for its serum half-life of approximately 2 h. It has a low affinity for serum proteins, and as a result, it is rapidly distributed in all body fluids. The cerebrospinal fluid concentration of chloramphenicol is approximately 50% of the simultaneous serum level. Friedman et al. [16] found that the presence or absence of bacterial meningitis had minimal effect on cerebrospinal fluid (CSF) concentrations. Such observations are in accord with the concept that this antibiotic can attain efficacious levels in infections of the central nervous system caused by susceptible organisms and the maintenance of good CSF levels in the absence of inflammation means that a full treatment course can be completed with oral antibiotics.

The introduction of chloramphenicol more than 30 years ago was greeted as a major advance in antimicrobial therapy, but it rapidly fell into disrepute because of its adverse effects on the bone marrow. It is now recognized as the commonest antimicrobial cause of aplastic anemia. Wallerstein et al. [43], from epidemiologic studies conducted in California, found that this often fatal adverse reaction to this drug is encountered in one of every 36 000 patients treated and that the incidence of chloramphenicol-induced aplastic anemia was 13 times that observed in the general population. They indicated that aplastic anemia may be encountered at any time during therapy with this antibiotic. Their figures lead one to believe that this form of chlorampenicol toxicity may be more common than expected in younger patients. Chloramphenicol, however, engenders two patterns of adverse effects on cells originating in the bone marrow. One results from inhibition of mitochondrial protein synthesis and is exemplified by suppression of erythropoiesis. It is reversible and dose-related. This form of bone marrow toxicity is characterized by suppression of the erythroid cells as evidenced by transient anemia, a decrease in the number of reticulocytes and elevated serum iron levels. Neutropenia and thrombocytopenia may also be observed. The bone marrow morphology is normocellular, but cytoplasmic vacuolization of the erythroid precursors is a prominent feature of this form of drug toxicity. The other adverse effect of chloramphenicol on cells originating from the bone marrow is rare but of more serious import. Bone marrow aplasia may occur, but the mechanism by which this is induced has not been established. Yunis [64] considers that it results from an inborn susceptibility of DNA synthesis to the antibiotic or one of its metabolites. The possibility that this entity has a genetic basis has been postulated by Dameshek [13] and Nagao and Maver [25] who reported chloramphenicol-induced bone marrow aplasia in identical twins. It was suggested by these investigators that bone marrow aplasia is due to the inability of congenitally defective stem cells to handle chloramphenicol. Morley et al. [24] consider that this idiosyncrasy associated with chloramphenicol therapy results from undue sensitivity of the pluripotent stem cells to the antibiotic. These investigators used an experimental animal model in which they had induced bone marrow damage with busulfan. They demonstrated a progressive reduction in the number of stem cells of the animals after low dose administration of chloramphenicol. In their control animals, they found that oral administration of the antibiotic had no demonstrable effect on the bone marrow. They concluded that such observations are in accord with the theory that congenital or acquired overt bone marrow damage may be accentuated by this antimicrobial agent.

Weisburger et al. [45] suggested that chloramphenicol reduction metabolites may be the cause of the aplastic anemia. Pazdernik and Corbett [31] were unable to demonstrate by in vitro studies that the nitrogenous metabolites of this antibiotic were directly toxic to femoral bone marrow cells obtained from mice. They reported that in vivo studies showed that the metabolites were more toxic than the parent compound to bone marrow and immunopoietic precursor cells. They suggest, because their studies showed that the immunopoietic cells were more sensitive to the toxic effects of chloramphenicol metabolites, that aplastic anemia induced by this antibiotic in some individuals may be due to an immunologic imbalance.

It has been postulated, although never substantiated, that chloramphenicol-induced aplastic anemia is due to hypersensitivity because this entity resembles a drug-induced immunologic disease since it is not dose-dependent and is more frequently encountered after multiple exposure. Chloramphenicol-induced marrow aplasia is not related to the total dosage of the drug administered and cannot be anticipated by prospective hematologic studies since the aplastic anemia may not be apparent until long after drug therapy has been discontinued. Polak et al. [32] reported that a pancytopenia may become evident as long as a year after chloramphenicol administration and that in patients where aplastic anemia develops two or more months after cessation of therapy, the prognosis is poor. As seemingly unrelated compounds have been incriminated as etiologic agents in aplastic anemia, it is not surprising to note that suppressor T cells have been implicated in some cases.

Ascensao et al. [1] have demonstrated that cells from patients with aplastic anemia are capable of suppressing granulocyte presursors *in vitro* and that pretreatment of bone marrow cells from such patients with anti-thymocyte globulin and complement enhanced the precursor cell population. Such findings indicate that further studies are needed in order to ascertain whether an immunologic mechanism is responsible for chloramphenicol-induced aplastic anemia. Pazdernik and Corbett [31] in their studies with mice with busulfan-induced bone marrow damage were unable to demonstrate that the oral administration of chloramphenicol significantly altered the hypoplastic marrow failure. They found that the nitrogenous reduction metabolites of this antibiotic were most suppressive to antigen-reactive cells as determined by in vitro hemopoetic precursor cell assays. They suggest that in their animal model both busulfan and chloramphenicol were able to suppress immune components of the hemic cell regenerative system. These investigators postulate that in chloramphenicol-induced aplastic anemia abnormally high levels of reduction metabolites of the drug can undermine immune competence and place an increased load on the myeloid-lymphoid system in an attempt to combat any infectious illness. Such an increased burden on the hemic cell renewal system can accentuate any genetic predisposition to aplastic anemia in some patients. Despite numerous studies, the mechanism whereby chloramphenicol or its metabolites cause aplastic anemia remains to be delineated. Although most of the cases of chloramphenicol-induced aplastic anemia have occurred after the oral administration of this drug, it may follow parenteral therapy. It is unfortunate that many of the cases of fatal aplastic anemia have occurred in patients who have had this antibiotic for dubious indications. Although this adverse effect is rare, the prudent physician reserves this antibiotic for use in the seriously ill patient and never prescribes it for trivial infections.

Chloramphenicol can cause hemolytic anemia in patients with erythrocyte glucose-6-phosphate deficiencies. This type of hemolysis occurs in patients with less than 30% of the normal amount of glucose-6-phosphate in their erythrocytes and can be induced by other antimicrobial agents such as sulfonamides and nitrofurantoins. Therefore, in patients with erythrocyte glucose-6-phosphate deficiency, chloramphenicol therapy is contraindicated.

Premature infants presumably because of hepatic immaturity are liable to develop the 'gray baby syndrome' as an adverse reaction to chloramphenicol therapy. The clinical manifestations of the 'gray baby syndrome' include shallow irregular respirations, hypothermia, abdominal distension, circulatory collapse, anemia, and ashen gray cyanosis. The mortality in neonates so afflicted is about 40%. Most of the cases reported in the past were the result of excessive dosage. It is rarely seen today because it does not occur where the total daily dosage of chloramphenicol is less than 25 mg/kg body weight.

Hodgman and Burns [20] reported that the serum half life of this antibiotic was prolonged in the neonate. On the first day of life, it ranged from 15 to 22 h and decreased by the end of the second week to between 8 and 15 h. Friedman et al. [16] studied the pharmacokinetics of chloramphenicol following its intravenous administration as the sodium succinate ester to 54 infants and children. Included in this study were eight neonates of which five were premature. The drug was administered to the neonates in doses of 12.5 to 25 mg/kg body weight/day, divided into one to four doses. They measured the serum biologically active chloramphenicol levels by a microenzymatic method and found that the serum half-life of this drug ranged from 2.49 to 14.8 h with a mean of 8.01 h in the neonates. They concluded that there is a marked variation in chloramphenicol pharmacokinetics in infants and that blood concentrations should be monitored during therapy with this potentially toxic antimicrobial agent.

As chloramphenicol is one of the few antibiotics that is mainly metabolized prior to its elimination from the body, Suhrland and Weisberger [39] considered that the toxic effects of this drug in the neonate are due to unconjugated drug rather than to its metabolites. Chloramphenicol is primarily inactivated by glucuronidation in the liver. Although inadequate glucuronidation plays an important role in the etiology of the 'gray baby syndrome', Lietman [23] is of the opinion that it cannot account for all the clinical manifestations. This investigator considers that since neither high serum concentrations nor failure of Glucuronidation of the drug provide an adequate explanation for the unique cardiovascular toxicity observed in this syndrome, some other action of the drug must be involved. As chloramphenicol is known to inhibit mitochondrial protein synthesis which is necessary for mitochondrial biogenesis, he suggests that this may be the mechanism by which the cardiovascular toxicity is induced. Although this drug is rapidly transmitted across the placenta, there is no documentation that maternal chloramphenicol therapy in late pregnancy has caused the 'gray baby syndrome' in an infant exposed to this antimicrobial agent during intrauterine life.

Chloramphenicol is known to have adverse reactions to other drugs. It is now well recognized that two drugs administered in close sequence may interact to accentuate or reduce the intended effect of one or other therapeutic agent or may interact to cause an unintended reaction. As chloramphenicol is metabolized in the liver, it can by inhibition of hepatic microsomal enzyme activity affect the metabolism of such drugs as tolbutamide, diphenylhydantoin, and dicumarol. Christensen and Skovsted [12] found that chloramphenicol in a daily dosage of 2.0 g for several days caused a marked elevation in the steady state serum concentrations of these drugs and prolonged their half-life threefold. Ballek et al. [2] reported nystagmus in a patient who was on diphenylhydantoin therapy and was receiving chloramphenicol for an infectious illness. Although these adverse interactions are uncommon, it is preferable to use an alternative antimicrobial agent to treat bacterial infections in patients on oral anticoagulant therapy or epileptics on diphenylhydantoin.

Chloramphenicol has a broad spectrum of antimicrobial activity. It is an effective agent for the treatment of infections caused by a wide range of Gram-positive and Gram-negative bacteria as well as most strains of mycoplasma, chlamydia, and rickettsiae. This antibiotic is, however, not effective against many strains of *Staphylococcus aureus*, *Serratia marcescens*, *Pseudomonas aeruginosa* and indole-positive *Proteus* species.

During the past several years because of a resurgence of interest in this antibiotic combined with its indiscriminate use, many enterobacteria, staphylococci, some strains of streptococci, and *Haemophilus influenzae* have been found to be resistant to this antimicrobial agent. In some bacterial species, resistance may result from relative impermeability to the drug, but it is most frequently due, as reported by Shaw [36], to inactivation of the antibiotic by *O*-acetylation. The enzyme chloramphenicol acetyltransferase was originally found in *Escherichia coli* and other enterobacteria as well as isolates of *Staphylococcus aureus*. It is now well recognized that the chloramphenicol acetyltransferases are plasmid linked and generally inducible in Gram-positive but are components of many Gram-negative bacterial species. *Streptococcus pneumoniae* which is the responsible agent for the majority of cases of bacterial pneumonia in otherwise healthy humans has been shown to be capable of inactivating this drug. The same mechanism of resistance has been reported by Shaw et al. [37] in some strains of *Haemophilus parainfluenzae*, and as a result, the antimicrobial efficacy of chloramphenicol in the treatment of respiratory infection due to this organism has been reduced. The resistance exemplified by staphylococci to chloramphenicol is also under plasmid control. Shaw [35] demonstrated, however, that naturally occurring strains of staphylococci do not synthesize chloramphenicol acetyltransferase and do not form resistant mutants that produce the enzyme. The emergence of chloramphenicol resistant strains of many bacterial species as well as the toxicity of this antimicrobial agent has drastically reduced its use in clinical practice. Even infectious illnesses caused by those organisms that are susceptible are frequently more effectively treated with other antimicrobial agents. In general, chloramphenicol has until recently remained the drug of choice for the treatment of typhoid fever and for serious infections caused by *Bacteroides fragilis*. This antibiotic is also recommended as an alternative drug of choice for various rickettsial infections as well as tularemia and plague when the causative organisms are resistant to streptomycin.

Chloramphenicol is still considered by many to be the drug of choice for the treatment of typhoid fever. Vazquez et al. [42] and Brown et al. [7] have reported chloramphenicol resistant strains of *Salmonella typhi* in various parts of the world, and they appear to have resulted in a marked increase in the incidence of endemic typhoid fever. It is apparent from these reports that there is a direct correlation between the widespread use of this antibiotic and the emergence of resistant strains of *Salmonella typhi*. Olarte and Galindo [29] reported, in an epidemic of typhoid fever involving more than 10 000 patients, that the majority of isolates of *Salmonella typhi* were resistant to chloramphenicol. They considered that resistance to the drug was associated with a single R factor. Butler et al. [10] reported R-factor mediated chloramphenicol resistance in four isolates of *Salmonella typhi* from patients with typhoid fever in Vietnam. These chloramphenicol resistant isolates of the infectious agent were susceptible in vitro to trimethoprim-sulfamethoxazole and to ampicillin. Trimethoprim-sulfamethoxazole therapy in these patients proved highly efficacious. Although chloramphenicol remains the drug of choice for typhoid fever except for those associated with resistant strains of *Salmonella typhi*, further therapeutic studies involving trimethoprim-sulfamethoxazole may indicate that this drug combination may displace chloramphenicol as the first choice antimicrobial agent for this disease.

During the past decade, chloramphenicol is one of the few antimicrobial agents that has played an important role in the therapy of life-threatening polymicrobial infections involving *Bacteroides fragilis*. As this drug is an effective antianaerobic agent, it is still considered by many to be the first choice drug in the initial treatment of serious anaerobic infections where the identity and/or antimicrobial sensitivity of the obligate anaerobic organisms have not been established. Bodner et al. [5] reported that chloramphenicol was the most efficacious agent available for treatment of bacteremia due to *Bacteroides species*. Sutter and Finegold [40] reported that chloramphenicol was as active in vitro as any other antimicrobial agent against obligate anaerobes. Finegold [15] regards chloramphenicol as the drug of choice for the initial therapy of serious anaerobic infections prior to microbiologic identification of the causative organisms. Ledger et al. [22] found chloramphenicol and clindamycin to be equally effective in the treatment of severe pelvic sepsis. In their comparative study, they indicated that the 102 patients who received either of these antibiotics represented the most serious forms of pelvic soft tissue infection encountered on their gynecologic service during a period of two years. All patients received penicillin and an aminoglycoside in addition to either chloramphenicol or clindamycin. Fifty-three patients received chloramphenicol and 49 received clindamycin. Both groups of patients had similar infections such as pelvic inflammatory disease, septic abortion, puerperal sepsis, or postoperative sepsis. Microbiologic documentation of bacteremia was established in six of the chloramphenicol-treated patients, but none of these had *Bacteroides fragilis* isolates, but strains of *Peptococcus* were isolated from two of this group. Of the six patients with bacteremia who received clindamycin, two had blood cultures which yielded *Bacteroides fragilis* and a further two had isolates of *Bacteroides* species. None of the patients in this study had any evidence of any underlying fatal disease, and consequently, it was considered that a good prognosis should be attained with adequate antimicrobial therapy. The study failed to demonstrate any superiority of either chloramphenicol or clindamycin. These investigations emphasized that the most crucial factor in the cure of serious pelvic sepsis is operative intervention and that antimicrobial therapy plays a secondary role. These views are in accord with those expressed by Fry et al. [17] who consider that the clinical efficacy of chloramphenicol and clindamycin in the treatment of *Bacteroides* species is much less convincing than the in vitro sensitivity data would lead one to believe. The low oxidation-reduction potential that is essential for the growth and viability of the *Bacteroides fragilis* group of anaerobes makes purulent collections and devitalized tissues their natural habitat. These investigators state that the poor blood supply in areas that have a redox potential that supports the proliferation of obligate anaerobes may be inadequate for the delivery of antimicrobial agents in sufficient dosage to the site of infection. They consider that anaerobic infections, to a greater extent than aerobic infections, require both appropriate surgical intervention and the choice of an antimicrobial agent consonant with the demonstrated or anticipated sensitivities of the infectious agent. To date, neither chloramphenicol nor clindamycin administered as the sole antimicrobial agent has been evaluated in prospective studies for the treatment of anaerobic infections.

In patients with anaerobic bacteremia, it is important that the physician realize that there is a high probability that aerobic bacteria are also involved in the septic illness. Fry et al. [17] reported the isolation of aerobic species in all but six of 80 cultures of the primary focus of infection in such patients. The most common aerobe isolated from both the primary site of infection and blood was *Escherichia coli*. These investigators state that once surgical drainage of any purulent collection has been achieved, antimicrobial therapy directed against the aerobic species is highly successful in the majority of patients. In a review of the records of 98 consecutive patients with positive blood cultures for *Bacteroides* species, the investigators demonstrated the importance of surgical drainage. In the 77 patients whose primary infectious focus was amenable to eradication by surgical measures, the mortality was 43%, but in ten patients where surgical drainage and debridement were not performed, no patients survived.

These investigators were able to obtain 39 isolates of *Bacteroides* species from these patients and antimicrobial sensitivity studies revealed that all strains were susceptible to chloramphenicol and 97% were sensitive to clindamycin. Despite these in vitro observations, neither drug, when administered in appropriate dosage, played a statistically significant role as regards patient survival. Eight of their patients with Bacteroides bacteremia had obstetric or gynecologic infections, all of these patients survived despite the fact that five of them received antimicrobial therapy which was inappropriate for *Bacteroides* species.

Gibbs et al. [18], in a study of 160 patients who developed post-operative pelvic infection following Cesarean section, recorded a cure rate of 78% by the use of penicillin and kanamycin. Most of the remaining patients, presumably because of the presence of *Bacteroides fragilis*, had a prompt response to chloramphenicol or clindamycin. Surgical drainage was necessary in only 11 patients, of which ten were patients who failed to respond to penicillin-kanamycin therapy. Despite their observation that there was a highly significant association between the isolation of *Bacteroides* fragilis and failure of the combination therapy with penicillin and kanamycin, 13 of the 105 (12%) who did respond to this antibiotic combination did have isolates of this obligate anaerobe. These investigators found that of the 19 patients who had isolates of *Bacteroides fragilis* and failed to respond to the combination therapy, only ten (53%) had a good response to chloramphenicol or clindamycin. They found that a number of the patients who failed to respond to penicillin and kanamycin had wound abscesses or hematomas. In seven of eight patients with wound complications, *Bacteroides* species were isolated from the uterine cavity. In the latter patients, it is possible that surgical drainage of the wound may have been curative without additional antimicrobial therapy with chloramphenicol or clindamycin. The latter concept is in accord with the opinion of Stone et al. [38] who consider that the results of treatment by mechanical measures and appropriate antimicrobial agents for aerobic species are not improved by the addition of antibiotics directed against obligate anaerobic organisms in post-operative polymicrobial sepsis.

Despite the marked reduction in the incidence of septic abortion in general hospitals, the most important factor in the management of this entity is the expeditious removal of the septic focus. Evacuation of the retained products of conception should be carried out within 6 h from the time the patient is admitted to hospital. Such infections are usually polymicrobial due to aerobic, microaerophilic and anaerobic species. Although antimicrobial therapy is an essential component of treatment, there is no unanimity as regards the preferred choice of antibiotics. The evaluation of a particular agent is complicated by the fact that multiple therapeutic measures are simultaneously instituted in order to improve the patient's ability to combat infection. Chow et al. [11] reported that penicillin and chloramphenicol is the antibiotic combination which is usually prescribed by gynecologists for the treatment of septic abortion. These investigators conducted a randomized double blind study in 77 patients with a clinical diagnosis of septic abortion that compared treatment with penicillin and chloramphenicol with clindamycin alone. Clindamycin was selected because of its efficacy against *Bacteroides fragilis* and other obligate anaerobes as well as aerobic Gram-positive cocci, except for *Streptococcus faecalis*. Thirty-seven patients received clindamycin and 40 were treated with penicillin and chloramphenicol. The severity of the infection, the incidence of bacteremia and the bacteria isolated from the uterine cavity and blood were comparable in each group. They found that, although the fever index and duration of hospital stay were similar in both groups, significantly more major complications were encountered in the patients who received clindamycin. These investigators ascribed these complications to the fact that enteric organisms such as *Escherichia coli* are not susceptible to clindamycin. They also found that in the clindamycin group early evacuation of the products of conception was more important than the antibiotic in the resolution of the sepsis. Two of the patients in the clindamycin group developed tubo-ovarian abscesses at a later date. Their results indicate that penicillin combined with chloramphenicol was more effective in the treatment of septic absorption than clindamycin because of the broad spectrum of antimicrobial activity of this antibiotic combination. They considered that if clindamycin is to be used empirically in the treatment of the septic abortion, it should be used in combination with an aminoglycoside for the treatment of the aerobic Gram-negative bacilli which are an important component of this polymicrobial infection. The exact role of obligate anaerobes in these infections as in other serious forms of sepsis involving the female genital tract has not, however, been clarified.

Controversy still exists concerning the acceptability of chloramphenicol for routine use in serious polymicrobial infections because of its unique form of adverse reaction, namely aplastic anemia. Despite this, many recent in vitro and clinical studies continue to demonstrate the continued susceptibility of obligate anaerobes to this drug. Bawden et al. [3] compared the antimicrobial susceptibility patterns of 92 clinical isolates of *Bacteroides fragilis* and found that the level of resistance to chloramphenicol was in general lower than that of clindamycin. They postulate that this may be due to the infrequent use of chloramphenicol in their hospitals or that resistance to this antimicrobial agent develops at a slower rate. Although the clinical significance of drug-resistant anaerobes has not been thoroughly evaluated, the demonstration by Saunders [34] of conjugative resistance from *Bacteroides species* to *Escherichia coli* indicates that with the availability of anaerobic susceptibility testing, minimal inhibitory concentrations should be determined for isolates from serious infections.

Tytgat [41] tested 152 strains of *Bacteroides fragilis* by an agar dilution method against seven antimicrobial agents and found that chloramphenicol at

8 μg/ml inhibited all the strains of this organism. This investigator considers that this antibiotic is the most active antibiotic against anaerobic species. Brown and Waatti [8] found that chloramphenicol was the most effective antibiotic in vitro against 1 266 clinical isolates of anaerobic bacteria tested in their laboratory. Twelve of their 231 strains of *Bacteroides fragilis* indicate that this species is uniformly susceptible to chloramphenicol and the majority of strains are inhibited by a concentration of 6.2 μg/ml. Chloramphenicol resistance has, however, been observed in numerous species of bacteria and during the past several years reports have appeared which indicate that strains of obligate anaerobes are resistant to this antibiotic. Data derived from in vitro studies as well as animal and clinical studies, attest to the fact that chloramphenicol resistant strains of *Bacteroides* species could pose serious problems in patient management.

Weinstein et al. [44] reported the use of an experimental animal model for the study of anaerobic infections. They implanted gelatin capsules containing an inoculum of cecal contents and barium sulfate into the peritoneal cavity of Wistar rats. By this means they were able to simulate the polymicrobial intra-abdominal sepsis that is encountered in clinical practice. During the ensuing five days, all animals developed peritonitis and those that survived this initial infection subsequently developed intra-abdominal abscesses. Onderdonk et al. [28] demonstrated that *Escherichia coli* and enterococci were the predominant species responsible for the peritonitis in this animal model. In the animals who survived and developed an intra-abdominal abscess, they found that the predominant bacteria present were the *Bacteroides fragilis* group of obligate anaerobes and *Fusobacterium varium*, although *Escherichia coli* and enterococci were still isolated but in lower concentrations. Such studies indicated that *Escherichia coli* was primarily responsible for the initial peritonitis and obligate anaerobes were the causative agents of intra-abdominal abscess formation in the experimental animal. Onderdonk et al. [26] by use of this animal model were able to compare the pathogenicity of encapsulated and non-encapsulated strains of the *Bacteroides fragilis* group of organisms. They found that the encapsulated strains were responsible for the intra-abdominal abscesses due to the presence of a capsular polysaccharide constituent. Onderdonk et al. [27] reported that chloramphenicol, despite its effectiveness in vitro against obligate anaerobes, did not protect against intra-abdominal abscess formation. They administered chloramphenicol by intramuscular injection to the animals 4 h after intraperitoneal implantation of a cecal inoculum or a combination of bacterial species. Chloramphenicol administration was continued thereafter at eight hourly intervals for ten days. When the rats were sacrificed 48 h after the completion of therapy, 34 of the 58 animals (59%) had intra-abdominal abscesses. The dose of chloramphenicol was 16 mg/animal. Such therapy resulted in a mean serum peak concentration of 22 μg/ml which far exceeded the minimal inhibitory concentration of chloramphenicol for *Bacteroides fragilis*, *Fusobacterium varium* and *Escherichia coli*. This inconsistency between in vitro and in vivo data implied that these anaerobic species may be capable of inactivating chloramphenicol. In order to assess the aptitude of *Bacteroides fragilis* and *Clostridium perfringens* to inactivate this antibiotic, these investigators added known concentrations of the drug to 18 h broth cultures of the organisms. After 6 h incubation, *Bacteroides fragilis* reduced the concentration of biologically active drug by two-thirds while *Clostridium perfringens* decreased it fifty-fold. The strains of these organisms did not, however, develop chloramphenicol resistance in vitro, but these investigators demonstrated that filtrates of the broth cultures of these organisms were capable of inactivating this antibiotic. They reported that as chloramphenicol resistance did not occur in vitro, it was probable that acetylation was not involved in the inactivation of the drug. In order to elicit the mechanism which resulted in the inactivation of this antibiotic, they demonstrated by gas-liquid chromatography that an inactive aminophenyl derivative of chloramphenicol was present in the bacterial cultures 3 to 6 h after addition of this antibiotic. Such data implies that chloramphenicol is reduced in vivo by such obligate anaerobes as *Bacteroides fragilis* and *Clostridium perfringens*.

Britz and Wilkinson [6] reported the isolation of chloramphenicol resistant strains of *Bacteroides fragilis* from stool specimens. Drug resistance was due to the acetylating enzyme acetyltransferase. The stool specimens from which the chloramphenicol resistant strains of *Bacteroides fragilis* strains were isolated also contained resistant strains of *Escherichia coli*. The acetyltransferase enzymes produced by the chloramphenicol strains of both organisms were similar but differed in specific activity. These investigators postulated that in vivo transfer of a plasmid-associated chloramphenicol acetyltransferase gene occurred between the bacteria. Although chloramphenicol resistance has been observed in numerous species of bacteria, this report by Britz and Wilkinson [6] is the first which demonstrates chloramphenicol resistance in a clinical isolate of *Bacteroides fragilis* due to the acetylating enzyme, chloramphenicol acetyltransferase.

Berman et al. [4] reported the failure of intravenous chloramphenicol, despite adequate serum concentrations, to eradicate *Bacteroides fragilis* from the cerebrospinal fluid of a neonate with meningitis. Bacteriologic cure occurred only after the initiation of metronidazole therapy. Chloramphenicol levels in the cerebrospinal fluid are about 50% of the serum levels, but as the minimal inhibitory concentration of this drug for *Bacteroides fragilis* ranges from 4 to 6 μg/ml, administration of maximum doses of this antibiotic is necessary. Although these investigators postulate that continued chloramphenicol therapy may have eradicated the organism from the cerebrospinal fluid, it is possible in the absence of relevant microbiologic studies that the strain of *Bacteroides fragilis* causing the meningitis could have been resistant to chloramphenicol. Although chloramphenicol readily diffuses into the cerebrospinal fluid, resistance to the drug has been described in cases of meningitis due to Gram-negative bacilli. Bryan et al. [9] described two patients with *Bacteroides fragilis* meningitis where treatment with chloramphenicol alone or in combination with nafcillin was unsuccessful. In one of the patients a blood culture yielded a strain of *Bacteroides fragilis* which was sensitive in vitro to chloramphenicol and *Streptococcus intermedius* which reacted with Lancefield Group F antiserum and was not susceptible in vitro to nafcillin. Despite treatment with chloramphenicol in a daily dosage of 6.0 g and nafcillin 12.0 g daily in divided doses for 12 days, the patient's condition deteriorated. Lumbar puncture yielded a purulent sample of cerebrospinal fluid which on culture yielded the identical bacterial isolates to those obtained on blood culture before the institution of antibiotic therapy. The minimal inhibitory concentration of chloramphenicol against the strain of *Bacteroides fragilis* isolated from the blood and cerebrospinal fluid was 3.9 μg/m. The other patient had multiple blood and cerebrospinal fluid cultures which yielded *Escherichia coli* and *Bacteroides fragilis*. Despite intravenous nafcillin 4.0 g, chloramphenicol 4.0 g, and gentamicin 240 mg/day in divided doses for seven days, the blood and cerebrospinal fluid cultures still grew the identical pathogens. The minimal inhibitory concentration of chloramphenicol against this strain of *Bacteroides fragilis* was 4.0 μg/ml. Such studies imply that the failure of chloramphenicol to eradicate the pathogen may have resulted from its inactivation in vivo by the obligate anaerobe. Most susceptible Gram-negative bacteria are inhibited by chloramphenicol concentrations of 5 to 15 μg/ml, and such serum levels must have been attained in both patients in the dose regimen prescribed. Furthermore, this report substantiates the often reiterated concept that the susceptibility of an organism in vitro to an antimicrobial agent does not necessarily mean that the drug will be efficacious in the treatment of clinical infections due to the specific bacterium.

The major selective force favoring the emergence of antibiotic resistance in hospital practice is the extensive use of antibiotics. Chloramphenicol, however, has had restricted usage because of its potential to cause serious and sometimes fatal aplastic anemia. Consequently, resistance of anaerobes to this antibiotic is infrequently encountered in clinical practice, and as a result, it is still highly efficacious in the treatment of serious anaerobic polymicrobial infection. Although this antibiotic is available in both oral and parenteral forms, available data suggests that fatal or reversible chloramphenicol-induced aplastic anemia occurs almost exclusively with oral administration of the drug and rarely with parenteral therapy. Parenteral administration should be the route of choice for the treatment of serious polymicrobial infections. It should be administered in the form of the succinate in a total daily dosage of 4.0 g in divided doses every 6 h for a maximum of five days. When administered in high dosage for severe sepsis, aplastic anemia is not a dose-related adverse reaction. The author has frequently used the intravenous formulation in a total daily dosage of 6.0 g in patients with *Bacteroides* bacteremia with no evidence of any adverse drug toxicity. In such cases, repeated evaluation of the peripheral blood picture is mandatory in order to detect at the earliest opportunity any deleterious effects of this antimicrobial agent. A significant reduction in hemoglobin concentration, leukocyte or platelet count is an indication to discontinue therapy to reverse the bone marrow depression. After conclusion of chloramphenicol therapy, all patients should have periodic evaluations of their hematologic status during the ensuing 12 months as aplastic anemia may not be evident until several months after cessation of chloramphenicol therapy. If it is used for a few specific indications, chloramphenicol will retain its current status as a most effective anti-anaerobic antibiotic, since the benefits of the drug in the treatment of life-threatening polymicrobial infections far outweigh the risks of its inherent toxicity.

REFERENCES

1. Ascensao J, Kagan W, Woore M, Pahwa R, Hansen J, Good R: Aplastic anaemia: Evidence for an immunological mechanism. Lancet 1:669–671, 1976
2. Ballek RE, Heidenberg MM, Orr L: Inhibition of diphenylhydantoin metabolism by chloramphenicol. Lancet 1:150, 1973
3. Bawdon RE, Rozmiej E, Palchaudhuri, S, Krakowiak J: Variability in the susceptibility pattern of *Bacteroides fragilis* in four Detroit area hospitals. Antimicrob Agents Chemother 16:664–666, 1979
4. Berman BW, King FH, Jr, Rubenstein DS, Long SS: *Bacteroides fragilis* meningitis in a neonate successfully treated with metronidazole. J Pediatr 93:793–795, 1978
5. Bodner SJ, Koenig MG, Goodman JS: Bacteremic bacteroides infections. Ann Intern Med 73:537–544, 1970
6. Britz ML, Wilkinson RG: Chloramphenicol acetyltransferase of *Bacteroides fragilis*. Antimicrob Agents Chemother 14:105–111, 1978
7. Brown JD, Mo DH, Rhoades ER: Chloramphenicol resistant *Salmonella typhi* in Saigon. J.A.M.A. 231:162–166, 1975
8. Brown WJ, Waatti PE: Susceptibility testing of clinically isolated anaerobic bacteria by an agar dilution technique. Antimicrob Agents Chemother. 17:629–635, 1980
9. Bryan CS, Huffman LJ, Del Bene VE, Sanders CV, Scalcini MC: Intravenous metronidazole therapy for *Bacteroides fragilis* meningitis. South Med J 72:494–497, 1979
10. Butler T, Linh NN, Arnold K, Pollack M: Chloramphinicol resistant typhoid fever in Vietnam associated with R factor. Lancet 2:983–985, 1973
11. Chow AW, Marshall JR, Guze LB: A double-blind comparison of clindamycin with penicillin plus chloramphenicol in treatment of septic abortion. J Infect Dis 135:535–539, 1977
12. Christensen LK, Skovsted L: Inhibition of Drug Metabolism by Chloramphenicol. Lancet 2:1397–1399, 1969
13. Dameshek W: Chloramphenicol aplastic anemia in identical twins: a clue to pathogenesis. N Engl J Med 281:42–43, 1969

14. Dupont HL, Hornick RB, Weiss CF, Snyder MJ, Woodward TE: Evaluation of chloramphenic acid succinate therapy of induced typhoid fever and Rocky Mountain fever. N Engl J Med 282:53–57, 1970

15. Finegold SM: Therapy for infections due to anaerobic bacteria: an overview. J Infect Dis 135:525–529, 1977

16. Friedman CA, Lovejoy FC, Smith AL: Chloramphenicol disposition in infants and children. J Pediatr 95:1071–1077, 1979

17. Fry DE, Garrison RN, Polk HC: Clinical implications in bacteroides bacteremia. Surg Gynecol Obstet 149:189–192, 1979

18. Gibbs RS, Jones PM, Wilder CJ: Antibiotic therapy of endometritis following Cesarean section. Obstet Gynecol 52:31–37, 1978

19. Hansen SL: Variation in susceptibility patterns of species within the *Bacteroides fragilis* Group. Antimicrob Agents Chemother 17:686–690, 1980

20. Hodgman JE, Burns LE: Safe and effective chloramphenicol dosages for premature infants. Am J Dis Child 101:140–148, 1961

21. Konin CM, Craig WA, Kornguth M, Monson R: Influence of binding on the pharmacologic activity of antibiotics. Ann NY Acad Sci. 226:214–224, 1973

22. Ledger WJ, Gee CL, Lewis WP, Bobitt JR: Comparison of clindamycin and chloramphenicol in treatment of serious infections of the female genital tract. J Infect Dis 135:530–534, 1977

23. Lietman PS: Pharmacologic effect on developing enzyme systems. Fed Proc 31:62–64, 1972

24. Morley A, Trainor K, Remes J: Residual marrow damage: possible explanation for idiosyncrasy to chloramphenicol. Brit J Haematol 32:525–531, 1976

25. Nagao T, Mauer AM: Concordance for drug-induced aplastic anemia in twins. N Engl J Med 281:7–11, 1969

26. Onderdonk AB, Kasper DL, Cisneros RL, Bartlett JG: The capsular polysaccharide of *Bacteroides fragilis* as a virulence factor: comparison of the pathogenic potential of encapsulated and unencapsulated strains. J Infect Dis 136:82–89, 1977

27. Onderdonk AB, Kasper DL, Mansheim BJ, Lovie TJ, Gorback SL, Bartlett JG: Experimental animal models for anaerobic infections. Rev Infect Dis 1:291–301, 1979.

28. Onderdonk AB, Weinstein WM, Sullivan NM, Bartlett JG, Gorback SL: Experimental intra-abdominal abscess in rats: quantitative bacteriology of infected animals. Infect Immun 10:1256–1259, 1974

29. Olarte J, Galindo E: *Salmonella typhi* resistant to chloramphenicol, ampicillin and other antimicrobial agents: Strains isolated during an extensive typhoid fever epidemic in Mexico. Antimicrob Agents Chemother. 4:597–601, 1973

30. Pazdernik TL, Corbett MD: Effects of chloramphenicol reduction products on hemopoietic precursor cells in vitro. Pharmacol 19:191–195, 1979

31. Pazdernik TL, Corbett MD: Role of chloramphenicol reduction products in aplastic anemia. Pharmacol 20:87–94, 1980

32. Polak BCP, Wesseling H, Dien S, Herxheimer A, Meyler L: Blood dyscrasias attributed to chloramphenicol. A review of 576 published and unpublished cases. Acta Med Scand 192:409–418, 1972

33. Pongs O, Bald R, Erdmann VA: Identification of chloramphenicol-binding protein in *Escherichia coli* ribosomes by affinity labelling. Proc Natl Acad Sci 70:2229–2233, 1973

34. Saunders JR: Anaerobes and transferable drug resistance. Nature 274:113–114, 1978

35. Shaw WV: Evolution of plasmid mediated chloramphenicol acetyltransferase. Proc Soc Gen Microbiol 4:93–96, 1977

36. Shaw WV: Chloramphenicol acetyltransferase from chloramphenicol resistant bacteria. Methods Enzymol 43:737–755, 1975

37. Shaw WV, Bouanchaud DH, Goldstein FW: Mechanism of transferable resistance to chloramphenicol in *Hemophilus parainfluenzae*. Antimicrob. Agents Chemother 13:326–330, 1978

38. Stone HH, Kolb LD, Geheber CE: Incidence and significance of intraperitoneal anaerobic bacteria. Ann Surg 181:705–715, 1975

174

39. Suhrland LG, Weisberger AS: Chloramphenicol toxicity in liver and renal disease. Arch Intern Med 112:747–754, 1963
40. Sutter VL, Finegold SM: Susceptibility of anaerobic bacteria to 23 antimicrobial agents. Antimicrob Agents Chemother 10:736–752, 1976
41. Tytgat F: Activité de sept antibiotiques sur *Bacteroides fragilis*. Ann Microbiol (Inst. Pasteur) 131:39–44, 1980
42. Vazquez V, Calderon E, Rodriquez RS: Chloramphenicol resistant strains of *Salmonella Typhosa* N Engl J Med 286:1220, 1972
43. Wallerstein, RO, Conduit PK, Kasper CK, Brown JW, Morrison RR: Statewide study of chloramphenicol therapy and fatal aplastic anemia. JAMA 208:2045–2050, 1969
44. Weinstein WM, Onderdonk AB, Bartlett JG, Gorbach SL: Experimental intra-abdominal abscesses in rats: development of an experimental model. Infec Immun 10:1250–1255, 1974
45. Weisburger JH, Shirasu Y, Grantham PH, Weisburger EK: Chloramphenicol, protein synthesis, and the metabolism of the carcinogen N-2-fluorenyldiacetamide in rats. J Biol Chem 242:372–378, 1967
46. Yunis, AA: Chloramphenicol-induced bone marrow suppression. Semin Hematol 10:225–234, 1973

CLINDAMYCIN

This semisynthetic bacteriostatic antibiotic is a derivative of lincomycin. It is better absorbed after oral administration and produces substantially higher blood levels than the parent compound. When it was initially introduced into clinical practice it was heralded as the drug of choice for Bacteroides infections and, despite its association with pseudomembranous colitis, it still remains a valuable antimicrobial agent in the therapy of polymicrobial infections involving *Bacteroides fragilis*.

Despite the fact that clindamycin bears no structural resemblance to the macrolide group of antibiotics, it has a similar antimicrobial spectrum to erythromycin in that it inhibits the growth of many Gram-positive organisms including many strains of penicillinase producing staphylococci. It is active both in vitro and in clinical settings against *Streptococcus pyogenes* and *Streptococcus pneumoniae*. However, in contradistincton to erythromycin, enterococci, *Haemophilus* and *Neisseria* species as well as mycoplasma are generally resistant to this antibiotic. There is evidence that cross resistance occurs between erythromycin and clindamycin. It is inactive against Gram-negative enterobacteria but possesses the ability to inhibit many of the Bacteroides group of organisms, more especially *Bacteroides fragilis*. The Gram-positive anaerobe *Actinomyces israelii* is susceptible to this antibiotic but many of the clinically important members of the *Clostridium* species are resistant. Clindamycin has a limited spectrum of effectiveness because it lacks efficacy against many important pathogenic organisms in clinical practice.

The oral formulation of clindamycin hydrochloride hydrate is readily absorbed from the gastrointestinal tract and attains therapeutic blood levels which persist for 6 to 8 h. Garrod et al. [21] reported that an oral dose of 120 mg of this antibiotic attains a serum peak level of 4.7 μg/ml within 2 h. Administration of the drug after a meal, unlike its congener lincomycin, does not impair its absorption. Rimmer and Sales [42] in a study of 22 normal adults who received 300 mg of the oral preparation every 12 h for five doses immediately after food found that the average serum peak concentration was 3.80 μg/ml, 1.5 h after the final dose of the drug. In a further study in the same group of individuals using an oral dosage of 150 mg every 6 h for ten consecutive doses, they found that the average serum concentration and the time of the peak concentration were comparable to those noted in their initial study.

The phosphate ester of clindamycin which is available for parenteral administration is rapidly hydrolysed in the body to the active form. De Haan et al. [15] showed that after the intramuscular administration of 300 mg of clindamycin phosphate serum peak levels of approximately 5.5 μg/ml were attained in about 3h. The recommended parenteral dosages provide effective antimicrobial activity for 6 to 8 h.

Despite the fact that clindamycin is about 90% bound to the glycoprotein component of the globulin fraction of serum it is widely distributed in many body fluids and tissues. Clindamycin, however, does not reach therapeutic levels in the cerebrospinal fluid and for this reason chloramphenicol and metronidazole are the drugs of choice for the treatment of intracranial suppuration and meningitis caused by *Bacteroides* species.

Wagner et al. [59] found that the serum half-life of this drug was 2.38 h in normal subjects following the oral administration of a single dose of 250 mg. Eastwood and Gower [18] in a similar study found that the serum half-life of clindamycin was 2.15 h following the oral administration of 150 mg of the drug. These investigators demonstrated that blood levels are not affected by hemodialysis and that this antibiotic was readily excreted in patients with chronic renal failure. Consequently, little adjustment of dosage is necessary for individuals with impaired renal function. Novak et al. [37] studied the urinary excretion patterns and found that only about 6% of the dose administered is excreted unchanged in the urine. Their findings indicate that most of the drug is metabolized as only minimal amounts are found in the feces. The major portion of any dose of this drug is metabolized in the liver and excreted in the bile and urine.

The most serious untoward effect of clindamycin therapy is the propensity of this drug to cause pseudomembranous colitis. Diarrhea, which is usually self-limited, has been recognized for many years as a common accompaniment of antibiotic therapy. Less frequently antibiotic-induced colitis occurs as a potentially life-threatening complication of therapy with broad spectrum antibiotics. Reiner et al. [40] drew attention to the relationship of aureomycin and chloramphenicol to this clinical entity. Since their report antibiotic-associated pseudomembranous colitis has been found to occur in conjunction with the administration of almost every class of antimicrobial agent. It has been associated with the use of penicillin, ampicillin, amoxicillin, indanyl carbenicillin, cephalothin, cephalexin, tetracycline, lincomycin as well as bactericidal and bacteriostatic antimicrobial agents with diverse spectra of antibacterial activity.

Clindamycin was originally introduced into clinical practice in an attempt to circumvent the increased incidence of gastrointestinal adverse effects associated with its parent compound lincomycin. This goal was not attained and the use of this compound has been associated with severe colitis which on occasion does not resolve on cessation of therapy. On occasion clindamycin-induced pseudomembranous colitis has resulted in the demise of the patient and some severe cases of colitis have been encountered several weeks after cessation of therapy. The high incidence of colitis associated with clindamycin is due to the selective suppression of the ecosystem of the large bowel which allows bacterial species that are resistant to the antibiotic to flourish. Bartlett et al. [6] demonstrated that toxin-producing strains of *Clostridium difficile* were the cause of clindamycin-induced colitis in hamsters. Larson et al. [29] found that the feces from a patient with penicillin-induced pseudomembranous colitis contained a cytopathic toxin produced by a strain of *Clostridium* species. In a further communication, Larson and Price [30] reported that the toxin was neutralized by *Clostridium sordellii* antitoxin. The toxin was not, however, present in the stools of patients with diarrhea from other forms of colitis. Rifkin et al. [41] reported the presence of a heat labile toxin which had a cytopathic effect on cells in tissue culture which could be neutralized by *Clostridium sordellii* antitoxin from the stools of patients with antibiotic-induced colitis. From such studies it became apparent that toxin-producing *Colostridia* were implicated in the pathogenesis of antibiotic-induced colitis.

The neutralization of the putative cytopathic toxin by *Clostridium sordelli* antitoxin linked this organism with the etiology of antibiotic induced colitis although bacteriologic fecal studies implicated *Clostridium difficile* as the pathogen. Clarification of this issue, however, was soon forthcoming when it was observed that the cytopathic toxin produced by *Clostridium difficile* was also neutralized by *Clostridium sordellii* antitoxin.

In a further communication, Bartlett et al. [7] reported that the administration of vancomycin protected hamsters against the development of clindamycin-induced enterocolitis due to strains of *Clostridium* species. Similar observations were reported by Browne et al. [10] using the same animal model. Bartlett et al. [2] demonstrated the presence of *Clostridium difficile* or its toxin in the cecal contents of 547 hamsters with antibiotic-induced lethal enterocolitis.

The clinical relevance of these observations in the animal model became apparent when Bartlett et al. [1] reported the recovery of *Clostridium difficile* from the stools of four patients with antibiotic-induced pseudomembranous colitis. Further confirmation of the role of *Clostridium difficile* in this clinical entity was the report of Larson et al. [31] who isolated this organism from four of their five patients and George et al. [21a] who recovered this Gram-positive spore-forming obligate anaerobe from the stools of 24 of their 25 patients. Although *Clostridium difficile* may not be the only *Clostridium* species capable of elaborating a toxin that is responsible for antibiotic-induced colitis, it is the only organism to date that has been conclusively implicated in the etiology of this entity. (Although *Clostridium difficile* was originally described by Hall and O'Toole [25] as a potential human pathogen which had the ability to produce a toxin which was lethal to laboratory animals, it did not appear to be a clinical problem.) This organism is now considered an enteric pathogen with the particular property to produce a toxin which induces a somewhat unique form of colitis in the presence of antibiotic exposure.

The usual clinical presentation of antibiotic-associated pseudomembranous colitis is the acute onset of profuse, watery diarrhea without any macroscopic evidence of blood or mucus. Most patients have abdominal pain, fever and a leukocytosis. In some patients, nausea, vomiting and abdominal distension may be associated clinical manifestations of this condition. Marked abdominal distension due to colonic dilatation in some patients may simulate toxic megacolon. This clinical entity can, however progress to produce toxic megacolon, peritonitis and death. This disease requires early recognition and prompt cessation of therapy with the offending antimicrobial agent is imperative. Tedesco et al. [55] consider that the more severe complications have occurred predominantly in patients who continued to receive the antibiotic after the development of diarrhea. Symptoms may commence at any time during antimicrobial therapy and for extended periods after cessation of such treatment. The range in the temporal relationship with antibiotic administration may be from a few hours from the initiation of antibiotic administration to several weeks after its discontinuation. In most instances the diarrhea persists for as long as six weeks after the offending drug has been discontinued. In a small percentage of patients the symptoms may subside in a matter of a few days, especially in individuals with the milder and more limited form of the disease. On occasion there have been no symptoms during the period of time during which antibiotics were administered but the disease became manifest in the form of profuse diarrhea two or three weeks after cessation of therapy. It is, therefore, essential that physicians adopt a more circumspect approach to antibiotic therapy and acquire knowledge of the effects of such drugs on the gastrointestinal tract.

A diagnosis of antibiotic-induced pseudomembranous colitis should be based on the history and sigmoidoscopic or colonoscopic findings. The extent of the abnormalities seen on endoscopy usually can be correlated with the severity of the disease. Although the disease is usually confined to the colon, Bartlett and Gorbach [5] have reported involvement of the small bowel. Totten et al. [58] reported their preference for colonoscopy because this procedure revealed involvement of the colon by the inflammatory process to at least the splenic flexure in seven of their 11 patients. The abormalities observed ranged from edema of the colonic mucosa with marked frIability and ulceration to diffuse or discrete, raised pale yellow-white plaques of pseudomembrane adherent to hyperemic ulcerated mùcosa. Kappas et al. [27] reported that all patients on their surgical service who had three or more stools per day in relation to antibiotic therapy had a sigmoidoscopic examination even if they had had a recent colonic resection. They consider that sigmoidoscopy is imperative in all patients with suspected antibiotic-related colitis and should not be delayed even if the patient is seriously ill.

Radiologic evaluation by barium enema is all too often of little diagnostic value. Stanley et al. [46] consider that the radiographic findings are not specific and quite variable in patients with this disease. Furthermore, as toxic megacolon can occur in patients with antibiotic-induced pseudomembranous colitis, Tedesco [54] considers that radiologic evaluation of patients with severe pseudomembranous colitis by barium enema should be avoided. Stanley et al. [47] reported that a plain abdominal film could often furnish valuable information for the elucidation of the illness. They noted in severe cases of this disease mucosal edema, thickening and distortion of the haustra of the colon and a pattern termed 'thumb printing' due to edema of the haustra. Sigmoidoscopy or colonoscopy are, however, far superior to any radiographic studies in substantiating a diagnosis of pseudomembranous colitis.

Price and Davies [38] consider that a biopsy should always be obtained when sigmoidoscopy reveals the presence of the characteristic pseudomembrane. They state that the histologic features of a well directed biopsy which includes the pseudomembrane and the underlying mucosa are diagnostic of this entity. The microscopic appearance of the pseudomembranous lesion reveals the presence of a fibrin-laden leukocytic exudate attached to crypts of glandular epithelium. The exudate is mixed with mucin which emanates from the lamina propria on to the mucosal surface. The mucin, desquamated epithelial cells and polymorphonuclear leukocytes appear as linear strands. There is no destruction of the deep layers although there is lymphocytic as well as polymorphonuclear leukocytic infiltration of the lamina propria. In most instances there is no evidence of vasculitis. The development of a membrane which is adherent over ulcerated mucosa differentiates this condition from other varieties of inflammatory lesions of the colon.

The diagnostic feature of pseudomembranous colitis is the formation of the diffuse or patchy pseudomembrane formation. Bartlett and Gorbach [5] state that this entity has been found in patients with uremia, heavy metal poisoning, intestinal obstruction, ischemic cardiovascular disease and after intestinal surgery. Such observations indicate that pseudomembranous colitis is not specifically a disease which is antibiotic-induced, although the vast majority of cases reported during the past decade has been associated with antibiotic therapy. In cases of pseudomembranous colitis unrelated to antimicrobial therapy the role of *Clostridium difficile* and its toxin have not been evaluated although other intestinal diseases do not appear to be associated with an increased risk of pseudomembranous colitis when antibiotics are administered. Bartlett et al. [4] reported the presence of the cytopathic toxin of *Clostridium difficile* in stool samples from 42 of 43 patients with antibiotic associated pseudomembranous colitis and from 12 of 78 patients with antibiotic-associated diarrhea. In a control group of patients, such as individuals with ulcerative colitis, neonates with necrotizing enterocolitis as well as healthy subjects, they failed to identify the toxin by means of tissue culture assays. Such findings implicated *Clostridium difficile* as the major cause of antibiotic-associated pseudomembranous colitis and indicate that the tissue culture assay for the detection of the toxin can play an important role in the diagnosis of this clinical entity. These investigators recommend that toxin assays be conducted in all patients with antibiotic-associated diarrhea which does not resolve on cessation of antibiotic therapy.

Therapy of antibiotic-associated pseudomembranous colitis depends on recognition of the disorder and prompt cessation of therapy with the implicated agent. In most instances this will result in prompt amelioration of the patient's symptoms. In moderate to severe cases proper maintenance of electrolyte and fluid balance is essential as the majority of the lethal forms of the illness are associated with shock from dehydration and electrolyte imbalance. If stool losses become excessive, infusions of albumin may be required to correct the resultant hypoproteinemia.

There is no data to indicate that the systemic administration of corticosteroids is efficacious in the treatment of pseudomembranous colitis. Totten et al. [58] administered prednisone in a dosage of 20–40 mg daily to three of their patients with no apparent benefit.

Anion binding resins have been used to treat pseudomembranous colitis. Burbige and Milligan [11] reported that cholestyramine resulted in rapid resolution of the illness in two patients. Chang et al. [12] demonstrated that cholestyramine appears to have the ability to bind to the toxin of *Clostridium difficile* and thereby have a beneficial effect in the treatment of pseudomembranous colitis. To date, however, there are no controlled studies which demonstrate the efficacy of this form of therapy. In the hamster model, Bartlett et al. [3] reported that the oral administration of colestipol to animals with clindamycin-induced pseudomembranous enterocolitis was of no value and did not prevent the death of the animals. Colestipol is an anion exchange resin which is a more effective agent than cholestyramine as regards its ability to bind anions.

The oral administration of vancomycin has been advocated for the management of patients with antibiotic-associated pseudomembranous colitis. Vancomycin is poorly absorbed from the gastrointestinal tract and Geraci et al. [22] found high concentrations after oral administration in the stools of patients with enterocolitis. Bartlett and Gorbach [5] reported that this fact together with its poor absorption from the gastrointestinal tract was the rationale for its use in the treatment of antibiotic-associated pseudomembranous colitis. Bartlett et al. [7] found that this antimicrobial agent was efficacious in animals with clindamycin-induced typhlitis. They found that oral vancomycin prevented death of the animals only during the time it was administered. Cessation of vancomycin treatment resulted in death of the animals within one week, even if the drug had been administered for as long as 12 weeks. Larson et al. [31] ascribed such deaths to recolonization of the intestinal tract of the animals with toxin-producing clostridia from the environment. Fekety et al. [20] support such a concept. They compared two groups of ten hamsters; one group was housed in one cage and the others in individual cages in a clean facility. Each animal received vancomycin for 21 days and 48 h after discontinuation of the drug the animals were given a lethal dose of clindamycin. All of the animals in the conventional facility died within seven days while only two of the group in the clean facility succumbed to typhlitis.

There is good evidence dating back for over a decade that oral vancomycin is efficacious for the treatment of antibiotic-associated colitis. Hall and Kahn [26] reported the successful treatment of what was considered to be antibiotic-induced *Staphylococcus aureus* enterocolitis, but in retrospect was probably pseudomembranous colitis, with oral vancomycin. Stalons and Thornsberry [45] demonstrated by in vitro studies that vancomycin inhibits enterococci and other facultative anaerobes as well as many obligate anaeorobes such as peptostreptococci, which complete with *Clostridium difficile*. This fact may explain the failure of vancomycin to cure one case of pseudomembranous colitis reported by Keighley et al. [28] and the acute exacerbation of symptoms in one case reported by Marrie et al. [35] after discontinuing vancomycin therapy. Keighley et al. [28] in a limited controlled study where nine patients received vancomycin and seven were given placebo demonstrated the therapeutic efficacy of this drug in terms of clinical response and elimination of *Clostridium difficile*. These investigators administered vancomycin in an oral dosage of 125 mg every 6 h. Tedesco et al. [56] reported the successful treatment of nine patients with pseudomembranous colitis with oral vancomycin. All of the patients had persistent diarrhea after discontinuation of the offending antibiotic which resolved during vancomycin therapy and the stool content of clostridial toxin was rapidly reduced. Bartlett et al. [4] administered oral vancomycin in a dose of 500 mg four times a day for at least seven days to 13 patients who had 10 to 20 stools/day following discontinuation of the antibiotic which had induced the colitis. There was a prompt response to vancomycin therapy and 12 of the 13 patients had no detectable toxin in their stools by the seventh day after initiation of treatment with this drug. None of the patients had any recurrence of their illness on cessation of therapy. Such results indicate that treatment with vancomycin of antiobiotic-induced pseudomembranous colitis that persists after discontinuation of the responsible antibiotic is highly successful. To date, despite the absence of any large series of cases treated with oral vancomycin, it is the drug of choice for patients who do not promptly improve after discontinuation of the offending antmicrobial agent. In some instances parenteral vancomycin has been used and at this time there is conflicting evidence as to the efficacy of this drug when it is administered by the intravenous route. Tedesco et al. [56] reported that one of their patients who received the drug parenterally had no reduction in the amount of toxin or evidence of vancomycin in the effluent from the colostomy. Ledger and Puttler [33] reported a lethal case of pseudomembranous colitis despite parenteral vancomycin therapy. Donta et al. [17] found that their patient with antibiotic-associated colitis improved after several days of intravenous vancomycin in a dose of 500 mg every 6 h. During parenteral vancomycin therapy they found that the toxin disappeared from the stool. The diagnosis was confirmed prior to treatment with vancomycin by sigmoidoscopy and radiographic studies. Sigmoidoscopy, one week after the initiation of parenteral vancomycin therapy, revealed only an edematous mucosa which was confirmed by biopsy. These investigators indicate from in vitro studies that it is unlikely that vancomycin directly interferes with the toxin's activity. While the basis of the efficacy of vancomycin may be due to its anticlostridial activity, other mechanisms may be involved. Be that as it may, further studies are necessary before the relative efficacies of the various routes of vancomycin administration are known.

Pseudomembranous colitis is the major adverse reaction associated with clindamycin therapy. As yet no dose relationship has been established. This therapeutic complication has occurred with both the oral and parenteral forms of the drug. There is apparently a slightly increased incidence of pseudomembranous colitis in female patients. Although the incidence of antibiotic-associated pseudomembranous colitis is unknown, the antibiotics which have been predominantly implicated are clindamycin and ampicillin. Tedesco et al. [55] reported the occurrence of diarrhea in up to 20% of patients on clindamycin therapy and about 10% developed pseudomembranous col-

182

itis. Swartzberg et al. [51] reported that only 6.6% of their 1000 patients who received clindamycin developed diarrhea. They found that the incidence of this side effect was more common following oral administration the drug and was also more common in female patients. Neu et al. [36] in a study of 200 patients who received clindamycin noted that 13.5% had diarrhea and 2.5% had colitis. They found that the incidence of gastrointestinal symptoms was greater in patients who received the drug parenterally. These investigators noted that twice as many females as males had protracted diarrhea and more female patients developed gastrointestinal symptoms than did the males. Such studies indicate that clindamycin therapy is associated with an increased risk of diarrhea and colitis but similar observations probably apply to other antibiotics but they have been less extensively studied.

In addition to gastrointestinal tract side effects, clindamycin can cause cutaneous eruptions, pruritus, proctitis and vaginitis. Less commonly, abnormal liver function tests, jaundice, leukopenia and neutropenia may be encountered during clindamycin therapy. This antibiotic also potentiates the neuromuscular blockade of such agents as D-tubocurarine and succinylcholine and it is therefore important that the anesthesiologist be alerted to the fact that the patient is on clindamycin therapy if surgical treatment is required.

Clindamycin, because of its gastrointestinal side effects, is no longer used for trivial infections but it will continue to have a role in the treatment of anaerobic infections and selected cases of staphylococcal infections, specifically those occurring in patients who are allergic to penicillin.

It is in the realm of polymicrobial infections involving the *Bacteroides fragilis* group of organisms that clindamycin has its maximum clinical usage. Sutter and Finegold [50] in evaluating the in vitro susceptibility of obligate anaerobes to antimicrobial agents found that clindamycin inhibited all strains of *Bacteroides fragilis* at 8 μg/ml and that 96% of the strains were inhibited at concentrations of 4 μg/ml. They also found that 96% of isolates of other *Bacteroides* species were susceptible to this antibiotic, but some strains of *Peptococcus* and *Clostridium* species were clindamycin resistant. Sutter [49] considered that this antibiotic was still an effective antimicrobial agent against most anaerobic bacteria and despite its widespread use found no trend toward greater resistance by such organisms. This investigator noted that although resistance in strains of *Peptococcus* and *Clostridium* species exist, they were no more prevalent than when clindamycin was initially introduced into clinical medicine. Bawdon et al. [9] found considerable variation in the susceptibility patterns of clinical isolates of *Bacteroides fragilis* as regards clindamycin. Of their 92 isolates, 11 (12%) were found to have minimum inhibitory concentrations of more than 8 μg/ml and six of the isolates required 250 to 512 μg. Although the clinical significance of antibiotic resistant anaerobes has not been adequately evaluated, these investigators consider that the emergence of strains with resistance to clindamycin is clinically important. Their findings may reflect the extensive use of the antibiotic which produces conditions which are favorable for the emergence of resistance among anaerobic bacteria. Plasmid-mediated transferable resistance to this antimicrobial agent has been observed in strains of *Bacteroids fragilis* by Tally et al. [53] and such findings may be a reflection of the extensive use of clindamycin during the past decade. Privitera et al. [39] reported multiple antibiotic resistance among subspecies of *Bacteroide fragilis*. From their in vitro studies they demonstrated that resistance to clindamycin and erythromycin is transferable to sensitive strains and this observation is suggestive of an extrachromosomal location of the genetic determinants of the antibioic resistance. The recognition of plasmid-mediated antimicrobial resistance in anaerobic bacilli could compromise therapy of infections due to these pathogens. Transference of clindamycin resistance to other strains of *Bacteroides fragilis* could curtail the choice of antimicrobial agents for the treatment of serious infections due to this pathogen. Currently, the level of clindamycin resistance among clinical isolates is low but susceptibility testing of this pathogen so as to detect resistant strains is important in hospital practice.

Favorable therapeutic results have been obtained in patients receiving clindamycin for intra-abdominal and pelvic infections due to anaerobic bacteria. Ledger et al. [32] compared the therapeutic efficacy of clindamycin and chloramphenicol in 102 patients with severe pelvic sepsis. All, except one who was postmenopausal, were young women with intact host defenses and no underlying malignant disease Forty-nine received intravenous clindamycin, 600 mg every 6 h, and 53 patients 1.0 gm of chloramphenicol intravenously every 6 h. The choice of antibiotic was made by random selection and both groups of patients were similar as regards age, race and type of infection. Six of the patients in each group had a bacteremia. The isolates from blood cultures of the patients who received clindamycin were *Bacteroides fragilis*, *Bacteroides* species, *Clostridium* species and *Escherichia coli*. The investigators reported that although bacteremia was only proven in 12% of the total study group it was most commonly associated with septic abortion. Patients with infected abortions rapidly recovered after initiation of antibiotic therapy and evacuation of the retained products of conception. It is of interest that 58 of the 102 patients required some form of surgical intervention in order to obliterate the suppurative process. Although the authors state that operative treatment was unrelated to the antibiotic therapy, it does emphasize the role of surgical drainage or ablation of any nidus of infection in the treatment of serious pelvic infections. Clindamycin therapy was discontinued in seven patients because of diarrhea and in a further patient because of a rash. Pseudomembranous colitis was not encountered in any of the women who received clindamycin. The study however failed to demonstrate that clindamycin was superior to chloramphenicol for the treatment of severe anaerobic pelvic sepsis. They encountered no cases of aplastic anemia in the 53 patients who received chloramphenicol. They concluded that clindamycin was their preference for serious anaerobic pelvic sepsis in patients with no symptoms referable to the gastrointestinal tract. In patients who develop diarrhea, they consider that chloramphenicol can be substituted for clindamycin if the anaerobic infection persists.

Levison et al. [34] treated 16 patients with severe intra-abdominal and pelvic infections with this antibiotic. Two of the 16 patients had *Bacteroides fragilis* bacteremia and seven of the patients had failed to respond to parenteral therapy with other antimicrobial agents. Thirteen of the patients, however, developed further abscesses during treatment with this antibiotic. All three patients had polymicrobial infections and all responded to further therapy, one to surgical drainage alone, another to surgical drainage and ampicillin therapy, and the remaining patient to surgical drainage and further clindamycin therapy. Lack of response in serious pelvic infections associated with anaerobes shown to be sensitive in vitro to specific antibiotics is well recognized. In most instances this is due to failure to eradicate any purulent collection by surgical measures. These investigators record the fact that six of their 16 patients became afebrile within 24 h after evacuation of an abscess. Such findings are in accord with the time-honored principle that the primary therapeutic modality for patients with readily identifiable suppuration is prompt surgical drainage. Many of these infections are caused by a combination of aerobic, microaerophilic and anaerobic organisms which act synergistically to cause serious suppurative disease, especially when the tissues are devitalized by surgery or other underlying disease. In such patients antimicrobial therapy has to be intitiated prior to the availability of a definitive microbiologic diagnosis. It is common practice, in view of the polymicrobial nature of the infection, to initiate antimicrobial therapy with a combination of antibiotics. The rationale for a combination of antibiotics emanates from the fact that currently there is no antibiotic available that has an antimicrobial spectrum which encompasses all the pathogens observed in these polymicrobial infections. The combination of clindamycin with an aminoglycoside has proven to be highly efficacious in such cases.

Chow et al. [14] reported that the parenteral administration of clindamycin and gentamicin eradicated polymicrobial infections in 56 (93%) of their 60 patients. Such therapy was highly successful in 16 (84%) of their 19 patients with bacteremia. In this study surgical drainage of abscesses and extirpation of any necrotic tissue was performed when indicated. Clindamycin-associated pseudomembranous colitis was not observed in any of the patients who received this antibiotic combination regimen. Swenson and Lorber [52] reported that the intravenous administration of clindamycin in a dosage of 300 to 450 mg and gentamicin in a dosage of 1.0 to 1.65 mg/kg weight every 8 h was highly efficacious in 115 (87.8%) of 131 patients with severe intra-abdominal or pelvic sepsis. Fourteen (10.6%) of the patients developed diarrhea which was severe enough in three (2.3%) to warrant discontinuation of clindamycin therapy. Two of the latter patients developed clindamycin-induced pseudomembranous colitis which was confirmed by endoscopy and biopsy. Fass et al. [19] reported that this antimicrobial combination furnished excellent results in 29 patients with polymicrobial infections which had been unresponsive to other antimicrobial regimens. Two of their patients with intra-abdominal sepsis had failed to respond to chloramphenicol. Such reports indicate that a combination of clindamycin and gentamicin, together with surgical intervention when necessary, is effective therapy for patients with polymicrobial sepsis. The administration of clindamycin is particularly efficacious when *Bacteroides fragilis* is known to be a major pathogen. When, however, *Bacteroides fragilis* is not the predominant anaerobic pathogen, regimens such as a combination of penicillin and an aminoglycoside is preferable. As the exact role of anaerobic species in pelvic sepsis has not been determined, controversy still persists as to whether or not antibiotics with antimicrobial spectra predomiantly against anaerobic organisms are important in the therapy of such infections. Stone et al. [48] administered an aminoglycoside to 405 patients with serious surgical infections. Of 176 patients in their study who had polymicrobial infections, eleven succumbed to bacterial sepsis. They concluded that elimination of the aerobic species will result in the eventual death of the obligate anaerobic organisms in such infections. The poor blood supply in areas of suppurative necrosis that have a redox potential compatible with replication of anaerobic bacteria may be impaired so that adequate antibiotic levels are not attainable at the site of infection in such patients. The latter may not only validate the importance of surgical measures but may explain why antibiotics which are effective against *Bacteroides* species do not significantly influence the prognosis when compared with agents which are efficacious against *Enterobacteriaceae*. Gorbach and Thadepalli [24] however reported that clindamycin when used in polymicrobial infections results in prompt eradication of the anaerobic bacteria, in spite of the persistance of the aerobic and facultative Gram-negative rods against which this antibiotic is ineffectual.

Chow and Guze [13] demonstrated that in patients with serious sepsis associated with *Bacteroidaceae* bacteremia, when therapy included surgical drainage, there was a negligible difference in the mortality rates whether or not appropriate antibiotics were administered. On the other hand, if surgical drainage was not instituted the mortality rate was significantly increased in patients who received inappropriate antimicrobial therapy. The choice of an appropriate antibiotic plus surgical and supportive measures constitute optimal care and result in a diminished fatality rate in patients with serious intra-abdominal or pelvic sepsis.

Bartlett et al. [8] reported on the use of the antibiotic combination of clindamycin and gentamicin on an empiric basis to treat 107 seriously ill patients with suspected polymicrobial sepsis. They emphasize that the physician cannot delay the initiation of antimicrobial therapy in such patients until microbiologic information is available pertaining to the causative organisms. These investigators chose the combination of clindamycin and gentamicin because of the predicted activity of these agents against the dominant pathogens encountered in serious mixed aerobic – anaerobic infections.

Fifty-seven of the patients had intra-abdominal sepsis and cure was obtained in 51 (89%). Five deaths occurred from the infectious process in this group, three had septicemia and two were hypotensive when antimicrobial therapy was instituted. The bacterial isolates from the blood cultures from the patients with lethal septicemia were *Bacteroides fragilis*, *Clostridium perfringens* and *Klebsiella* species.

A further 30 patients who received this combination of antibiotics had hospital-acquired aspiration pneumonia. The diagnosis was made on the basis of such features as: radiologic evidence of an infiltrate in a dependent pulmonary segment, clinical evidence of sepsis with no extrapulmonary focus of injection or a predisposition to aspirate due to altered consciousness and pulmonary findings such as bronchospasm or atelectasis. Cultures of transtracheal aspirates were obtained from 21 of the 30 patients prior to the initiation of antimicrobial therapy. Eleven of 21 patients had aerobic and anaerobic organisms, nine had aerobes and the remaining patient had only anaerobes isolated from transtracheal aspirates. The predominant isolates were *Enterobacteriaceae*, anaerobic Gram-negative rods other than *Bacteroides fragilis*, anaerobic Gram-positive cocci and *Staphylococcus aureus*. Resolution of the clinical and radiologic features of the infection occurred in 23 of the 30 patients on this antibiotic regimen. Four patients had demonstrable improvement of their pulmonary infection at the time of their demise from such causes as myocardial infarction, cardiac arrythmia, pulmonary embolism and gastrointestinal hemorrhage. In the remaining three patients the pulmonary infection contributed to their demise. These three patients were severly debilitated and had diffuse pulmonary involvement by the infection. Death occurred within three days of treatment with clindamycin and gentamicin. The cultures from these patients yielded mixed aerobic – anaerobic flora and all isolates were found to be susceptible in vitro to one or both of the antibiotics used.

The remaining 20 patients in this report had cutaneous and soft tissue infections. Five of the patients had bacteremia and blood cultures yielded

Bacteroides fragilis from two patients and peptostreptococci, *Clostridium paraputrificum, Serratia marcescens*, respectively, were isolated from the other three individuals. Eighteen of the 20 patients responded to the antibiotic regimen. One patient who was considered to be a therapeutic failure had *Bacteroides fragilis* bacteremia and died on the initial day of antimicrobial therapy. The other patient had diabetes mellitus and severe cellulitis. The organisms isolated were *Proteus mirabilis* and *Pseudomonas aeruginosa* and, although both of these pathogens were reported to be susceptible to genta-micin, no clinical improvement was observed in the patient's infection.

In the final evaluation of the efficacy of combined therapy with clinda-mycin and gentamicin in polymicrobial infections, it should be noted that this antibiotic regimen achieved a cure in 92 (90%) of the 102 patients in this study. Although there were, in theory, ten therapeutic failures, almost all the pa-thogens were susceptible to either clindamycin or gentamicin. These inves-tigators consider that the antibiotic regimen was ineffectual in these ten patients because of the fulminant course of their infectious illness. No men-tion is made in this report of clindamycin resistant anaerobic species or gentamicin-resistant enterobacteriaceae which could have been responsible for some of the therapeutic failures.

Sharpe et al. [44] reported a patient who developed *Bacteroides fragilis* bacteremia following vaginal hysterectomy. A pure growth of *Bacteroides fragilis* was isolated from cultures of the postoperative pelvic abscess which in in vitro was found to be sensitive to clindamycin. Oral administration of this antibiotic in a dosage of 300 mg every 6 h for five days failed to prevent the development of Bacteroides bacteremia. They conducted further in vitro susceptibility studies which demonstrated that the strain of *Bacteroides fra-gilis* was sensitive to clindamycin but despite further therapy with this anti-biotic the patient's infectious illness did not resolve until treatment with metronidazole was instituted. These investigators offer no explanation for the failure of clindamycin to attain a cure in their patient. Clinical studies that report the value of different antibiotics in the treatment of intra-abdominal and pelvic sepsis have usually been difficult to accurately interpret because of the presence of uncontrollable variables in the host. The unavoidable lack of untreated controls further confuses the interpretation of the pathophysiolo-gic processes that are associated with the inception of these infections. To date, no prospective studies are available pertaining to clindamycin in such infections. For such reasons debate continues concerning which antibiotic or antimicrobial regimen should be used for optimal clinical results. Further-more, as exemplified by the case report of Sharp et al. [45] in vitro suscep-tibility studies do not always portray that a clindamycin sensitive strain of *Bacteroides fragilis* will respond to this antibiotic in the clinical setting.

Warner et al. [60] reported two cases of *Bacteroides fragilis* bacteremia which failed to respond to intensive intravenous clindamycin therapy despite in vitro sensitivity of the infecting strains of this organism to this drug. The clindamycin minimum inhibitory concentration for the strain of *Bacteroides fragilis* isolated from the blood of one patient was <0.1 μg/ml and for the other patient it was 1.6 μg/ml. Both patients promptly responded to treatment with metronidazole. Rissing et al. [43] have also reported a patient with a life treatening infection due to *Bacteroides* species which failed to respond to clindamycin as well as other antimicrobial agents but responded to treatment with metronidazole.

Postpartum endomyometritis of polymicrobic etiology is now frequently encountered in obstetric practice because of the steady increase in the Cesarean section rate. In order to circumvent this infectious complication many clinicians have used antibiotic prophylaxis. As the wound is the most common focus of infection in any surgical patient, satisfactory levels of the antimicrobial agent within the wound are necessary for prophylaxis. The concentrations achieved in the wound may play a significant role in the efficacy of the antibiotic in prophylaxis and/or treatment of wound infections. Gibbs and Weinstein [23] administered immediately prior to Cesarean section, and eight hours after delivery, clindamycin intravenously in a dose of 600 mg and gentamicin, 80 mg intramuscularly, to 54 patients. Despite this combined antibiotic prophylaxis regimen, eight (14.8%) of the patients developed postpartum endometritis. The polymicrobial nature of the infections in these patients were confirmed by transcervical aerobic and anaerobic cultures. These investigators reported an increased incidence of isolates of *Escherichia coli* and Enterococci but a decrease in *Bacteroides* species as well as both aerobic and anaerobic streptococci in the eight patients with puerperal endometritis. They failed, however, to demonstrate that clindamycin – gentamicin was superior to the prophylactic administration of ampicillin and kanamycin. DiZerga et al. [16] reported that the treatment of postpartum endomyometritis with the combination of clindamycin and gentamicin prevented progression of the infectious process. They consider that the time of initiating such therapy is critical as undue delay will not prevent serious sepsis. They are in accord with other investigators that antibiotic prophylaxis reduces postoperative febrile morbidity but does not prevent serious puerperal infections in all women who are delivered by Cesarean section. These investigators state that the early inception of therapy with clindamycin and gentamicin for postoperative endomyometritis is preferable to administering potent antibiotics to all women undergoing abdominal delivery.

Clindamycin should not be used in prophylaxis because it may be followed by serious pseudomembranous colitis. Likewise, despite its useful Gram-positive aerobic spectrum of activity, it should rarely be prescribed for infections caused by clindamycin susceptible gram-positive aerobic cocci. This antibiotic is not effective against many strains of peptococci and certain *Clostridium* species other than *Clostridium perfringens*. Most of these organisms are susceptible to penicillin G. Consequently, clindamycin in combination with penicillin G is a rational theapeutic regimen in a number of serious anaerobic pelvic infections where peptococci and *Clostridium* species may be encountered. Such a regimen does not cover the *Enterobacteriaceae* and, as a result, triple antimicrobial therapy in the form of penicillin G, clindamycin and an aminoglycoside has been found highly efficacious in such serious polymicrobial infections. Clindamycin should never be administered for simple pelvic infections if the *Bacteroides fragilis* group of organisms are not involved in the infectious process. Less potentially toxic antimicrobial agents should be used if the infection is judged to be non life-threatening. One of the features that characterize pelvic sepsis involving *Bacteroides fragilis* is the proclivity of these organisms to form abscesses. The relative ineffectiveness of antimicrobial agents in the presence of extensive suppuration and abscess formation is well recognized. In such cases polypharmacy is not a substitute for surgical drainage. Antimicrobial agents should be assigned a secondary role, namely to localize the infectious process and assist the host defense mechanisms.

In conclusion, clindamycin still remains one of the most effective antimicrobial agents for the treatment of serious or life-threatening infections associated with the *Bacteroides fragilis* group of organisms. Now that physicians are aware of the propensity of this antibiotic to induce pseudomembranous colitis the incidence of this adverse reaction has markedly decreased, mainly because the clinician has paid greater attention to antibiotic induced gastrointestinal symptoms and no longer prescribes clindamycin for trivial non life-threatening infections.

REFERENCES

1. Bartlett JG, Chang TW, Gurwith M, Gorbach SL, Onderdonk AB: Antibiotic associated pseudomembranous colitis due to toxin producing colostridia. N Engl J Med 298:531–534, 1978
2. Bartlett JG, Chang TW, Moon N, Onderdonk AB: Antibiotic-induced lethal enterocolitis in hamsters: studies with eleven agents and evidence to support the pathogenic role of toxin producing clostridia. Amer J Vet Res 39:1525–1530, 1978
3. Bartlett JG, Chang TW, Onderdonk AB: A comparison of five regimens for treatment of experimental clindamycin-associated colitis. J Infect Dis 138:81–86, 1978
4. Bartlett JG, Chang TW, Taylor NS, Onderdonk, AB: Colitis induced by *Clostridium difficile*. Rev Infect Dis 1:370–378, 1979
5. Bartlett JG, Gorbach SL: Pseudomembranous colitis (antibiotic-related colitis). In: GH Stollerman, (ed.). Advances in internal medicine. Chicago: Yearbook Medical Publishers, 1977, pp. 455–476
6. Bartlett JG, Onderdonk AB, Cisneros RL, Kasper DL: Clindamycin-associated colitis due to a toxin-producing species of *Clostridium* in hamsters. J Infect Dis 136:701–705, 1977

190

7. Bartlett JG, Onderdonk AB, Cisneros RL: Clindamycin-associated colitis in hamsters: protection with vancomycin. Gastroenterology 73:772–776, 1977
8. Bartlett JG, Miao PVW, Gorbach SL: Empiric treatment with clindamycin and gentamicin of suspected sepsis due to anaerobic and aerobic bacteria. J Infect Dis 135:s80–s85, 1977
9. Bawdon RE, Rozmiej E, Palchaudhuri S, Krakowiak J.: Variability in the susceptibility pattern of *Bacteroides fragilis* in four Detroit area hospitals. Antimicrob. Agents Chemother. 16:664–666, 1979
10. Browne RA, Fekety R, Silva J, Boyd DL, Work CO, Abrams GD: The prospective effect of vancomycin on clindamycin-induced colitis in hamsters. Johns Hopkins Med J 141:183–192, 1977
11. Burbige EJ, Milligan FD: Pseudomembranous enterocolitis associated with antibiotics and therapy with cholestyramine. JAMA 231:1157–1158, 1975
12. Chang TW, Onderdonk AB, Bartlett JG: Anion-exchange resins in antibiotic-associated colitis. Lancet 2:258–259, 1978
13. Chow AW, Guze LB: Bacteroidaceae Bacteremia: clinical experience with 112 patients. Medicine 53:93–126, 1974
14. Chow AW, Ota JK, Guze LB: Clindamycin plus gentamicin as expectant therapy for presumed mixed infections. Can Med Assoc J 115:1225–1229, 1976
15. De Haan RM, Metzler CM, Schellenberg D: Pharmacokinetic studies of clindamycin phosphate. J Clin Pharmacol. 13:190–209, 1973
16. DiZerga G, Yonekura L, Roy S, Nakamura RN, Ledger WJ: A comparison of clindamycin-gentamicin and penicillin-gentamicin in the treatment of post-Cesarean section endomyometritis. Am J Obstet Gynecol. 134:238–242, 1979
17. Donta ST, Lamps GM, Summers RW, Wilkins TD: Cephalosporin-associated colitis and *Clostridum difficile*. Arch Inter Med 140:574–576, 1980
18. Eastwood JB, Gower PE: Study of the pharmacokinetics of clindamycin in normal subjects and patients with chronic renal failure. Postgrad. Med J 50:710–712, 1974
19. Fass RJ, Ruiz DE, Gardner WG, Rotilie CA: Clindamycin and gentamicin for aerobic and anaerobic sepsis. Arch Intrn Med 137:28–38, 1977
20. Fekety R, Silva J, Toshniwal R, Allo M, Armstrong J, Browne R, Ebright J, Rifkin G: Antibiotic-associated Colitis: effects of antibiotics on *Clostridium difficile* and the disease in hamsters. Rev Infect Dis 1:386–397, 1979
21. Garrod LP, Lambert HP, O'Grady G: In: Antibiotic and chemotherapy. Edinburgh: Churchill Livingston, 1973 p. 208
21a. George RH, Symonds JM, Dimock F, Brown JD, Arabi Y, Shinagawa N, Keighley NRB, Alexander-Williams J, Burdon DW: Identification of *Clostridium difficile* as a cause of pseudomembranous colitis. Br Med J 1:695–697, 1978
22. Geraci JE, Heilman FR, Nichols DR, Wellman WE, Ross GT: Some laboratory and clinical experiences with a new antibiotic, vancomycin. Proc Staff Meetings Mayo Clin. 31:564–582, 1956
23. Gibbs RS, Weinstein AJ: Bacteriologic-effects of prophylactic antibiotics in Cesarean section. Am J Obstet Gynecol 126:226–229, 1976
24. Gorbach SL, Thadepalli H: Clindamycin in the treatment of pure and mixed anaerobic infections. Arch Intern Med 134:87–92, 1974
25. Hall IC, O'Toole E: Intestinal flora in newborn infants with description of a new pathogenic anaerobe, *Bacillus Difficile*. Amer J Dis Child 49:390–402, 1935
26. Hall MY, Kahn WH: Staphylococcal enterocolitis – treatment with oral vancomycin. Ann Intern Med 65:1–8, 1966
27. Kappas A, Shinagawa N, Arabi Y, Thompson H, Burdon DW, Dimock F, George RH Alexander-Williams J, Keighley MRB: Diagnosis of pseudomembranous colitis. Br Med J 1:675–678, 1978
28. Keighley MRB, Burdon DW, Arabi Y, Alexander-Williams J, Thompson H, Young D, Johnson M, Bentley S, George RH, Mogg GAG: Randomized controlled trial of vancomycin in pseudomembranous colitis and postoperative diarrhoea. Br Med J 2:1667–1669, 1978

29. Larson HE, Parry JV, Price AB, Davies DR, Dolby J, Tyrrell DAJ: Undescribed toxin in pseudomembranous colitis. Br Med J 1:1246–1248, 1977
30. Larson HE, Price AB: Pseudomembranous colitis presence of clostridial toxin. Lancet 2: 1312–1314, 1977
31. Larson HE, Price AB, Honour P,Borriello SP: *Clostridium difficile* and the aetiology of pseudomembranous colitis. Lancet 1:1063–1066, 1978
32. Ledger WJ, Gee CL, Lewis WP, Bobitt JR: Comparison of clindamycin and chloramphenicol in treatment of serious infections of the female genital tract. J Infect Dis 135:s30–s34, 1977
33. Ledger WJ, Puttler OL: Death from pseudomembranous colitis. Obstet Gynecol 45:609–613, 1975
34. Levison ME, Santoro , Bran JL, Ries K, Rubin W: In vitro activity and clinical efficacy of clindamycin in the treatment of infections due to anaerobic bacteria. J Infect Dis 135: s49–s53, 1977
35. Marrie TJ, Falkner TS, Bradley BWD, Hartlen MR, Comeau SA, Miller HR: Pseudomembranous colitis: isolation of two species of cytotoxin clostridia and successful treatment with vancomycin. Can Med J 119:1058–1060, 1978
36. Neu HC, Prince A, Neu CO, Garvey GJ: Incidence of diarrhea and colitis associated with clindamycin therapy. J Infect Dis 135:s120–s125, 1977
37. Novak E, Wagner JG, Lamb DJ: Local and systemic tolerance, absorption and excretion of clindamycin hydrochloride after intramuscular administration. Int J Clin, Pharmacol 33: 201–208, 1970
38. Price AB, Davies DR: Pseudomembranous colitis. J Clin Pathol 30:1–12, 1977
39. Privitera G, Dublanchet A, Sebald M: Transfer of multiple antibiotic resistance between subspecies of *Bacteroides fragilis*. J Infect Dis 139:97–101, 1979
40. Reiner L, Schlesinger MJ, Miller GM: Pseudomembranous colitis following aureomycin and chloraphenicol. Arch Pathol 54:39–67, 1952
41. Rifkin GD, Fekety R, Silva J, Browne RA, Ringler DH, Abrams GD: Antibiotic induced colitis, implication of a toxin neutralized by *Clostridium sordellii* antitoxin. Lancet 2:1103–1106, 1977
42. Rimmer DMD, Sales JEL: Lincomycin and clindamycin antibiotics. Chemother 25:204–216, 1978
43. Rissing JP, Moore WL, Newman C, Crockett JK, Buxton TB, Edmondson HT: Treatment of anaerobic infections with metronidazole. Current Ther Res 27:651–663, 1980
44. Sharp DJ, Corringham RET, Nye EB, Sagor GR, Noone P: Successful treatment of *Bacteroides* bacteremia with metronidazole after failue with clindamycin and lincomycin. J Antimicrob Chemother 3:233–237, 1977
45. Stalons DR, Thornsberry C: Broth-dilution method for determining the antibiotic susceptibility of anaerobic bacteria. Antimicrob. Agents Chemother 7:15–21, 1975
46. Stanley RJ, Melson GL, Tedesco FJ: The spectrum of radiographic findings in antibiotic-related pseudomembranous colits. Radiology 111:519–524, 1974
47. Stanley RJ, Melson GL, Tedesco FJ, Saylor JL: Plain-film findings in severe pseudomembranous colitis. Radiology 118:7–11, 1976
48. Stone HH, Kolb LD, Geheber CE, Dawkins JE: Using aminoglycosides in surgical infections. Ann Surg 183:660–666, 1976
49. Sutter VL: In vitro susceptibility of anaerobes: comparison of clindamycin and other antimicrobial agents. J Infect Dis 135:s7–s12, 1977
50. Sutter VL, Finegold SM: Susceptibility of anaerobic bacteria to 23 antimicrobial agents. Antimicrob Agents Chemother 10:736–752, 1970
51. Swartzberg JE, Maresca, RM, Remington JS: Clinical study of gastrointestinal complications associated with clindamycin therapy. J Infect Dis 135:s99–s103, 1977
52. Swenson RM, Lorber B: Clindamycin and carbenicillin in treatment of patients with intra-abdominal and female genital tract infections. J Infect Dis 135:s40–s48, 1977
53. Tally FP, Snydman DR, Gorbach SL, Malamy MH: Plasmid-mediated, transferable resistance to clindamycin and erythromycin in *Bacteroides fragilis*. J Infect Dis 139:83–88, 1979

54. Tedesco FJ: Clindamycin and colitis: a review. J Infect Dis 135:s95–s98, 1977
55. Tedesco FJ, Barton RW, Alpers DH: Clindamycin-associated colitis. A prospective study. Ann Intern Med 81:429–433, 1974
56. Tedesco FJ, Markam R, Gurwith M, Christie D, Bartlett JG: Oral vancomycin therapy of antibiotic-associated pseudomembranous colitis. Lancet 2:226–228, 1978
57. Tedesco FJ, Stanley RJ, Alpers DH: Diagnostic features of clindamycin-associated pseudo-membranous colitis. N Engl J Med 290:841–843, 1974
58. Totten MA, Gregg JA, Freemont-Smith P, Legg M: Clinical and pathological spectrum of antibiotic-associated colitis. Am J Gastroenterol 69:311–319, 1978
59. Wagner JG, Northam JI, Sokoloski WT: Biological half-lives of the antibiotic lincomycin observed in repetitive experimets in the same subjects. Natura 207:201–202, 1965
60. Warner JF, Perkins RL, Cordero L: Metronidazole therapy of anaerobic bacteremia, meningitis and brain abscess. Arch Intern Med 138:167–169, 1979

METRONIDAZOLE

Metronidazole is a nitroheterocyclic compound (Fig. 1) and the first of the nitroimidazole derivatives to be introduced into clinical practice. It has been extensively used for the treatment of vaginal trichomoniasis as well as infections due to *Giardia lambia* and *Entamoeba histolytica*. Since the chance observation of Shinn [44] that it was efficacious in the treatment of Vincent's stomatitis, it has become the drug of choice for fuso-spirochetal infections. Subsequent studies have shown that metronidazole has a bactericidal effect on anaerobic organisms but faculatative anaerobes are resistant to it. This

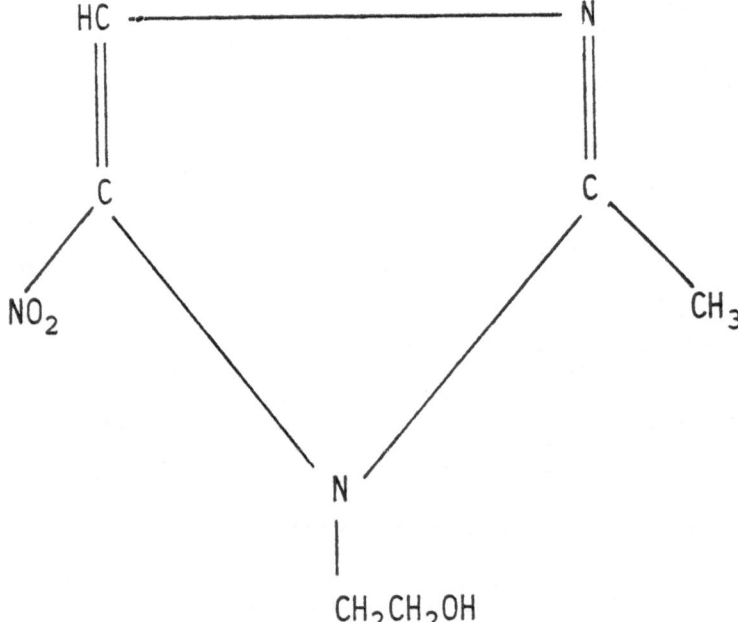

Fig. 1. Chemical structure of metronidazole.

compound is much less active against microaerophilic streptococci and such anaerobic Gram-positive bacilli as *Propionibacterium* species. Although in vitro studies have shown that metronidazole is bactericidal to obligate anaerobes, Chow et al. [7] reported activity against some microaerophilic bacteria such as *Campylobacter fetus* which is a well recognized cause of epidemic infectious enteritis and *Gardnerella vaginalis* which is believed by many to be the causative agent of nonspecific vaginitis. Metronidazole is, however, not active in vitro against most microaerophilic and aerobic bacteria, even at concentrations of up to 100 μg/ml.

To date, metronidazole is the only available antimicrobial agent that has selective anaerobic microbicidal properties. Other nitroimidazole derivatives such as tinidazole have been shown by Wise et al. [57] to have a similar antimicrobial spectrum of activity. From in vitro studies these investigators concluded that tinidazole was twice as active as metronidazole against *Bacteroides fragilis*.

The mode of action of metronidazole remains to be delineated. Ings et al. [24] postulated that the trichomonicidal properties of this compound was due to its reduction to a reactive intermediate in the cell which reacts with the dexoyribonucleic acid (DNA) of the cell to form a DNA complex which fails to function as an effective primer for DNA and RNA polymerases. As a result, nucleic acid and protein synthesis ceases and cell death occurs. Lindmark and Muller [31] have shown that the reduction of the nitro group at the 5-position on the imidazole ring is responsible for the antimicrobial activity of metronidazole. As the spectrum of activity of this compound is limited to those organisms whose metabolism is anaerobic it appears that the drug or its metabolites affect a biochemical reaction which is unique to anaerobes. Edwards [11] is in accord with the view that the microbicidal properties of metronidazole is due a reduction product or products which as yet have not been isolated or characterized because of their inherent instability. He considers that metronidazole is selectively active against anaerobic organisms because only anaerobes have electron transfer proteins of low enough redox potential to reduce the nitro group of the compound. The reduction product in turn binds to DNA resulting in strand brakage, disintergration of helix formation and degradation of the macromolecule. Such effects result in disruption of DNA replication and transcription and cell death.

Much speculation has been engendered as to the safety of metronidazole because reports have indicated that this drug may have both mutagenic and carcinogenic properties. Rosenkrantz and Speck [41] reported that both the parent compound and its metabolites are mutagenic in bacteria. Metronidazole is not, however, mutagenic under conditions where it is not reduced. As mammalian cells are incapable of reducing the drug, it is highly likely that the mutagenicity data pertaining to bacteria does not apply tO the therapeutic use of this drug in humans. Rusting and Shubik [42] reported an increased incidence of lung tumors in male and female Swiss mice as well as malignant lymphoma in mice which had been given prolonged high doses of the drug in their diet. The dosage administered to these animals was about 500 times that required for the treatment of vaginal trichomoniasis. Roe [40] considers that since both types of neoplasia commonly occur in these specific laboratory animals, the increased incidences reported could be achieved by simple manipulation of their diet over an extended period of time. This investigator found that carcinogenicity studies in hamsters failed to demonstrate that metronidazole had carcinogenic properties. Brodgen et al. [4] in a retrospective study of 767 women who received this compound on at least one occasion for the treatment of vaginal trichomoniasis failed to document an increased incidence of genital tract carcinoma. The age of the patients who received the drug in a total dosage of 7.5 g over a ten day period ranged from 10 to 81 yr. The follow-up studies represented a total period of 7442 patient yr. During this time, 13 patients developed carcinoma in situ and 23 developed invasive carcinoma of the cervix. The authors point out that the incidence of invasive malignant disease following metronidazole therapy was in accord with the expected incidence computed by the Connecticut Tumor Registry and the Third National Cancer Survey, Minneapolis, for the age-specific rates for cervical cancer. The only malignancy found at a statistically significant higher rate than expected was lung cancer. Four cases of lung cancer were recorded, three in women over the age of sixty years. The authors considered that the four cases of lung cancer could have been the result of heavy smoking. Beard et al. [2] in a similar retrospective study observed no appreciable incidence of malignant disease following metronidazole therapy for vaginal trichomoniasis. Despite these reassuring reports the cancer risk from metronidazole in humans will not be evaluated until the data are divided according to different exposure periods 20 yr after therapy. Beard et al. [2], because of the small number of gravid patients who were treated with this drug in the first trimester of pregnancy, were unable to confirm or deny the suggestion that metronidazole may have teratogenic properties. In their study, 23 women had received metronidazole in the first trimester, three of the pregnancies ended in spontaneous abortion and of the 20 births, five were associated with congenital anomalies. Two of the progeny had a hydrocele, one had congenital dislocation of the hip, one had unilateral metatarsus varus and one was mentally retarded. The child who was mentally retarded was born to mentally retarded parents. Dunn et al. [10], in a discussion of the Fetal Alcohol Syndrome, state that drugs such as disulfiram which inhibit aldehyde dehyrogenase should not be used in pregnancy. As metronidazole has a similar action to disulfiram, they feel that although they are unaware of any cases of the Fetal Alcohol Syndrome in association with metronidazole the drug should be avoided during pregnancy, or if used, the patient should be given strict instructions to avoid alcohol. The reports that metronidazole is a mutagenic and carcinogenic agent should be put into perspective as the clinical relevance of the microbiologic and animal studies has not been determined. The marked benefit of this anaerobic bactericidal agent in severe clinical infections has been adequately demonstrated and the benefit-risk ratio is at present highly in favor of its continued use in serious anaerobic infections.

Experience of the past 20 yr has shown that the toxicity of metronidazole is low. Occasional side effects noted when it is used for the treatment of vaginal trichomoniasis include nausea, anorexia, vomiting, an unpleasant taste in the mouth, lethargy and, on rare occasions, vertigo. Despite the marked effect that this compound can have on the anaerobic ecosystem of the colon, diarrhea is rarely a side effect and as yet only one case of metronidazole related enterocolitis has been reported. Willson [56] has reported reversible granulocytopenia in some patients but there have been no reports of any serious blood dyscrasia. Ingham et al. [20] reported the development of a sensory peripheral neuropathy in a patient with impaired renal function after prolonged therapy of an intracranial abscess. All signs and symptoms disappeared on cessation of therapy. There is no evidence to indicate that this drug is nephrotoxic and only after prolonged therapy in the presence of renal disease is there any evidence that the drug can accumulate in the body. Sprott and Ingham [45] state that after ingestion, about one-third of the drug is metabolized in the liver and excreted in the urine. No hepatotoxicity has been reported.

Before reviewing the role of metronidazole in the treatment and prevention of anaerobic infections, some comment is necessary pertaining to its use in patients with vaginal trichomoniasis and *Gardnerella vaginalis* infections.

TRICHOMONAL VAGINITIS

Metronidazole seems to have maintained its efficacy in the treatment of vaginal trichomoniasis although clinical failures using standard doses have been reported. In most cases, failure to eradicate the protozoon can be ascribed to poor absorption of the drug, inactivation of metronidazole by vaginal flora, failure to treat the sexual partner or lack of compliance by the patient. Poor absorption of the drug following oral administration is rarely a cause of treatment failure. This compound is usually readily absorbed from the gastrointestinal tract and Melander et al. [33] showed that its bioavailability is not significantly altered by the ingestion of food. These investigators failed to observe any significant variation in peak serum levels when the drug was administered during a fasting state or after a meal.

McFadzean et al. [32] reported that several organisms commonly found in the vagina, such as *Escherichia coli, Streptococcus faecalis, Klebsiella, Proteus* and *Mimae* are able to inactivate metronidazole. This metronidazole inactivation effect is rare but it may be responsible for a few therapeutic failures. This effect is apparently due to the absorption of the drug by metronidazole-insensitive organisms in the vagina. As these organisms are able to reduce the compound, their viability is not affected but the drug concentration in the vagina is reduced below that which is required to kill the protozoon.

Thurner and Meingassner [52] have suggested that metronidazole resistant clinical strains of *Trichomonas vaginalis* do occur. DeCarneri et al. [8] and DeCarneri and Gionnane [9] were able by in vitro and in vivo experiments to induce metronidazole resistance in some strains of *Trichomonas vaginalis*. These investigators found that after passage of the protozoon on media containing increasing concentrations of metronidazole, the minimum trichomonicidal concentration of the drug for the original strain had increased almost four-fold. In five strains of *Trichomonas vaginalis* injected into a mouse treated with suboptimal doses of metronidazole and then enriched in culture in drug free media and subjected to 20 of these alternated passages, the in vivo resistance was increased by about ten-fold.

The sexual partners of patients with vaginal trichomoniases, although usually asymptomatic, should be treated as high reinfection rates have been observed in women whose sexual partners remain untreated.

The failure rate is influenced by the type of patient and whether they in fact swallow all the tablets as prescribed. Various dosage schedules have been used but the most common course of treatment until recently was one 250 mg tablet by mouth, three times a day for seven to ten days. This regimen results in a clinical cure in about 90% of patients. Such multiple dosage regimens depend on patient compliance and one method of overcoming the discrepance between treatment prescribed and that actually taken is to give a single 2 g dose of metronidazole. Morton [34] demonstrated that the single dose regimen was highly efficacious for the treatment of trichomoniasis in women and their sexual partners. Fleury et al. [13] administered a single 2 g dose of metronidazole to 243 women with symptomatic vaginal trichomoniasis. These investigators re-evaluated 203 of the patients seven to ten days following drug administration and noted that 13 were still infected by the protozoon. Three of the treatment failures were considered to have been reinfected because of multiple exposure to untreated sexual partners but they did respond to a second single dose of metronidazole. These investigators did not evaluate the sexual partners and relied on the presence of the protozoon in wet smears to substantiate their clinical diagnosis of trichomonal vaginitis. Their results indicate that 193 (95%) of the 203 women who attended for follow-up studies were cured. The relatively innocuous nature of a two gram single dose regimen deserves acceptance as the physician can ensure the drug is taken by the patient, an assurance that is not possible with prolonged multiple dose therapy. Patients should be warned of the possibility of nausea and cautioned to avoid all alcohol in the subsequent 24 h because of the disulfiram-effect of metronidazole. Sexual intercourse should be prohibited after treatment until tests of cure have been performed to establish that the patient is free of the parasite. Patients should be followed for three months and repeated tests carried out to confirm that the parasite has been eradicated.

Treatment of the gravid patient with metronidazole during the first trimester is best avoided, as the potential effects of the drug on organogenesis have not been defined. In view of the very high serum levels involved with the large single dose form of therapy, it would seem unwise at the present time to use this regimen during pregnancy. If, however, the gestation is more than 16 weeks duration and other measures have been ineffectual and the patient has a profuse, frothy vaginal discharge and swelling and soreness of the vulva due to vaginal trichomoniasis, a seven day course of metronidazole, 250 mg three times a day, should be prescribed. Concomitant infections are, however, not infrequent and demand evaluation and appropriate therapy. Metronidazole has no effect on gonococcal or candidal infections of the lower genital tract, therefore, it is important that all patients complaining of a vaginal discharge have proper microbiologic studies before initiating therapy. Metronidazole is not a cure-all for all vaginal infections and the empiric use of this drug is to be deprecated. Vaginal trichomoniasis and gonorrhea frequently occur together in the same patient and the symptoms may be entirely due to the protozoal infection. If empiric therapy with metronidazole is prescribed, the trichomonal vaginitis will be cured but the gonococcal infection will remain quiescent until complications such as salpingitis develop or until the sexual partner is reinfected with the diplococcus. Acceptable standards of medical diagnosis require a careful history, clinical evaluation and laboratory investigations. Such standards must also be vigorously followed in women with suspected vaginal trichomoniasis if the correct treatment is to be prescribed.

GARDNERELLA VAGINALIS VAGINITIS

The term 'nonspecific vaginitis' has been applied to vulvovaginitis when no evidence of gonococcal, fungal or trichomonal infection, or an allergic cause is discernible. Most cases of nonspecific vaginitis present with a grayish-white, homogenous malodorous vaginal discharge which has a pH between 5.0 and 5.5. The onset of symptoms is unrelated to the menstual cycle and only in about 50% of the patients is pruritus vulvae a symptom of this clinical entity.

Gardner and Dukes [15] isolated a small Gram-negative coccobacillus which they termed *Haemophilus vaginalis* from patients with nonspecific vaginitis. Although the taxonomy of this organism is still a subject of debate, it is now currently referred to as *Gardnerella vaginalis*. Gardner and Dukes [15] reported the isolation of this organism from 123 (93%) of 138 women with profuse leukorrhea but not from vaginal cultures of 78 women who had no symptoms of lower genital tract infection. They found that when samples of vaginal secretions of women colonized with *Gardnerella vaginalis* were instilled in the vaginas of 15 women with no gynecologic symptoms, eleven (73%) developed a diffuse grayish-white homogeneous leukorrhea. On examination of wet mount preparations of vaginal aspirates from women with nonspecific vaginitis, these investigators noted epithelial cells stippled with bacteria which they termed 'clue cells' as well as an almost complete absence of polymorphonuclear leukocytes. Gram-stain of the vaginal discharge revealed not only the presence of the pleomorphic Gram-negative coccobacillus, but a scant number of lactobacilli. Gardner and Kaufman [16] consider that the presence of 'clue cells' in a wet mount preparation is all that is necessary to formulate a diagnosis of *Gardnerella vaginalis* vaginitis. Josey et al. [26] reported that wet mount preparations of vaginal secretions lack specificity and diagnostic accuracy.

Despite the controversy that has eeisted pertaining to the pathogenicity of *Gardnerella vaginalis*, recent studies have confirmed the association of this organism with nonspecific vaginitis. Pheifer et al. [39] conducted a prospective case-control study of the vaginal flora in order to define the causative agent of nonspecific vaginitis. They found that the presence of 'clue cells' in vaginal secretions and a 'fishy' amine-like odor released on mixing the secretions with a 10% solution of potassium hydroxide were commonly associated with this form of vaginitis. In their study they matched 18 patients for age, race, marital status and total number of sexual partners who were considered to have nonspecific vaginitis with 18 women with no evidence of vaginitis. *Gardnerella vaginalis* was isolated from 17 (94%) of the 18 women with clinical evidence of nonspecific vaginitis as compared to only one of the controls. They found that in patients with nonspecific vaginitis semi-quantitative anaerobic cultures yielded higher concentrations of anaerobic bacteria. Although they acknowledge that asymptomatic women may be colonized with *Gardnerella vaginalis*, they consider that many such women have clinical evidence of nonspecific vaginitis. In their report, the investigators confirm the sexual transmissibility of the infection. They found positive isolates of the organism from 27 (79%) of 34 male sexual partners of women with nonspecific vaginitis. In addition, they demonstrated that recurrent vaginal infections correlated with sexual re-exposure.

Balsdon et al. [1] from a study of 30 nongravid patients with nonspecific vaginitis concluded from their clinical, microscopic and culture findings that *Gardnerella vaginalis* may have a pathogenic role. In their Department of Genitourinary Medicine, a diagnosis of *Gardnerella vaginalis* vaginitis was made in 422 patients during a period of nine months. They reported that this form of vaginitis was almost as common as vulvovaginal candidiasis and more than three times as common as vaginal trichomoniasis. These investigators found that *Gardnerella vaginalis* vaginitis accounts for more than 90% of cases of nonspecific vaginitis.

The treatment of nonspecific vaginitis has long been unsatisfactory. This emanates from the fact that there are no universally accepted diagnostic criteria and antimicrobial agents such as ampicillin, tetracyclines and sulfonamides are often ineffectual. Pheifer et al. [39] reported that all patients in their study who used a triple sulfonamide vaginal had a recurrence of their symptoms within two weeks of cessation of such therapy. They found that although ampicillin is highly active in vitro against *Gardnerella vaginalis*, two-thirds of their patients who had positive vaginal cultures had persistent colonization by the organism during ampicillin therapy. Likewise, they found that doxycycline is of low efficacy for the treatment of this infection. They found that metronidazole in a dosage of 500 mg twice daily for seven days was the most efficacious form of therapy. All 81 women in their study who received mentronidazole had negative cultures and all except one had no leukorrhea on completion of the prescribed course of treatment. They emphasized that it is futile to treat the sexually active woman without treating her partner. These investigators state that the efficacy of metronidazole therapy is in accord with the concept that synergy between anaerobic organisms and *Gardnerella vaginalis* plays an important role in the etiology of nonspecific vaginitis. Balsdon et al. [1] conducted a double-blind randomized controlled trial of metronidazole and placebo therapy. Twenty-two patients received a seven day course of metronidazole in a daily dosage of 800 mg. Of the 17 patients who attended for follow-up four weeks after completion of the course of metronidazole, 15 women showed both clinical and bacteriologic cure, one was clinically cured but had a positive vaginal culture for *Gardnerella vaginalis* and the remaining patient who was clinically and bacteriologically cured ten days after therapy had a recurrence of her vaginitis. These results confirm that metronidazole is effective in curing this common form of vaginitis, but the investigators found difficulty in reconciling the efficacy of the drug with the relative in vitro insensitivity of *Gardnerella vaginalis*. They postulated that either the laboratory studies may not reflect that which pertains in vitro or that the drug may accumulate in the vagina to attain concentrations that are effective against the organism. The mechanism of action of metronidazole in the treatment of *Gardnerella vaginalis* vaginitis remains to be defined, but at present it appears to be the preferred drug for a troublesome complaint of many women.

PROHPHYLAXIS AND TREATMENT OF ANAEROBIC INFECTIONS

The availability of effective antimicrobial agents fostered hopes that wound infection could be banished from our midst. The results of early studies of antimicrobial prophylaxis in surgical procedures were generally disappointing. Carefully controlled prospective studies such as those of Ledger et al. [30] have conclusively shown that a short course of an antimicrobial agent selected for its efficacy against anticipated bacterial contaminants administered prior to the operative procedure can augment meticulous surgical technique in reducing the incidence of wound infection. The objective of antimicrobial prophylaxis is to reduce the number of bacterial species that may act synergistically to produce postoperative morbidity. The use of chemoprophylaxis for vaginal hysterectomy in premenopausal women has been advocated because of the high postoperative infection rate. The optimal drug and dosage schedule for prophylaxis remains to be determined.

Until recently prophylatic antimicrobial regimens have been directed almost exclusively against aerobic Gram-negative bacilli. Metronidazole prophylaxis has been shown to be highly efficacious in preventing postoperative sepsis caused not only by the metronidazole sensitive anaerobes, but also by aerobic Gram-negative bacilli which are resistant to this drug. Ingham et al. [21] have shown that some obligate anaerobes inhibit phagocytosis of aerobic bacteria in vitro and this phenomenon may be the clue to the extraordinary success of metronidazole prophylaxis in preventing postoperative sepsis. Another explanation for the efficacy of metronidazole in the prevention of postoperative sepsis is that anaerobic organisms convert the drug to active metabolites which are active against other microbes. Onderdonk et al. [37] demonstrated in an animal model that metronidazole prevented coliform bacteremia although they failed to demonstrate in vitro activity of this drug against *Escherichia coli*. From their data they concluded that metronidazole activity against *Escherichia coli* required the presence of *Baceroides fragilis* or similar anaerobic organisms. Ingham et al. [22] have shown that under anaerobic conditions metronidazole is active against *Escherichia coli*. They found that when *Escherichia coli* was incubated under anaerobic conditions in the supernatant of Robertson's cooked meat medium in the presence of metronidazole in a concentration of 10 mg/l, the viable count increased in the initial 6 h only to be followed by a thousand-fold decrease in the subsequent 18 hours. This effect of metronidazole on *Escherichia coli* was neither enhanced or reduced by the presence of *Bacteroides fragilis*. These investigators state that such studies furnish a better understanding of the fundamental aspects of the pathogenesis of infections but caution against correlating their in vitro findings to the use of metronidazole in the prevention or treatment of human infections.

The trauma of gynecologic operative procedures and the resultant devitalized tissues provide conditions which are favorable to the development of postoperative infections. Anaerobes have been implicated in the pathogenesis of these infections and it has been shown that the prophylactic administration of metronidazole decrases the incidence of such infections. The Study Group [46] reported their findings in 202 gynecologic surgical procedures where the patients received either placebo oral metronidazole. This prospective study involved all patients admitted for elective hysterectomy provided that they had no evidence of existing infection and no recent history of metronidazole or other antimicrobial therapy. The grup of patients who received oral metronidazole were given 2.0 g of the drug at the time of hospital admission and 200 mg three times a day when oral administration of the compound was feasible until the seventh postoperative day. In this study a total of 152 patients underwent hysterectomy and were evaluated for anaerobic infection during the subsequent 14 days. Bacteriologically, confirmed clinical infections due to obligate anaerobes occurred in 18 (23%) of the 78 patients who received placebo compared with one delayed infection in the 73 individuals who received metronidazole. Nine patients in the placebo group who developed pelvic infections due to non-clostridial anaerobes were successfully treated with oral metronidazole. The study indicated that the risk of infection following vaginal hysterectomy is higher than that associated with the abdominal operation. Although there were only seven patients in the placebo group who underwent vaginal hysterectomy, three developed postoperative infections. Seligman [43], in a review of this study, noted that in those patients with bacteriologically proven anaerobic infections, the septic process was almost always polymicrobial and in one-third facultative anaerobes such as *Escherichia coli* were isolated. He states that if anaerobes had Not been looked for, or isolated, the investigators would have grown pure cultures of facultative organisms which would have then been incriminated as the cause of the postoperative infections. This investigator reported that because of the good results obtained with metronidazole prophylaxis, the trial was discontinued because it was considered unethical to withhold such prophylaxis from patients who required a hysterectomy. It was then decided to ascertain the minimal effective course of metronidazole that would provide a bactericidal serum drug level at the time of the surgical procedure. Fifty patients received a single 2.0 g dose of metronidazole 12 h before operation and their postoperative course was compared with 50 patients who received the original metronidazole prophylaxis regimen. No case of bacteriologically proven infection of the abdominal wound or pelvic tissues was observed. When the two groups were compared as regards post-operative pyrexia as defined by a temperature in excess of 37.2° C, it was noted that 23 of the patients on the prolonged course remained afebrile as compared to only eight of the patients on the single dosage regimen. In 11 of the patients who had a single dose of metronidazole, the febrile morbidity was prolonged while the pyrexia did not persist for more than three days in any patient who had a seven day course of the drug. In view of these findings, a study was conducted to ascertain whether the administration of an oral dose of 2.0 g of the drug prior to surgery followed by 2.0 g at eight hourly intervals for the first 24 h following operation prevented postoperative infections. The postoperative drug prophylaxis was administered in the form of suppositories. This dosage regimen was more efficacious than the single preoperative dose prophylaxis but inferior to the extended course. A further trial was instituted which extended the post-operative period of drug administration to 48 h. During this time period suppositories were replaced by oral administration of the drug as soon as feeding of the patients was established. Seligman [43] reported that this prophylaxis regimen was highl efficacious in the prevention of postoperative sepsis. He indicated that in subsequent studies they have reduced the pre-operative dose of metronidazole to 1.2 g and found that this dosage attains a bactericidal level at the time of surgery in all patients. Willis [55] reported that therapeutic serum levels of metronidazole can be achieved by the rectal administration of the drug. He found that 1 h after administering 1.0 g of metronidazole in the form of a rectal suppository the mean serum level was 2.3 μg/ml. Peak serum levels occurred 4 h after rectal administration of the drug when the mean serum level was 10.5 μg/ml.

Despite the increased clinical use of metronidazole prophylaxis in gyne-cology, there is no evidence to indicate that short-term use of the drug leads to the emergence of resistant organisms. This does not mean to say that the continued use of metronidazole prophylaxis in gynecologic surgery will not lead to metronidazole resistant anaerobic organisms. Ever since the begin-ning of the antimicrobial era, the emergence of variants of infectious micro-organisms which are no longer susceptible to antimicrobial agents have been encountered. There are no simple or immediate solutions to this problem. In order to have any impact on prevention of human infections by antimicrobial resistant bacteria it is essential that clinicians, epidemiologists, microbiol-ogists and hospital administrators institute surveillance policies in respect to antimicrobial susceptibility of the pathogens in their respective areas of responsibility and define which drugs are being over-prescribed. Prophylactic use of an antimicrobial agent should only be prescribed when there is a known increased risk of postoperative sepsis but chemotherapeutic prophylaxis is not necessary in all patients requiring gynecologic surgery. The major indication for such measures is the premenopausal patient admitted for vaginal hysterectomy. Ohm and Galask [35] in a review of the records of 230 patients who underwent vaginal hysterectomy found that 52.3% had postoperative infections. As a result of these findings they conducted a prospective double-blind study using either a cephalosporin or placebo as prophylaxis in women admitted for vaginal hysterectomy. Endocervical cultures were obtained before the administration of the drug or placebo and the isolates compared with those from cultures obtained from the vaginal apex on the fifth postoperative day. Patients were classified as having postoperative morbidity if a temperature of 38° C or more was recorded on two successive occasions, 6 h apart after the initial 24 h or if there was clinical evidence of sepsis. All patients had an iodophore vaginal douche and perineal preparation on the night before surgery. The patients received the antimicrobial agent or placebo by intramuscular injection the night before surgery, on call to the operating room and, following the operative procedure at eight hourly intervals until oral administration at the same time interval was feasible. All patients received drug or placebo for the first five postoperative days. A total of 25 patients received the antimicrobial agent and 23 received the placebo. Eleven (48%) of the placebo group had postoperative morbidity while no patient who received the prescribed course of the antimicrobial agent had any evidence of sepsis. Five patients of the placebo group (21.7%) developed vaginal cuff infections which were confirmed by culture. One patient who received the antimicrobial agent was readmitted to hospital on account of a pelvic abscess, while three of the placebo group were readmitted because of pelvic cellulitis. Such studies imply that antimicrobial prophylaxis does not predispose patients to delayed onset postoperative sepsis. In a further communication which is a sequel to the previous report, Ohm and Galask [36] found that 72% of the patients who received the antimicrobial agent had six or more bacterial isolates in the preoperative endocervical culture, but only 12.5% had a similar number of isolates from postoperative vaginal cultures. Similar cultures from the patients who received the placebo revealed that 52% had six or more isolates prior to surgery and 50% had a similar number on the fifth postoperative day. They noted in both groups of patients in the postoperative cultures a trend towards an increased number of isolates of aerobic Gram-negative rods and *Bacteroides fragilis*, but a decrease in aerobic Gram-positive rods and *Staphylococcus epidermidis*. These investigators commented on the marked disparity between the number of isolates of aerobic Gram-negative rods from the postoperative cultures of the patients who received the cephalosporin compared to those who received the placebo. The most frequently isolated organism isolated from both groups of patients was *Escherichia coli*, although *Pseudomonas aeruginosa* and *Enterobacter* species which are cephalosporin-resistant Gramnegative rods, were isolated from the patients who received the antibiotic. Although they found *Bacteroides fragilis* in the postoperative cultures in both groups of patients, *Bacteroides* species were most frequently isolated from the placebo treated patients. These observations emphasize the necessity to identify and test for antimicrobial sensitivity organisms isolated from patients with postoperative infections.

The author, in a prospective Study of 25 perimenopausal patients who had received broad spectrum antibiotics, such as ampicillin for urinary tract or respiratory infections, within six weeks of hospital admission for vaginal hysterectomy, found that 16 developed postoperative pelvic sepsis. No patient received perioperative antimicrobial prophylaxis. This study was undertaken because of the possibility that recent antimicrobial therapy could alter the vaginal and cervical microflora and predispose such patients to an increased susceptibility to postoperative sepsis. Nine of the 16 patients developed low-grade pyrexia, pelvic pressure and painful defecation due to a vaginal cuff abscess between the fifth and seventh postoperative day. All nine of the vaginal cuff abscesses resolved after adequate drainage, hot vaginal douches with an iodophore solution and metronidazole in an oral dosage of 500 mg every 8 h for seven days. At the time of surgical drainage, aerobic and anaerobic cultures were obtained. Ampicillin resistant strains of *Escherichia coli* were isolated from six of the patients. Other aerobic organisms isolated were *Staphylococcus epidermidis*, diphtheroids and *Lactobacillus* species. Anaerobic Gram-negative bacilli were isolated from seven of the patients and anaerobic Gram-positive cocci from the remaining cultures. *Bacteroides fragilis* and *Bacteroides melaninogenicus* were isolated from five patients and *Bacteroides bivius* from the other two patients who had isolates of anaerobic Gram-negative bacilli. Low grade pyrexia developed in a further five patients. All of these patients had pelvic cellulitis but no clinical evidence of an associated vaginal cuff abscess. These patients rapidly became afebrile and symptom free on metronidazole therapy. Two patients who had an uneventful postoperative course were readmitted to hospital three weeks after the operative procedure. Both patients had an intermittent high fever, a palpable adnexal mass and evidence of peritoneal irritation. A diagnosis of tubo-ovarian abscess was substantiated in both patients at the time of laparotomy. Following surgical ablation of the tubo-ovarian abscess together with the contralateral tube and ovary and metronidazole therapy, both patients had an uneventful postoperative course. These observations suggest that the administration of antibiotics within six weeks of the operative procedure may selectively favor an antibiotic-resistant pathogenic organism such as *Escherichia coli*. Such a possibility emphasizes the necessity of identifying and testing for antimicrobial susceptibility any pathogen isolated from patients with postoperative infections. Because of the fact that 16 of the 25 patients

(64%) developed postoperative sepsis, the author is of the opinion that no patient who has received antimicrobial therapy within six weeks of hospital admission should have a vaginal hysterectomy unless preoperative cultures are obtained and adequate perioperative chemoprophylaxis instituted. Preliminary results indicate that combined chemoprophylaxis with a short perioperative course of a cephalosporin together with oral metronidazole in a dosage of 500 mg every 6 h for two days prior to surgery and for the second, third and fourth postoperative days is highly effective in the prevention of serious postoperative sepsis.

Antimicrobial prophylaxis has no role in normal obstetrics. Likewise it is of no value in the prevention of fetal infection in the presence of chorioamnionitis, as the fetal kinetics are such that adequate drug levels cannot be attained in the fetal lungs for the prevention of congenital pneumonia. Recently, much interest has been generated in the use of antimicrobial prophylaxis for Cesarean section. Sweet and Ledger [49] in their study of puerperal morbidity found that the incidence of endometritis following abdominal delivery was seven-fold that following vaginal delivery. Ledger et al. [29] reported that puerperal bacteremia was ten times as common following Cesarean section compared to delivery per via naturalis. Such studies clearly indicate that this operative procedure is associated with an increased risk of postpartum morbidity. Furthermore, studies such as those of Gibbs et al. [17] have clearly demonstrated that anaerobic organisms can be isolated from endometrial cultures from women with serious pelvic infections following abdominal delivery and that there is a positive correlation between the presence of *Bacteroides fragilis* and the severity of the infection. In view of such observations it is not surprising to note that metronidazole prophylaxis has been used in operative obstetrics. A report by a Study Group [41] analyzed the puerperal morbidity of a double-blind trial where 139 patients received either metronidazole or placebo at the time of induction of labor and for the first seven days of the puerperium. Among the 73 patients who received metronidazole, nine required Cesarean section but in no instance was puerperal infection recorded. Bacteriologically confirmed clinical infection developed in three (4.5%) of the 66 patients who received placebo. All three patients in this latter group were delivered by Cesarean section. Two had abdominal wound infections due to aerobic organisms (*Staphylococcus aureus* and *Escherichia coli*) and one had an anaerobic pelvic infection due to *Bacteroides fragilis*. In the same study six patients admitted for elective Cesarean section received prophylactic metronidazole and four received placebo. One of the patients who received placebo developed a peptostreptococcal wound infection but no postoperative sepsis was noted in the patients who received metronidazole. The dosage of metronidazole prescribed for the 73 patients who were admitted for induction of labor was 1000 mg in a rectal suppository at the time of artificial rupture of the membranes. This was repeated every eight hours until delivery when an oral dose of 200 mg three times a day was administered for seven days. Patients admitted for elective Cesarean section received an oral dose of 1000 mg 18 h before surgery and 200 mg every 8 h for seven days. Maternal and cord blood levels of metronidazole were determined in 56 of the patients. The maternal blood levels ranged from 0.1 to 36.7 μg/ml with a mean of 11.1 μg/ml. Although no data is furnished in respect of the pharmacokinetics of the drug, it is apparent that metronidazole readily traverses the placenta. In 17 patients breast milk levels were determined on the sixth day of the puerperium and the mean concentration of metronidazole was 4.7 μg/ml. Such findings make it mandatory that all infants exposed to the drug in utero and in breast milk be followed up for at least 15 yr in view of the animal data pertaining to the tumorigenic effect of metronidazole. Willis [55] reported that in a larger group of patients delivered by Cesarean section, the incidence of anaerobic postoperative sepsis was about 20% in women who did not receive metronidazole prophylaxis. No side effects from metronidazole prophylaxis have been noted in either the mothers or ther progeny, but no long term follow-up studies on the infants is incorporated in these reports.

The potential role of this drug in the treatment of anaerobic infections was delineated in the studies of Tally et al. [51], who found that 51 of 54 strains jof various anaerobic organisms were inhibited in vitro by 6.25 μg of metronidazole/ml. In their report they included preliminary clinical studies attesting to the efficacy of this anaerobic microbicidal drug in the treatment of serious bacteroides infections. Tally et al. [50] reported that adequate bactericidal levels are readily achieved in serum and at the sites of infection following oral administration. Eykyn and Phillips [12] in a report of 50 patients with severe anaerobic sepsis treated with metronidazole state that it is often difficult to assess the clinical response in such patients because the essential modality of therapy in severe abdominal and pelvic sepsis is surgical drainage of any abscess. They reported that ten (20%) of the patients failed to respond to metronidazole therapy. Severe underlying disease accounted for nine of the therapeutic failures and in the other patient, inadequate surgical drainage of an abscess was responsible for the poor response. Twenty (40%) of the patients who were successfully treated with this drug received no other antimicrobial agent. Ledger et al. [28] reported that 20 (80%) of 25 puerperal women with septic endometritis responded to oral metronidazole therapy. In the five treatment failures, anaerobic organisms were not isolated but all responded to other antimicrobial agents to which the aerobic species were susceptible. Willis [54] considers that as the therapeutic response of anaerobic Gram-negative rods to metronidazole is now well recognized, it should be prescribed empirically for all patients with suspected anaerobic infections. He is of the opinion that metronidazole combined with gentamicin is effective first choice therapy for patients with severe Gram-negative sepsis. As the Bacteroides group of organisms is considered to be the most frequently isolated from deep seated anaerobic infections, it is not surprising that metronidazole has become, because of its relative lack of toxicity, the drug of choice for the therapy of severe pelvic infections.

Although *Staphyloccus aureus* is the major pathogen isolated from patients with a puerperal breast abscess anaerobes are common pathogens in subareolar infections in non-puerperal women. Leach et al. [27] consider that the presence of a subareolar abscess associated with a retracted nipple in a non-puerperal women should alert the clinician to the presence of an anaerobic infection. This is readily confirmed by the presence of foul smelling pus on surgical drainage. They isolated anaerobes from eight of 15 patients with non-puerperal breast abscess seen in their hospital during one year. The anaerobes most frequently isolated were *Bacteroides melaninogenicus*, *Bacteroides bivius*, *Peptococcus* and *Peptostreptococcus* species. In two cases only *Bacteroides bivius* was isolated, but in the other cases up to four different anaerobes were recovered. These investigators drew attention to the fact that anaerobic breast abscesses tend to recur as exemplified by four of their patients from whom anaerobes were isolated. While surgical drainage is the primary treatment of subareolar breast abscess, antimicrobial therapy should also be prescribed. Six of the patients in the report of Leach et al. [27] received metronidazole therapy. In two patients the abscess recurred after intervals of four and 12 months, respectively, but further drainage and treatment with metronidazole resulted in resolution of the infection. These investigators recommend that if an antimicrobial agent is to be administered to a patient with a subareolar breast abscess at the time of surgical drainage, a drug with predictable anaerobic microbicidal activity such as metronidazole should be prescribed.

There is some evidence to indicate that anaerobic organisms may have a role in perinatal and neonatal infections. Chow et al. [6] reported that anaerobic bacteremia in neonates most frequently occur as a sequel to inoculation of such infants during parturition. Septicemia and meningitis caused by *Bacteroides fragilis* may occur in the neonate as the result of chorioamnionitis. Berman et al. [3] reported the successful treatment of a premature infant with *Bacteroides fragilis* meningitis with metronidazole after chloramphenicol had failed to eradicate the causative agent from the cerebrospinal fluid. Oral metronidazole was initially administered via a nasogastric tube in a daily dosage of 30 mg/kg body weight which was later increased to 35 mg/kg body weight. A sterile cerebospinal fluid culture was obtained six days after the commencement of metronidazole therapy. Because of the oncogenic effects in mice, mutagenic effects in bacteria and limited use in neonates, further studies are necessary to establish metronidazole pharmacokinetics and efficacy in infants.

Jokipii et al. [25] have shown that 90 min after the oral administration of 2400 mg of metronidazole to human volunteers, the cerebrospinal fluid concentrations were in the range of 6.0 to 22.7 μg/ml which approximate to 43% of the serum levels. Ingham et al. [23] treated nine patients who had an otogenic cerebral abscess with metronidazole. They found that the drug concentrations in the pus of the abscess cavity ranged from 21.0 to 35.0 μg/ml when metronidazole was administered in a dosage of 400 mg every 8 h. Eight of the nine patients recovered with no residual neurologic sequelae. The other patient had cerebellar ataxia. These investigators concluded since obligate anaerobic bacteria are commonly found in cerebral abscesses metronidazole therapy should reduce the high mortality which is associated with intracranial suppurative disease.

Since 1975 an intravenous preparation of metronidazole as the hydrochloride salt has been made available for the treatment of anaerobic infections on a trial basis, it is made up as an isotonic 0.5% weight to volume aqueous solution buffered with sodium bicarbonate in 100 ml bottles. This preparation can be administered over a period of about 30 min every 8 h. Eykyn and Phillips [12] reported no toxicity or thrombophlebitis from this preparation. From their preliminary trials they concluded that it was highly efficacious in the treatment of severe postoperative anaerobic infections. Galgiani et al. [14] consider that members of the *Bacteroides fragilis* group are the commonest anaerobic species isolated from patients with Bacteremia or refractory anaerobic infections. They state that the currently available antimicrobial agents are not always successful in the therapy of severe anaerobic infections even when the causative organism is susceptible in vitro to a particular drug. They reported the successful treatment of two patients with *Bacteroides fragilis* bacteremia with intravenous metronidazole. Both patients had initially received clindamycin but the bacteremia persisted despite the fact that the organism showed in vitro susceptibility to this antibiotic. Warner et al. [53] confirmed the efficacy of intravenous metronidazole in the treatment of *Bacteroides fragilis* bacteremia. One of their patients had a premature delivery of a stillborn infant and severe postpartum hemorrhage. She was found to have blast cells in her peripheral blood smear which resulted in a diagnosis of promyelocytic anemia. On the ninth postpartum day the patient developed a fever and repeated blood cultures grew *Bacteroides fragilis*. The bacteremia was thought to be the result of postpartum endometritis. As her platelet count was only 5000/ml^3; no surgical exploration of the uterus was undertaken. The patient was treated with intravenous clindamycin for eight days without any response. Because of persistent high fever and shaking chills, intravenous metronidazole in a dosage of 500 mg every 6 h was commenced. By the fifth day of metronidazole the patient was afebrile. This drug was administered to the patient for 25 days and no toxic effects attributable to metronidazole were recorded. A further patient who was known to have a leiomyosarcoma of the uterus for three and one-half years was admitted to hospital with fever, chills and right lower quadrant abdominal pain. Three of the four blood cultures obtained yielded *Bacteroides fragilis*. The patient was treated with intravenous and then oral metronidazole in a dosage of 500 mg every 6 h for 14 days. She also received cefazolin sodium 2.0 g intravenously every 8 h for ten days and tobramycin sulfate 85 mg intravenously every 8 h for eight days. After 24 h of antimicrobial therapy the blood cultures were sterile and the patient was afebrile by the fifth day. On cessation of the metronidazole therapy, her infection did not recur. These investigators also report the successful treatment of a patient who had a mixed bacteremia due to *Escherichia coli* and *Bacteroides fragilis* with a combination of metronidazole, cefazolin and gentamicin. The patient received metronidazole, 500 mg and cefazolin sodium 1.5 g intravenously every 6 h and gentamicin sulfate 115 mg intravenously every 8 h for 14 days. After cessation of therapy the patient was afebrile and asymptomatic. Included in this report is a further patient with *Bacteroides fragilis* bacteremia who failed to respond to treatment with intravenous clindamycin. On oral metronidazole in a dosage of 500 mg every 6 h the patient was afebrile within 48 h. The metronidazole therapy was continued for 14 days and no drug toxicity was noted.

These investigators also describe the successful use of intravenous metronidazole for the treatment of ventriculitis and meningitis due to a *Bacteroides* species in a premature infant. The child was initially treated for 17 days with intravenous penicillin G and chloramphenicol but, despite this therapeutic regimen, cultures of the cerebrospinal fluid continued to grow *Bacteroides* species. Intravenous metronidazole therapy was then instituted at a dose of 40 mg every 8 h and the chloramphenicol and penicillin G discontinued. When the treatment with metronidazole was commenced, the infant was reported to be moribund. On the fourth day of metronidazole therapy a sample of cerebrospinal fluid obtained by ventricular puncture was cultured and found to be sterile. Metronidazole therapy was continued for a further 24 days during which time repeated cultures of samples of cerebrospinal fluid remained sterile. Although the infant developed hydrocephalus as a complication of the meningitis which was successfully managed by a ventriculoperitoneal shunt, the child required no further antimicrobial therapy for the infection caused by *Bacteroides* species. The infant was discharged from hospital in good condition 47 days after cessation of metronidazole therapy.

In the same report these investigators confirmed that metronidazole was efficacious in the treatment of intracranial suppurative disease. They presented the history of a patient with a right frontal lobe abscess which had failed to respond to three neurosurgical procedures and extensive parenteral antibiotic therapy with ampicillin, penicillin G and chloramphenicol in the previous three months. Cultures of the drainage from the craniotomy wound yielded a beta-hemolytic *Streptococcus* which did not belong to group A, B or D, *Bacteroides* Species, *Fusobacterium naviforme* and *Peptostreptococcus* species. Further therapy was instituted with penicillin G potassium intravenously in a total daily dosage of 60 million units. After seven days the patient was still symptomatic and repeat cultures grew the same anaerobic organisms but no beta-hemolytic *Streptococcus*. Oral metronidazole, 500 mg every 6 h, was then commenced. By the third day of mentronidazole therapy the wound drainage had diminished and cultures yielded neither aerobic nor anaerobic organisms. Metronidazole therapy was continued for six weeks and the patient was asymptomatic at the time of discharge from hospital.

These clinical studies indicate that metronidazole, whether administered intravenously or orally, is a safe effective antimicrobial agent to treat serious infections caused by susceptible anaerobic bacteria. In many instances metronidazole has been effective when therapy with clindamycin or chloramphenicol was ineffectual despite in vitro sensitivity of the causative organisms to these antibiotics.

Perera et al. [38] reported the use of intravenous metronidazole in the prophylaxis and treatment of proven and presumed anaerobic infection in 149 patients. Fifty-nine patients received intravenous metronidazole prophylactically prior to surgery. This group of patients included 49 who had large bowel surgery and one who had bilateral leg amputation. Subsequent anaerobic infections occurred in only one patient who developed a superficial wound hematoma which became infected with *Bacteroides* species. The infected hematoma was successfully treated by surgical drainage without further antimicrobial therapy.

Ninety patients were treated with intravenous metronidazole for suspected anaerobic sepsis. Five of the 90 patients received two systemic courses of therapy with this drug. The total intravenous dose administered in a single course ranged from 1.0 g to 25.5 g Anaerobic sepsis was confirmed by microbiologic studies in 42 of the patients. One patient had two episodes of bacteremia and a further patient had both an aspiration pneumonia and a deep wound infection due to anaerobic organisms. *Bacteroides fragilis* was the most frequently isolated organism. It was the only organism isolated from four patients but was present in 31 (70%) of the cultures obtained from the 42 patients with anaerobic sepsis. All the isolates of *Bacteroides fragilis* were sensitive to metronidazole at a concentration of 5 μg/ml. Mixed infection with aerobes was noted in 35 of the infections. *Escherichia coli* was isolated on 27 occasions (61%). Thirty-three of the 43 courses of metronidazole treatment resulted in complete eradication of the infection. Metronidazole was administered in combination with other antimicrobials in 30 of these courses of treatment. In 27 instances such combination therapy was indicated because of the presence of aerobic isolates and in the three other cases combination therapy was prescribed in order to attain broad spectrum antimicrobial therapy. The agents used were gentamicin, ampicillin, flucloxacillin, penicillin and cotrimoxazole. Despite such treatment, anaerobic sepsis was a contributory factor in the death of six patients. Three deaths were due to *Bacteroides fragilis* septicemia.

Fifty-two courses of metronidazole were administered to patients with suspected anaerobic infection. In the majority of the patients metronidazole therapy produced prompt resolution of the infectious disease. Six of the patients who did not respond to metronidazole therapy were found to have septicemia due to aerobic organisms and a further patient had tuberculous salpingitis. These investigators also reported the successful use of intravenous metronidazole in the treatment of a gravid patient with acute Giardiasis. At the time of the illness the pregnancy was of 30 weeks duration and the patient received a total dose of 5.0 g of the drug by the intravenous route. The pregnancy continued until the 39th week when a normal infant was delivered.

The authors state that the drug and the chemicals used to buffer it in solution were well tolerated by all their patients. No vomiting was recorded with the intravenous formulation. Two patients developed a neutropenia but both were also receiving cotrimoxazole which is known to cause agranulocytosis. In one patient the white blood count recovered when the cotrimoxazole was discontinued. The other patient with profound neutropenia died of pseudomonas septicemia although some recovery of the bone marrow was observed after the cotrimoxazole was discontinued.

These investigators observed a reversible sensory neuropathy in a 13-year-old boy who initially received a total intravenous dose of 2.0 g followed by a daily oral dose of 57 mg/kg body weight. After ten weeks of metronidazole therapy and a total dose of 165 g, the patient noted paresthesia of his hands and feet. Physical examination revealed a sensory neuropathy affecting the hands and legs as well as wasting of the small muscles of the hands. Seven months after the cessation of therapy complete recovery occurred.

To date, this is the largest series of patients who have received intravenous metronidazole for serious anaerobic infection. Complete microbiologic and clinical cure was achieved in 76% with the treatment course prescribed for proven anaerobic sepsis. Other antimicrobials were given simultaneously to 90% of the patients because of the polymicrobial nature of their infections. The investigators state that although treatment of the anaerobic component of polymicrobial infections may suffice in effecting a clinical cure, they consider that except in a few instances the poor general condition of their patients did not permit them to rely solely on metronidazole for the eradication of the infection. From these studies they conclude that intravenous metronidazole can be recommended as safe and efficacious therapy for patients with serious anaerobic infections. In the therapy of polymicrobial infections it can be combined with such aerobic microbicidal agents as the penicillins and cephalosporins.

Treatment of anaerobic infections cannot be initiated unless the nature of the infectious process can be identified by the clinician and the microbiologic diagnostic laboratory. Identification of the causative organisms and antimicrobial sensitivity testing are essential so that patients can receive optimal therapy. Metronidazole has been shown to be consistently bactericidal against anaerobes but with its more extensive use in the treatment of serious anaerobic infections it is highly probable that metronidazole resistant strains of *Bacteroides fragilis* will emerge. The response of microorganisms to antimicrobial agents is their ability to develop resistance. Ingham et al. [19] reported the development of metronidazole resistance in *Bacteroides fragilis* in a patient who had received the drug for a prolonged period of time for the treatment of Crohn's disease. Without knowing the clinical and bacteriologic details, it is possible that the three patients who died from *Bacteroides fragilis* septicemia reported by Perera et al. [38] could have had a metronidazole resistant strain of this organism. Leach et al. [27] reported the isolation of a *Bacteroides* species which was not *Bacteroides fragilis* from a subareolar breast abscess which was resistant to metronidazole. The other anaerobic organisms isolated from the pus, namely *Bacteroides bivius*, *Bacteroides melaninogenicus* and *Peptococcus assachacrolyticus* were all sensitive to metronidazole and therapy with this drug in conjunction with surgical drainage was successful.

As exemplified by the various reports quoted in this review, metronidazole has proved efficacious in the treatment of anaerobic infections where clindamycin and chloramphenicol have been unsuccessful. Currently there is no standardized procedure for antimicrobial susceptibility testing for anaerobes. Sutter et al. [48] have recommended that the reference method proposed by the National Committee for Clinical Laboratory Standards Subcommittee on Antimicrobial Susceptibility Testing be accepted. This agar dilution reference method is not practical for daily use in clinical laboratories, but it might be appropriate for laboratories to determine susceptibility profiles for anaerobes isolated on a periodic basis by this method. Such information could be helpful to clinicians for the selection of appropriate antimicrobial therapy as well as identifying resistant strains of anaerobic organisms. Brown and Waatti [5] reported that the incidence of resistance of anaerobic bacteria to antimicrobial agents is greater than originally believed and indicated a need for reliable susceptibility testing methodology. These investigators in susceptibility testing of 231 strains of *Bacteroides fragilis* obtained from clinical isolates found that 5.2% were resistant to chloramphenicol and 44% were resistant to clindamycin. Hansen [18] compared the in vitro activity of cefoxitin clindamycin, chloramphenicol and metronidazole against members of the *Bacteroides fragilis* group of organisms. Of the 89 *Bacteroides fragilis* strains, more than 90% were susceptible to achievable serum levels of these antimicrobial agents. This investigator emphasized that meticulous identification and susceptibility testing of isolates of the *Bacteroides fragilis* group of anaerobes is important to the clinician because of variations in susceptibility patterns between species and between strains within species.

At this time it is not possible to define the relative therapeutic efficacy of metronidazole compared with clindamycin and chloramphenicol. Metronidazole is, however, an important anaerobic microbicidal agent that will be extensively used in the treatment of anaerobic septicemia and severe infections in obstetrics and gynecology in the next few years. Whatever views may be held about the prophylactic as opposed to the therapeutic use of metronidazole, experience to date indicates that this drug should now be considered the antimicrobial agent of choice for the prevention of these infections and for the treatment of those serious non-clostridial anaerobic infections that require antimicrobial therapy.

REFERENCES

1. Balsdon MJ, Taylor GE, Pead L, Maskell R: Corynebacterium vaginale and vaginitis: a controlled trial of treatment. Lancet 1:501–504, 1980
2. Beard CM, Noller KL, O'Fallon M, Kurkland LT, Dockerty MB: Lack of evidence for cancer due to use of metronidazole. N Engl J Med 301:519–522, 1979
3. Berman BW, King FH Jr, Rubenstein DS, Long SS: *Bacteroides fragilis* meningitis in a neonate successfully treated with metronidazole. J Pediatr 93:793–795, 1979
4. Brogden RN, Heel RD, Speight TM, Avery GS: Metronidazole in anaerobic infections: a review of its activity, pharmacokinetics and therapeutic use. Drugs 16:387–417, 1978
5. Brown WJ, Waatti PE: Susceptibility testing of clinically isolated anaerobic bacteria by an agar dilution technique. Antimicrob Agents Chemother 17:629–635, 1980
6. Chow AW, Leake RD, Yamauchi T, Anthony BF, Guze B: The significance of anaerobes in neonatal bacteremia, analysis of 23 cases and review of the literature. Pediatr 54:736–745, 1974
7. Chow AW, Patten V, Bednorz N: Susceptibility of *Campylobacter fetus* to 22 antimicrobial agents. 17th Interscience Conference on Antimicrobial Agents and Chemotherapy, October 1977, Abstract No. 59.
8. DeCarneri I, Achilli G, Monti G, Trane F: Induction of in vivo resistance of *Trichomonas vaginalis* to nitroimidazine. Lancet 2:1308–1309, 1969
9. DeCarneri I and Gionnane R: Drug resistance in *Trichomonas vaginalis*. Lancet 2:1152, 1971
10. Dunn PM, Stewart-Brown S, Peel R: Metronidazole and the fetal alcohol syndrome. Lancet 2:144, 1979
11. Edwards DI: Mechanism of antimicrobial action of metronidazole. J Antimicrob Chemother 5:499–502, 1979
12. Eykyn SJ, Philips I: Metronidazole and anaerobic sepsis. Br Med J 2:1403–1404, 1976
13. Fleury FJ, VanBergen WS, Prentice RL, Russel JG, Singleton JA, Standard JV: Single dose of two grams of metronidazole for *Trichomonas vaginalis* infection. Am J Obstet Gynecol 128:320–322, 1977
14. Galgiani JN, Busch DJ, Brass C, Rumans LW, Mangels JI, Stevens DA: Bacteroides fragilis endocarditis, bacteremia and other infections treated with oral or intravenous metronidazole. Am J Med 65:284–289, 1978

214

15. Gardner HL, Dukes CD: *Haemophilus vaginalis:* A newley defined specific infection pre-viously classified 'nonspecific' vaginitis. Am J Obstet gynecol 79:962–976, 1955
16. Gardner HL, Kaufman RH: Benign diseases of the vulva. The C.V. Mosby Company, St. Louis, 1969, pp 191–207
17. Gibbs RS, O'Dell TN, MacGregor RR, Schwarz RH, Morton H: Puerperal endometritis: a prospective microbiologic study. Am J Obstet gynecol 121:919–925, 1975
18. Hansen SL: Variation in susceptibility patterns of species within the *Bacteroides fragilis* group. Antimicrob Agents Chemother 17:686–690, 1980
19. Ingham HR, Eaton S, Venables CW, Adams PD: *Bacteroides fragilis* resistant to metroni-dazole after long-term therapy. Lancet 1:214, 1978
20. Ingham HR, Selkon JB, Hale JH: The antibacterial activity of metronidazole. J Antimicrob Chemother 1:355–361, 1975
21. Ingham HR, Selkon JB, Roxby CM: Bacteriological study of otogenic cerebral abscesses: chemotherapeutic role of metronidazole. Brit Med J 2:991–993, 1977
22. Ingham HR, Sisson PR Selkon JB: Current concepts of the pathogenetic mechanisms of non-sporting anaerobes: chemotherapeutic implications. J Antimicrob Chemother 6:173–179, 1980
23. Ingham HR, Sisson PR, Tharagonnet D, Selkon JB, Codd AA: Inhibition of phagocytosis in vitro by obligate anaerobes. Lancet 2:1252–1254, 1977
24. Ings RMJ, McFadzean JA, Ormerod WE: The mode of action of metronidazole in *Tri-chomonas vaginalis*, other microorganisms. Biochem Pharmacol 23:1421–1429, 1974
25. Jokopii AMM, Myllylä VV, Hokkanen E, Jokipii L: Penetration of the blood brain barrier by metronidazole and tinidazole. J Antimicrob Chemother 3:239–245, 1977
26. Josey WE, McKenzie WJ, Lambe DW:Corynebacterium vaginale (Haemophilus vaginalis) in women with leukorrhea. Am J Obstet gynecol. 126:574–578, 1976
27. Leach RD, Eykyn SJ, Phillips I, Corrin B: Anaerobic subareolar breast abscess. Lancet 1:35–37, 1979
28. Ledger WJ, Gee CL, Pollin PA, Lewis WP, Sutter VL, Finegold SM: A new approach to patients with suspected anaerobic postpartum pelvic infections. Transabdominal uterine aspiration for culture and metronidazole for treatment. Am J Obstet gynecol 126:1–6, 1976
29. Ledger WJ, Norman M, Gee C, Lewis W: Bacteremia on an obstetric-gynecologic service. Am J Obstet Gynecol 121:205–212, 1975
30. Ledger WJ, Sweet RL, Headington JT: Prophylactic cephaloridine in the prevention of postoperative pelvic infections in premenopausal women undergoing vaginal hysterectomy. Am J Obstet Gynecol 115:766–774, 1973
31. Lindmark DG, Muller M: Antitrichomonad action, mutagenicity and reduction of metroni-dazole and other nitroimidazoles. Antimicrob Agents chemother. 10:476–482, 1976
32. McFadzean JA, Pugh IM, Squires SL, Whelan JPF: Further observations on strain sensi-tivity of *Trichomonas vaginalis* to metronidazole. Brit J Vener Dis 45:161–162, 1969
33. Melander A, Kahlmeter G, Kamane C, Ursing B: Bioavailability of metronidazole in fasting and non-fasting healthy subjects and in patients with Crohn's disease. European J Clin Pharmacol 12:69–72, 1977
34. Morton RS: Metronidazole in the single-dose treatment of *Trichomonal vaginitis* in men and women. Brit J of Vener Dis 48:525–527, 1972
35. Ohm MJ, Galask RP: The effect of antibiotic prophylaxis on patients undergoing vaginal operations. I. The effect on morbidity. Am J Obstet Gynecol 123:590–596, 1975a
36. Ohm MJ, Glask RP: The effect of antibiotic prophylaxis on patients undergoing vaginal operations. II. Alterations of microbial flora. Am J Obstet Gynecol 123:597–604, 1975b.
37. Onderdonk AB, Lovie TJ, Tally FP, Bartlett JG: Activity of metronidazole against *Escher-ichia coli* in experimental intra-abdominal sepsis. J Antimicrob Chemother 5:201–210, 1979
38. Perera M, Chipping PM, Noone P: Intravenous metronidazole in the treatment and pro-phylaxis of anaerobic infection. J Antimicrob Chemother 6:105–112, 1980
39. Pheifer TA, Forsyth PS, Durfee MA, Pollock HM, Holmes KK: Nonspecific vaginitis. Role of *Haemophilus vaginalis* and treatment with metronidazole. N Engl J Med 298:1429–1434, 1978

40. Roe FJC: Metronidazole: Review of uses and toxicity. J Antimicrob Chemother 3:205–212, 1977
41. Rosenkrantz HS, Speck WT: Mutagenicity of metronidazole activation by mammalian liver microsomes. Biochem Biophys Res Commun 66:520–522, 1975
42. Rustin M, Shubik P: Induction of lung tumors and malignant lymphomas in mice by metronidazole. J Nat Cancer Institute 48:721–729, 1972
43. Seligman SA: Metronidazole in obstetrics and gynaecology. J Antimicrob Chemother 4 (Suppl. C) 51–54, 1978
44. Shinn DLS: Metronidazole in acute ulcerative gingivitis. Lancet 1:1191, 1962
45. Sprott MS, Ingham HR: Treatment of infections due to nonsporing anaerobes. Drugs 18:137–149, 1979
46. Study Group: An evaluation of metronidazole in the prophylaxis of anaerobic infections in obstetrical patients. J Antimicrob chemother 4 (Suppl.) 55–62, 1978
47. Study Group: An evaluation of metronidazole in the prophylaxis and treatment of anaerobic infections in surgical patients. J Antimicrob Chemother 1:393–401, 1975
48. Sutter VL, Barry AL, Wilkins TD, Zabransky RJ: Collaborative evaluation of a proposed reference dilution method of susceptibility testing of anaerobic bacteria. Antimicrob Agents Chemother 16:495–502, 1979
49. Sweet RL, Ledger WJ: Puerperal infections morbidity – A two year review. Am J Obstet Gynecol. 117:1093–1100, 1973
50. Tally FP, Sutter VL, Finegold SM: Treatment of anaerobic infections with metronidazole. Antimicrob Agents Chemother 7:672–675, 1975
51. Tally FP, Sutter VL, Finegold SM: Metronidazole versus anaerobes – in vitro data and initial clinical observations. Calif Med 117:22–26, 1972
52. Thurner J, Meingassner JG: Isolation of *Trichomonas vaginalis* resistant to metronidazole. Lancet 2:738, 1978
53. Warner JF, Perkins RL, Cordero L: Metronidazole therapy of anaerobic bacteremia meningitis, and brain abscess. Arch Intern Med 139:167–169, 1979
54. Willis AT: Metronidazole in anaerobic infections. Scot Med J 22:155–158, 1977
55. Willis AT: Metronidazole in the prevention and treatment of anaerobic sepsis. Scand J Infect Dis 19:98–104, 1979
56. Willson RL: Acute drug administration and cancer control. Lancet 1:810–811, 1974
57. Wise R, Andrews JM, Bedford KA: The activity of four antimicrobial agents, including three nitroimidazole compounds, against *Bacteroides Sp*. Chemother 23:19–24, 1977

SUMMARY

The introduction and widespread use of antibiotics has resulted in profound changes in the number and character of infections that are being encountered in clinical paractice. A great deal of emphasis has been placed on the role of anaerobic organisms in serious pelvic infections in obstetrics and gynecology. *Bacteroides fragilis*, although it is a relatively uncommon commensal in the lower female genital tract, is by far the most common anaerobic isolate from serous life-threatening bacteremias encountered in obstetrics and gynecology.

Although penicillin G and its congeners are active against almost all anaerobes, this group of antibiotics are ineffective against *Bacteroides fragilis* and should not be used alone in the treatment of serious infections of the female genital tract. The same applies to the cephalosporins as these antibiotics, like the penicillins, are inactivated by the β-lactamases of *Bacteroides fragilis*.

Several years ago tetracycline was the drug of choice for anaerobic infections involving *Bacteroides fragilis*, but because of the declining sensitivity of this organism to this antibiotic it is no longer of any value in the treatment of life-threatening infections. The same is true of its analogues, minocycline and doxycycline, and as a result the clinician until recently had to turn to chloramphenicol or clindamycin as the drugs of choice for the treatment of serious *Bacteroides fragilis* infections.

Chloramphenicol has excellent in vitro activity against most strains of *Bacteroides fragilis*, although of late resistant strains have been reported.

Therapeutic failures in patients with life-threatening sepsis associated with *Bacteroides fragilis* have been reported despite the fact that the clinical isolate was sensitive to chloramphenicol. Such failures may have resulted from in vivo inactivation of this antibiotic by chloramphenicol acetyltransferase produced by the organism. Although this antibiotic has proved to be highly efficacious in many serious *Bacteroides fragilis* infections, its clinical acceptance has been limited by its potential hematologic toxicity.

The activity of clindamycin against *Bacteroides fragilis* is similar to chloramphenicol. Plasmid-mediated transferable resistance to this antibiotic has been reported in clinical isolates of *Bacteroides fragilis* and, as a result, despite the well documented in vitro effectiveness of clindamycin against *Bacteroides* species, some treatment failures have been encountered in clinical practice. Concern still persists regarding the pseudomembranous colitis that may follow the administration of this antibiotic, but if the physician is alert to the possible association of any antibiotic with this clinical entity, serious forms of colitis can be circumvented.

Mentronidazole is at present the only anaerobic microbicidal agent that has been found to be highly efficacious in the treatment of serious infections involving obligate anaerobes. This nitroimidazole derivative is unaffected by β-lactamases and has no serious toxic properties. This drug has, however, been under close surveillance because it has been reported to be mutagenic in certain bacteria and carcinogenic in one animal species. Metronidazole has been available for the treatment of vaginal trichomoniasis for over twenty years and as yet there is no evidence that implicates this chemotherapeutic agent as a carcinogen in humans. In addition to the oral preparation a buffered isotonic aqueous formulation of metronidazole is available for intravenous administration in severe life-threatening infections involving *Bacteroides fragilis*. As yet it is not possible to clearly define the relative therapeutic efficacy of the parenteral preparation with that of clindamycin and chloramphenicol although it has been used successfully in the treatment of *Bacteroides fragilis* bacteremia and fulminant infections of the female genital tract. At present, tinidazole, another member of the imidazole group of chemotherapeutic agents, is undergoing clinical evaluation for serious anaerobic infections and preliminary reports indicate that it is as efficacious as metronidazole.

Since anaerobes have been strongly implicated in the pathogenesis of serious pelvic and intra-abdominal infections current research is being directed to finding agents which have none of the serious adverse reactions which may be encountered during chloramphenicol or clindamycin therapy. A new group of antimicrobial agents, the cephamycins which are closely related to the cephalosporins, have recently been made available for the treatment of anaerobic infections. The first of these compounds, cefoxitin, although effective against many anaerobic species, it is not active against all strains of *Bacteroides fragilis* and *Clostridium* species. Consequently, to date chloramphenicol, clindamycin and metronidazole still remain the drugs of choice for the treatment of serious infections involving *Bacteroides fragilis*.

The continuing problem of the β-lactamase mediated resistance of *Bacteroides fragilis* and other clinically important bacteria to β-lactam antibiotics has encouraged the search for more effective inhibitors of this enzyme. The first of such compounds is clavulanic acid which has the ability to inhibit the β-lactamases of staphylococci and Gram-negative bacteria and, as a result, in vitro studies have demonstrated that it can extend the antibacterial spectrum of ampicillin and amoxycillin. The enhancement of antibacterial activity by clavulanic acid has been reported for these antibiotics as well as the new cephalosporin, cefotaxime, against *Bacteroides fragilis*. Other β-lactamase inhibitors are also being investigated such as penicillanic acid sulphone which is potentiator of the activity of ampicillin against resistant bacteria including *Bacteroides fragilis*. Such compounds could have widespread clinical applicability and result in the penicillins and cephalosporins attaining the title of drugs of choice for serious polymicrobial infections involving *Bacteroides fragilis*. Until clinical trials have been undertaken with inactivators of β-lactamases the clinician has to rely on the potent and potentially toxic antibiotics chloramphenicol and clindamycin or the anaerobic bactericidal agent, metronidazole.

Author's address:
Department of Obstetrics and Gynecology
Marshall University School of Medicine
Huntington, West Virginia 25701
U.S.A.

9. CEPHALOSPORINS AND CEPHAMYCINS

RICHARD L. SWEET, M.D.

The clinician is faced with a veritable explosion in the investigation and introduction of cephalosporin and cephalosporinlike antibiotics. Although very little clinical and in vitro differences exist between the first generation cephalosporins (Fig. 1), there has been a steady proliferation of these agents. Although, the clinical efficacy of this versatile group of first generation cephalosporins, which are broad spectrum bactericidal beta lactam antibiotics, is well established, in fact, they are not the drug of choice for any specific infection. However, they have become the second choice drugs for many bacterial infections. This confusing situation will become even more complex, as the so-called second and third generation cephalosporins receive either widespread use or introduction into clinical medicine. This second generation and third generation of cephalosporins have enhanced broad

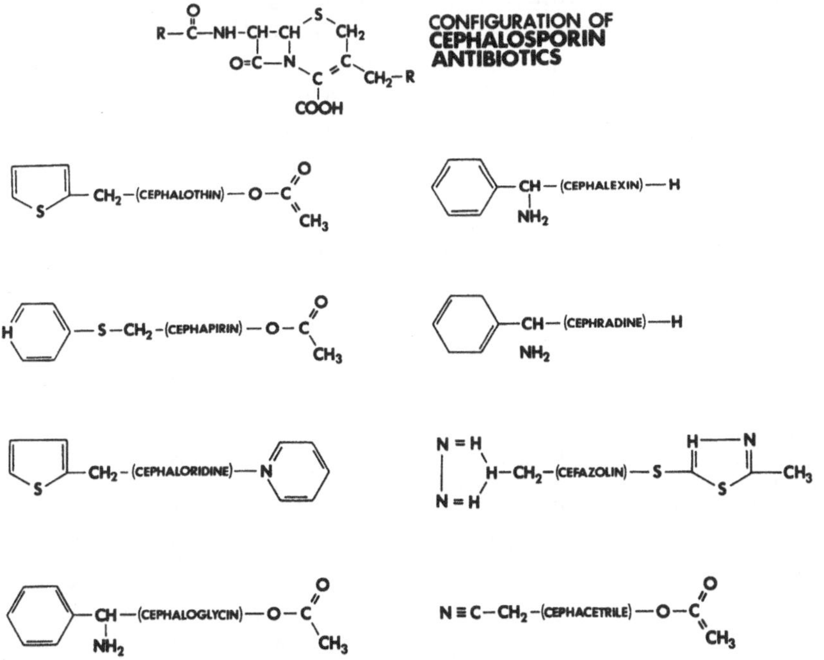

Fig. 1. Structures of first generation cephalosporins.

W.J. Ledger (ed.), Antibiotics in Obstetrics and Gynecology, 219–252. All rights reserved.
Copyright © 1982 by Martinus Nijhoff Publishers, The Hague/Boston/London. ISBN-13:978-94-009-7466-1

220

spectrum antimicrobial activity, which may be of clinical importance. The cephamycin group of antibiotics which are related to he cephalosporins also have come into being.

First Generation Cephalosporins

In 1945, Giuseppe Brotzu isolated a strain of *Cephalosporium acremonium* from the Mediterranean Sea off the island of Sardinia. He reported that thus fungus secreted antimicrobial substances. In 1948, Professor Brotzu sent a culture of his organism to Oxford University. The preliminary studies were undertaken by a group of scientists headed by E.P. Abraham, in an attempt to isolate the active antibacterial factors. Several different active antibiotic agents were isolated from these broth cultures. In 1953, Newton and Abraham discovered an antibiotic in the metabolic products of Brotzu's strain of cephalosporium which was named cephalosporin C, and found to have several remarkable properties [1]. Not only was it active against *Salmonella typhi*, *Escherichia coli* and the Oxford strain of *Staphylococcus aureus*, but it also proved resistant to penicillinase. This agent, cephalosporin C, is the parent substance from which the first cephalosporin for clinical use was derived. In addition to its very broad range of antimicrobial activity, it had the interesting features of being relatively acid stable and resistant to penicillinase. At present there are 12 preparations of ten different cephalosporins avalable for clinical use in Europe and the United States (Table 1).

Moellering has noted that as a class, the cephalosporins possessed a number of desirable properties [2]. First, like penicillins, cephalosporins are beta lactum antibiotics, which inhibit senthesis of the bacterial cell wall. The result of this activity is death of the cell rather than simple inhibition of growth; thus

Table 1. Cephalosporins currently available for clinical use in the United States.

Generic name	Trade name	Route of administration		
		IV	IM	PO
Cephalothin	Keflin	X	X	–
Cephaloridine	Loridine	X	X	–
Cefazolin	Ancef, Kefzol	X	X	–
Cephapirin	Cefadyl	X	X	–
Cephacetrile	Celospor	X	X	–
Cephradine	Velosef, Anspor	X	X	X
Cephaloglycine	Kafocin	–	–	X
Cephalexin	Keflex	–	–	X
Cefamandole	Mandol	X	X	–
Cefoxitin	Mefoxin	X	X	–

these are bactericidal agents. Second, as a class, the cephalosporins are relatively resistant to hydrolysis by beta lactamases produced by *S. aureus*. Hence, they are active against a number of strains of penicillin resistant staphylococci, except the methicillin resistant *S. aureus*, which does have cross resistance to cephalosporins. Third, cephalosporins possess broad spectrum activity and are effective against several species of penicillin resistant gram negative rods including *E. coli, Klebsiella pneumoniae*, and *Proteus mirabilis*. Fourth, these compounds possess a high therapeutic-toxic index. Indeed, serious side effects are relatively uncommon with the cephalosporins and consist primarily of local reactions to injection of infusion and hypersensitivity reactions. Allergic reactions are said to occur in 5% of recipients, but such figures include eosinophilia. Anaphalatic reactions to the cephalosporins appear to be very infrequent, but have been described. Fifth, despite extensive use of these antibiotics, there is little evidence to support the thesis that such utilization has resulted in widespread emergence of resistant organisms.

Unfortunately, the cephalosporins also possess a number of characteristics that are less than optimal. These agents are rapidly and efficiently excreted by the kidneys resulting in a relatively short serum half-life. Thus, they must be administered at frequent intervals to maintain adequate blood levels. Of the currently available first generation cephalosporins, cefazolin has the longest serum half-life. With the exception of cephaloridine both glomerular filtration and tubular secretion are involved in the renal excretion of these compounds. For cephaloridine, the amount of drugs subjected to tubular secretion is negligible. Unlike the penicillins, the cephalosporins do not penetrate well into the cerebrospinal fluid, even in patients with meningitis. The lack of activity of the first generation cephalosporins against certain bacteria is an additional drawback [3]. None of the first generation cephalosporins is effective against enterococci, and the majority of strains of *Haemophilus influenzae, Enterobacter* species, indole positive *Proteus* species, *Providencia* species, *Pseudomonas aeruginosa, Serratia marcescens*, and *Bacteroides fragilis* are resistant as well. In the case of enterococci, the resistance appears to be intrinsic since no beta-lactamase activity has been identified in these organisms. Many of the gram-negative organisms are capable of producing beta-lactamases (cephalosporinases), which mediate the hydrolysis of various cephalosporins. Dose-relaed nephrotoxicity of the cephalosporins in experimental animals has been demonstrated [4]. Only cephaloridine has been definitely linked with nephrotoxicity in humans [5], but the potential probably exists for the other agents as well. Foord [6] summarized the experience with cases of renal damage due to cephaloridine (96 cases). He concluded that most cases with cephaloridine resulted from excessive dosage and/or abnormal renal function and that the renal lesion produced by cephaloridine is most likely the result of a direct toxic effect upon the kidney, especially occuring with large doses (usually greater than 4 to 6 g/day) of drug given. On the other hand cephalothin-related nephrotoxicity is uncommon even with large doses. Foord [6]suggested most cases resulted from use of a dose excessive for the state of renal function or to use of concurrent agents which were potentially nephrotoxic. Barza stated that the most logical explanation for cephalothin nephrotoxicity is that of a phenomenon related to hypersensitivity – similar to that seen with penicillins [7]. The possibility that combinations of cephalosporins with aminoglycosides may be associated with enhanced nephrotoxicity in humans has been raised, but no proof exists.

Many of the currently available first generation cephalosporin antibiotics were introduced in the hope of overcoming some of the above noted deficiences and of producing enhanced therapeutic efficacy [2]. Unfortunately, it has been difficult thus far to document truly important differences among the first generation cephalosporins in any parameters other than their pharmacokenetics. This similarity is reflected in the recommendation that a single drug (cephalothin) be used to represent all first generation cephalosporins in disc diffusion susceptibility testing.

Except for the previously noted nephrotoxicity of cephaloridine, there is no evidence for important differences in toxicity among the present cephalosporins. Many studies have attempted to find differences in phlebitis producing potential among these agents, but in general these studies have shown little difference in the incidence of phlebitis caused by any of these agents [2].

Only in pharmacological parameters do significant differences occur among the currently available first generation cephalosporins. Table 2 provides a summary of the data derived from the use of injectable cephalosporins. The peak serum levels of cephalothin, cephapirin, and cephacetrile are comparable. Cephaloridine produces serum levels approximately twice as high in cefazolin and three to four times as high as the other three injectable compounds. The blood levels of cephradine after parenteral administration are consistently lower than those for any of the other five drugs. Significant differences in the serum half-life. and protein binding for these compounds are noted in Table 2. The shortest $t\frac{1}{2}$ values are seen with cephalothin and the longest with cefazolin and cephaloridine. The protein binding of cephalosporins ranges from a low level of 15% with cephalexin and cephradine to 85% with cefazolin. The mean serum $t\frac{1}{2}$ of each cephalosporin progressively increases as the rate of creatinine clearance decreases (Table 3). A suggested dosage schedule for impaired renal function is presented in Table 3. The pharmacokinetics of cephalosporins in patients with reduced renal function has been recently reviewed by Andriole [8].

Table 2. Comparative pharmacology of selected cephalosporins.

Drug	Peak serum level (1gm IM)	Serum half-life (minutes)	Total daily dose (grams)	Dosage interval (hours)	Protein binding (Percent)
Cephalothin (Keflin)	15–20 mcg/ml	37	4–12	4–6	65
Cephapirin (Cephadyl)	15–20	37	4–12	4–6	70
Cefazolin (Kefzol; Ancef)	50–70	100	2–6	6–12	85
Cefamandole (Mandol)	20–30	75	4–12	4–6	70
Cefoxitin (Mefoxin)	22	40	4–12	4–6	60
Cephalexin* (Keflex)	13–18	45	1–4	6	15
Cephradine* (Anspor; Velosef)	13–18	45	1–4	6	15

* Oral preparations. Serum levels based on 0.5 g orally.

Table 3. Cephalosporin dosage adjustment in renal failure*

Drug	Moderate	Severe	Post hemo-dialysis dose**
Cephalothin (Keflin)	1–1g q 6–12h	1gm q 12h	1g
Cephapirin (Cephadyl)	1–1g q 1–12 h	1gm q 12h	1g
Cefazolin (Kefzol, Ancef)	0.5g q 12h	500mg q 24h	0.5g
Cefamandole (Mandol)	1g q 12 h	1gm q 24h	0.5g
Cefoxitin (Mefoxin)	1g q 6–12h	1gm q 24h	1g
Cephalexin (Keflex)	0.25–0.5g q 8–12h	0.25–0.5g q 24h	0.5g
Cephradine (Anspor, VeloseF)	0.25–0.5g q 8–12h	0.25–0.5g q 24h	0.5g

* No adjustment necessary in mild renal failure.
  Mild = creatinine clearance 50–80 ml/min.
  Moderate = creatinine clearance 10–50 ml/min.
  Severe = creatinine clearance less than 10 ml/min.
** Hemodialyzed patients should receive dosage schedule as in 'severe' renal failure *plus* additional dose as listed.

Second Generation Cephalosporins

Although the currently available first generation cephalosporin antibiotics are active against a wide range of bacteria, these agents have limited activity against a number of important pathogens, especially those seen with increased frequency as nosocomial infections. None of the first generation cephalosporins is effective against enterococci and the majority of strains of *Hemophilis influenzae*, *Enterobacter* species, indole-positive *Proteus* species, *Providencia* species, *Pseudomonas aeruginosa*, *Serattia marsescens*, *Citrobacter* species, and the anaerobe *Bacteroides fragilis* are resistant as well [3]. Many of the Gram-negative organisms are capable of producing beta-lactamases (Cephalosporinases) which mediate the hydrolasis of various cephalosporins [9, 10]. This is the major mechanism for the resistance of Enterobacteriaceae, *Pseudomonas*, and *B. fragilis*. The Enterococci do not produce beta-lactamases and are inherently resistant to the first generation cephalosporins.

This lack of activity of the first generation cephalosporins in certain bacteria was a major drawback to their use and resulted in a major effort to develop cehpalosporins which are less readily inactivated by beta-lactamases and which thus have a broader spectrum of antibacterial activity. These efforts have resulted in the introduction of the so-called 'second generation' cephalosporins. This group includes cefamandole, cefaclor, and cefuroxime. In addition, the cephamycin antibiotic, cefoxitin, has also been introduced. Cefamandole, cefoxitin and cefaclor have recently been introduced into clinical practice in the United States, while cefuroxime, although available in Europe, is an investigational drug in the United States.

CEFAMANDOLE

Cefamandole nafate is a semisynthetic derivative of 7-amino-cephalosporanic acid (Fig. 2). This agent, the first of a series of second and third generation cephalosporins, is the first new cephalosporin introduced into clinical medicine which provides more than simple pharmacokinetic advantages over the previously available cephalosporins. Prior to the introduction of cephalomandole, the antibacterial spectrum of the cephalosporins remained unchanged from 1963, when cephalothin was introduced. The formula of cephalomandole and its relationship to cephalothin are shown in Fig. 2. Only with the development of agents modified at position 7 of the beta-lactam nucleus was a significant increase in the antibacterial spectrum of cephalosporins achieved. Cephalmandole has a D-Mandelamido function at Carbon-7 and a Methyltetrazole-thiomethylene group at Carbon 3.

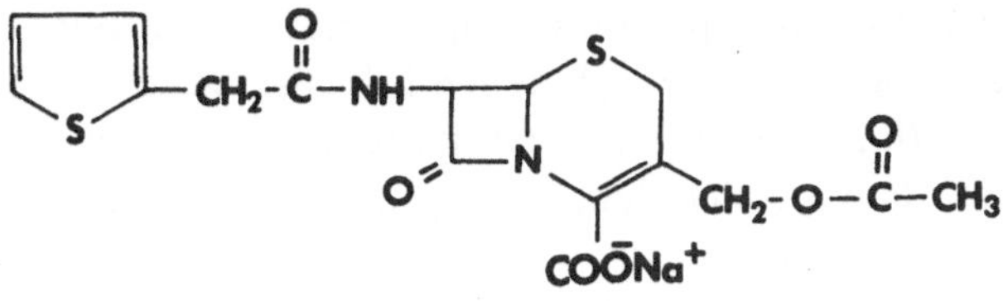

CEPHALOTHIN

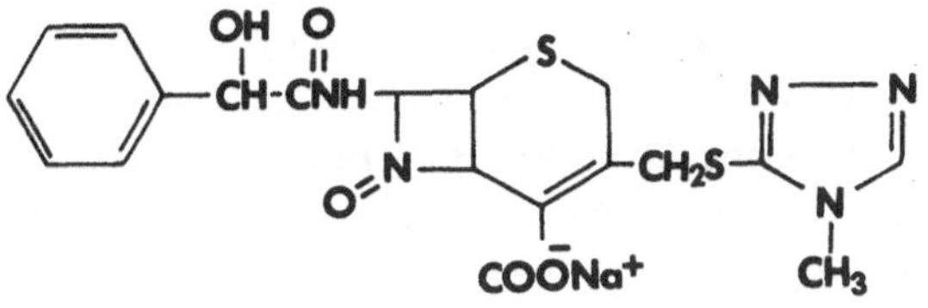

CEFAMANDOLE SODIUM

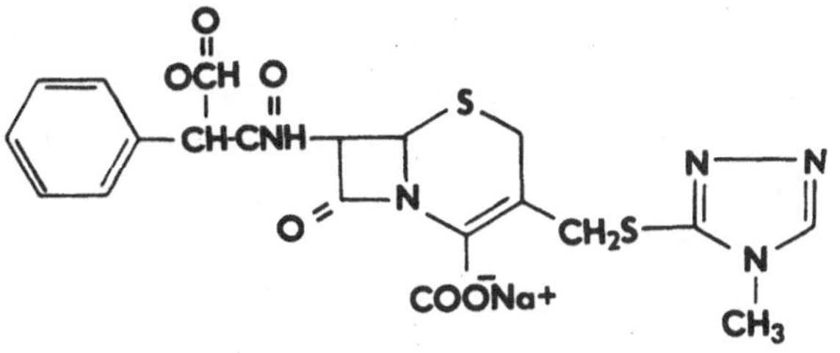

CEFAMANDOLE NAFATE

Fig. 2. Structure of cefamandole compared with cephalothin.

Initial in vitro studies revealed that Cefamandole had activity against *S. aureus* similar to that of first generation cephalosporins and was a more potent compound against gram-negative organisms and inhibited a wider spectrum of organisms [14, 15]. Cefamandole was active against strains of *Enterobacter* and indole-positive *Proteus* that had traditionally been resistant to cephalosporins. It also showed excellent potency against *Haemophilus influenzae*.

Following these initial encouraging findings, subsequent in vitro and clinical microbiological studies were undertaken [16–29]. In general, cefamandole was found to be active against a wide variety of Gram-positive and Gram-negative bacteria. In vitro studies showed that cefamandole was more active on a weight basis than cephalothin, cephaloridine, cefazolin, or cephalexin against Gram-negative bacteria, but slightly less active against Gram-positive bacteria [16–27]. Although the Gram-positive cocci are less susceptible to cefamandole than cephalothin, therapeutic levels of cefamandole are achieved in the blood after the administration of the drug. Because of its broader antimicrobial spectrum of activity, it has been recommended that a cefamandole disc be used to test sensitivity to this agent [18].

Gram-positive cocci, except Streptococcus *fecalis* (Enterococci), were exceptionally susceptible to cefamandole. Meyers and Hirschman [26] noted that *Streptococcus pyogenes* (Group A) were very susceptible and that all strains were inhibited at·concentrations less than 0.125 μg/ml. *Streptococcus pneumoniae* were very susceptible as well, and 100% of strains were inhibited by less than 1.2 μg/ml cefamandole. In addition, *Viridans streptococci* also were inhibited at low concentrations. For most Gram-positive cocci, the MICs and the MBCs of cefamandole were equal. Cefamandole was highly active against penicillin G susceptible and penicillinase-producing strains of *S. aureus* and that in vitro activity was equal against the two groups. The MBCs were either equal to or one tube dilution different from the MIC [26]. Methicillin-resistant strains of *S. aureus* were susceptible to cefamandole when standard inoculum of 10^4 dilutions of an overnight culture were used. The MBCs were two to four times greater than the MICs. However, if the inoculum was increased to 10^5 colony forming units per ml, the MICs were generally higher, two to three times increased [26]. An increase in inoculum size of methicillin resistant *S. aureus* caused a greater than ten-fold increase in the MIC. Most strains of *E. coli*, *Klebsiella* species, and *Proteus* species were inhibited by low concentrations of cefamandole. Strains of *Haemophilus influenzae* were very susceptible. *Salmonella typhi*, including ampicillin and chloramphenicol resistant strains, were inhibited by low levels of cefamandole. Cefamandole was active against a wide variety of Gram-negative bacteria. Indole-positive strains of *Proteus* were susceptible to cefamandole and had a mean MIC of 3.35 μg/ml. Fu and Neu reported that the activity of *Proteus morganii*, *Proteus rettgeri*, and *Proteus vulgaris* seemed to be bimodal with a sensitive group and a highly resistant group [28]. Most strains of *E. coli* tested were susceptible and the mean MIC was 4.43 μg/ml. However, some strains of *E. coli* showed a marked resistance with larger inoculum. *Enterobacter* species are varied in their susceptibility to cefamandole with some being resistant. Serratia species were resistant to cefamandole. *Pseudomonas aeruginosa* strains were highly resistant and the MIC was greater than 50.

Fu and Neu [28] compared the in vitro activity of cefamandole with that of other cephalosporins against the *Enterbacteriaceae* and *S. aureus* that possess beta-lactamases. They noted that cefamandole had distinct advantages over many of the other cephalosporins. This agent inhibited greater than 85% of the beta-lactamases producing *E. coli* at concentrations of less than or equal to 25 μg/ml and 60–70% of cephalothin resistant isolates of *E. coli*. The MICs of cefamandole for cephalothin resistant *Klebsiella* were 20–50 μg/ml. Against *Enterobacter* and *Citrobacter*, cefamandole was most active with MICs in the range of 1.6–6.3 μg/ml. Shigella that produced beta-lactamase were well-inhibited by cefamandole, but poorly by cephalothin. Eykin et al. noted that *Neisseria gonorrhoeae* were susceptible to cefamandole [22]. Cefamandole was active in vitro against *N. gonorrhoeae* that are penicillin sensitive or penicillin resistant.

Several investigations have looked at cefamandole's in vitro activity against anaerobic bacteria [18, 19, 29–34]. In vitro, cefamandole has been shown to be effective against 98–100% of the strains of *Bacteroides* species, *Clostridium, Fusobacterium, Eubacterium, Lactobacillus, Peptococcus,* and *Peptostreptococcus* tested at minimum inhibitory concentrations of 32 μg or less, although at 64 μg/ml cefamandole was effective against 76% of 412 isolates of *Bacteroides fragilis* [18, 19, 29–33]. Only 2 to 48% of *Bacteroides fragilis* group are susceptible at 16 μg/ml or less of cefamandole. In general, bacterial isolates are considered susceptible to cefamandole if the MIC is not more than 16 μg/ml and they are considered resistant if the MICs are greater than 32 μg/ml. However, it should be noted that the pharmacokinetics of cefamandole (as will be discussed in the following section) do result in extremely high levels which have peak concentrations that far exceed the upper limit of MICs for the majority of strains of *Bacteroides fragilis*.

Several investigators have noted that with increasing inoculum size, susceptible bacteria became increasingly resistant to cefamandole [26]. Farran and O'Dell noted that cefamandole is not completely stable to the beta-lactamases of Gram-negative bacilli. Richmond and Wooton have demonstrated that cefamandole is hydrolyzed at a substantial rate by both type III. a. (plasma mediated) and IV. c. (chromosomely mediated) enzymes [9]. Thus, the decreasing sensitivity with increasing bacterial inocula may be related to destruction of the antibiotic by beta-lactamases.

Pharmacokinetics of Cefamandole

Attempts to prepare cefamandole sodium in a crystalline form suitable for commercial use were unsuccessful. Cefamandole nafate is the O-formyl ester of cefamandole and is the preferred clinical formulation for reasons of crystalinity and stability [37]. Rapid hydrolysis of cefamandole nafate to cefamandole in vivo occurs, as does partial hydrolysis of cefamandole in vitro before administration (caused by sodium bicarbonate in the formulation). Thus, cefamandole is the major circulating antibiotic (85–89% of total plasma concentration) after IV administration of cefamandole nafate [35]. In normal clinical microbiologic determinations and in experimental infections in mice, cefamandole nafate and cefamandole sodium show the same potency [36]. In the artificially acidic medium required to keep the ester function of cefamandole nafate intact, cefamandole sodium appears to have greater potency [36]. However, the conversion of cefamandole nafate to cefamandole in humans is so rapid ($T\frac{1}{2}$, 13 min) that the availability of cefamandole is assured [35].

Clinical use of antibiotics should be correlated with both the vitro MIC data and the pharmacokinetics of the agent. The half life of cefamandole is similar to cephalothin (32 min see Table 2). Cefamandole is approximately 70% bound protein [20]. The drug is excreted unchanged in the urine. Serum levels are 20–36 μg/ml after a 1 g IM dose [20, 37, 38]. These concentrations greatly exceed the MICs and MBCs for all Gram-positive bacteria studied except for the enterococcus. The mean serum level of 1.9 μg/ml found at 6 h post 1 g doses by Meyers et al. [38] still exceeded the MICs for these organisms. Many Gram-negative species would be inhibited as well at these serum concentrations. The serum level of 4.56 μg/ml obtained at 4 h post – 1 g dose is higher than the MICs for 90% of the strains of *H. influenzae*, 78% of *E. coli*, 86% of *Klebsiella* species, 100% of *Proteus mirabilis* and 67% of indole positive – *Proteus* tested [38]. They noted that serum levels after a 1 g IV attained a peak of 103 μg/ml at 15 min, but declined to 47 μg/ml at 45 min, and to 29 μg/ml by 1 h. These concentrations would be sufficient to inhibit most Gram-negative bacteria, including all strains of *Salmonella typhi*, many strains of *Enterobacter* species and some of *Serratia* species. The urinary levels of Cefamandole are high as the compound is excreted by tubular mechanisms. The administration of probenicid elevates peak levels in serum and prolongs excretion in a manner similar to that seen with other cephalosporins and penicillins.

In considering the enteric bacteria, peak serum levels after a 1 g IM dose would be adequate for many strains of *Klebsiella* and *Proteus mirabilis*, but not for the less common species, such as *Enterobacter*, *Providencia*, or the indole-positive *Proteus*. Indeed, after a 1 g IV dose given for 10–30 min, there would be adequate concentrations with free drug to clear the serum of bacteria for only 1 h, and it is questionable whether organisms such as Enterobacter would be eliminated [20]. Thus, Neu recommended that in the serious lifethreatening infections, it would be wise to give cefamandole in 2 g IV doses at least every 4 h [20].

The high urinary concentrations of cefamandole will inhibit most of the enterobacteriaceae and enterococci, but not Serratia and Pseudomonas [20]. However, since 60% of the drug is cleared in the first two hours in situations of high flow rates, there may be periods in which organisms such as Enterobacter or indole-positive Proteus could grow and fail to be eradicated.

Based on the knowledge of the pharmacokinetics and the MIC data for cefamandole, it is apparent that the administration of this agent by IM injection provides adequate serum levels to treat most infections with Gram-positive organisms, except enterococci, and provides adequate urinary levels for most infections due to enterobacteriacieae. When cefamandole is administered IV the rapid clearance of the drug necessitates that it be given in doses of 1–8 g every 4 h, to treat septic states due to infections with enterobacteriaceae, if adequate serum levels are to be achieved [20].

As with other cephalosporins, the $T_{\frac{1}{2}}$ of cefamandole increased progressively as the rate of cratinine clearance decreased. The mean serum $T_{\frac{1}{2}}$ in moderate renal failure was 3.0 ± 0.3 h, which is an increase of $2_{\frac{1}{2}}$ times the $T_{\frac{1}{2}}$ value in patients with normal renal function [8]. The mean serum $T_{\frac{1}{2}}$ of cefamandole in severe renal failure was 7.95 h, or 6.7 times that in patients with normal renal function [8]. Patients on hemodialysis have only minimally influenced $T_{\frac{1}{2}}$ for cefamandole, and the same is true for peritoneal dialysis [8]. Similar to first generation cephalosporins in the presence of renal failure the dosage of cefamandole is adjusted is adjusted based on the cratinine clearance (see Table 3).

Clinical Experience with Cefamandole

A number of reports have documented the efficacy of cefamandole in daily doses of 4–16 g in the therapy of a variety of clinical infections [39–38] Perkins et al. noted that clinical cures were obtained in 48 (91%) of 53 patients with infections of skin and soft tissue and clinical, plus bacteriologic cures were obtain in 36 (68%) [41]. Levine and McCain reported that the use of 2–12 g daily of cefamandole resulted in satisfactory clinical response of 26 of 30 patients with serious bone and joint infections [48]. Plout and Perlino noted that cefamandole was effective in 50 of 58 patients with pneumonia due to *Streptococcus pneumoneae*; these results were similar to the penicillin regimen [42]. Gentry demonstrated that patients with severe Gram-negative bacterial infections were successfully treated with a combination of cefamandole nafate, plus either gentamicin or tobramycin in 31 patients [43]. All patients treated with this combination of therapy survived. All the patients were clinically and bacteriologically cured of their primary infections; bacteremia cleared in all patients within 24 h after combined antibiotic therapy was initiated. *E. coli* was the most common pathogen encountered, and was the etiologic agent in 28 patients. Two patients were infected with *Klebsiella pneumonieae* and the remaining patient had an infection with *Proteus vulgaris*.

Of pertinence to the obstetrician-gynecologist are studies with the use of cefamandole in the treatment of intra-abdominal, pelvic, and anaerobic infections. Levine et al. reported on a multicenter trial involving 147 patients treated for serious anaerobic infections with cefamandole at a dose of 1–16

230

g/day [45]. Treatment was successful in 122 of 133 patients (92%) evaluated for clinical response. All of 38 patients with skin and soft tissue infections responded satisfactorily. Six of eight patients with lower respiratory tract infections were cured completely. Bacteroides was observed n 53 instances, with 25 of these being identified as *Bacteroides fragilis*. Of these 25, 23 were treated successfully (clinically and bacteriologically cured). The MICs for 11 of the 22 cases of *B. fragilis* infections were 64–128 μg/ml, a satisfactory clinical response was obtained in ten of these 11 patients. The usual dose for these patients was 2 g IV q h; based on these data, the authors have suggested that cefamandole, when used in high doses, is effective in the treatment of infections caused by *B. fragilis*, even when the MIC is relatively high.

However, cefamandole is generally not recommended as an agent for treatment of *B. fragilis* infection. Although the effectiveness of cefamandole in the therapy of infections caused by anaerobes other than *B. fragilis* has been demonstrated [39, 40] the efficacy of the antibiotic in *B. fragilis* infections – even in high (12–16 g) daily doses – is uncertain, except in the instance of infections caused by strains demonstrated to be susceptible. Stone et al. studied cefamandole in the treatment of peritonitis [44]. It was evaluated as the sole antimicrobial agent used to treat bacterial peritonitis in 113 patients. The dosage varied between 1 and 2 g IV every 6 h. A good clinical response was obtained in 107 patients (95% of the total group). Bacteriologic studies reealed aerobic peritonitis in 99% of the patients, with anaerobic participation in 60% of these cases. The authors concluded from the results of this study, that it would appear that cefamandole is a reliable and effective antibiotic for use in the treatment of most forms of acute peritonitis. However, 99 of the 113 patients in this study required laparotomy for the excision of infected or gangrenous tissue, closure of GI perforation, or drainage of an abscess. In addition, although 91% of the Gram-negative rods were susceptible to cefamandole, only 61% of the anaerobes recovered from these patients were susceptible to cefamnole. Thus, this study should be viewed with caution, as to the role the antibiotic actually played in treatment, as compared to the surgical intervention.

Gibbs and Huff used cefamandole 12 g/day as sole treatment in 43 women with endomyometritis following Cesarean section [47]. The most common organisms were bacteroides species (88%) anaerobic cocci (63%) and *Bacteroides fragilis* (34%). Anaerobes were isolated in 98% of the patients. Six patients had bacteremias revealing *Bacteroides* species, *Peptococcus* species, *Group B streptococcus*, *Group A streptococcus*, *E. coli*, and *Enterobacter*. The clinical response was note to be good with cefamandole alone in 85% (34 of 43) of patients. Drug failures were explained by resistant organism in two patients and by a wound abscess in one. In three others, no clear explanation was available, and none of these had bacteroides fragilis. Of 14 patients with

Bacteroides fragilis isolated, two failed to respond. Cunningham and Gilstrap used cefamandole to treat 95 women admitted with a multitude of gynecologic and obstetric infections [46]. The initial dose was 2 gm every 4 h. The infections included metritis with pelvic cellulitis, following Cesarean section (49), severe acute pelvic inflammatory disease (24), post operative vaginal cuff abscesses (15), vulvar abscesses (4), and abdominal incision abscesses (3). Anaerobes accounted for 65% of the isolates. The majority were Grampositive cocci. Bacteroides species accounted for 11% of the anaerobes. Greater than 90% of the organisms were sensitive at less than 32 μg/ml; in approximately 10% of patients, surgical therapy and/or the addition of chloramphenicol was used. These authors concluded that reatment with cefamandole for obstetric and gynecologic infections appeared to be effective and safe [46, 47].

In these clinical studies [39–48], cefamandole was well tolerated. The most common side effects were eosinophilia (of no clinical significance), reversible hepatic enzyme elevation, and phebitis at the site of infusion. Thus, like other beta-lactam antibiotics, cefamandole is a safe antimicrobial with a high degree of selective toxicity aimed at microorganisms.

Stone et al. suggested that cefamandole, because of its broad spectrum of activity, may be an excellent prophylactic agent for abdominal and gynecologic surgery [44]. However, Slama and Fass reported the failure of a two-day course of high dose perioperative cefamandole prophylaxis to prevent serious infection due to *Bacteroides fragilis*, in patients undergoing elective colon resection or anastamosis [49]. This study in which 35% of the cefamandole group developed postoperative infection suggests that cefamandole has limited utility in prophylaxis against infection due to *Bacteroides fragilis*, and questions its utility in the treatment of infections in which *Bacteroides fragilis* may be involved. Similarly animal model work by Bartlett et al. has suggested that cefamandole as a sole agent or in combination with aminoglycosides does not prevent the abscesses due to anaerobic organisms in mixed aerobic/anaerobic intra-abdominal sepsis in the rat [50]. The explanation for this failure in the in vitro action of cefamandole in the animal model was the resistance of Bacteroides fragilis to this agent. The relevance of this animal model to disease processes in man is not clear at the present time. Kreutner and co-workers evaluated cefamandole as a prophylactic agent in patients undergoing primary cesarean section [51]. They noted that cefamandole levels were twice as high as cephalothin levels in serum and tissue. However, cefamandole was no more effective than cephalothin (both were significantly more effective than placebo) in reducing febrile morbidity and endometritis; cefamandole was effective in reducing the fever index while cephalothin was not. Recently, Long and colleagues reported that intrauterine irrigation with cefamandole nafate solution was effective in preventing endometritis [52].

Irrigation with cefamandole reduced the rate of endometritis to 0%; saline irrigation and no irrigation resulted in endometritis rates of 26.7% and 23.3%, respectively. This innovative approach must be varied by other investigators.

In summary, cefamandole in limited studies to date has been effective in 80–90% of obstetric and gynecologic infections when used in large dosages of 12 g/day [46, 47]. Cefamandole appears to be a significant advancement in the coverage against *Enterobacter, Indole-positive Proteus, Providencia*, and *H. influenzae. However, the lack of coverage against Bacteroides fragilis* should be kept in mind and because of the prevalence and importance of this organism in pelvic infections, cefamandole does not appear to be a first choice anim-crobial for severe obstetric and gynecologic infections. As a prophylactic agent, it appears no more effective than first generation cephalosporins and should, because of its costs, not be used in that role.

CEFOXITIN

Recently, another family of beta lactam antibiotics has been discovered – the cephamycins [11, 12, 53, 54]. These compounds are simiar in structure to cephalosporins, but differ in having a methoxy group in the 7 position on the beta lactam ring (Fig. 3). They also differ from cephalosporins as they are not

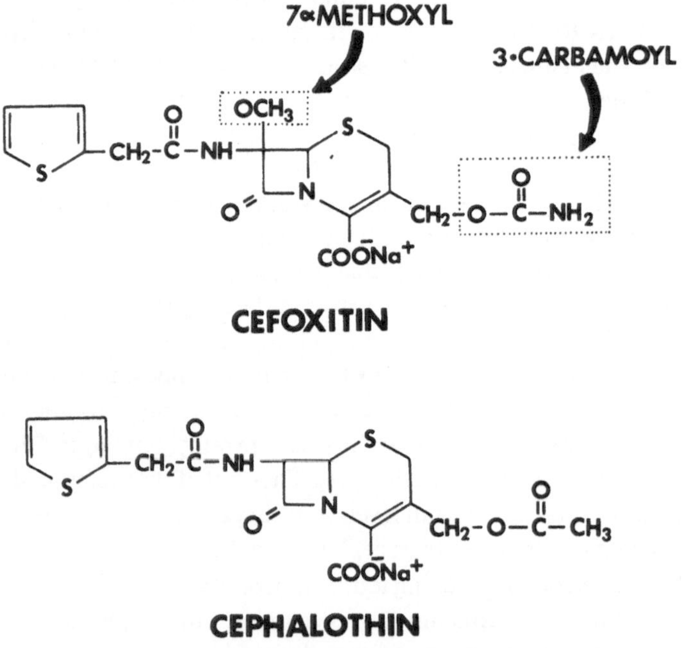

Fig. 3. Structure of cefoxitin as compared with cephalothin.

produced by fungi, but by actinomycetes – a filamentous bacteria. As do the penicillins and cephalosporins, the cephamycins lend themselves to removal of the side chain to give a nucleus from which semisynthetic cephamycins can be prepared. Cefoxitin is one such compound which is available and shows markedly increased stability to many of the beta-lactamases produced by Gram-negative bacilli [54]. Cefoxitin was the first of the semi-synthetic derivatives of cephamycins C to become available for laboratory and clinical use. This agent's activity has been summarized by Kass and Evans [13]. Because of its increased resistance to Gram-negative beta-lactamases, it has a wider spectrum of activity against the Gram-negative organisms than any cephalosporin or penicillin derivative currently available. The 7-alpha-methoxy group that places cefoxitin in the cephamycin family of antibiotics also appears to be crucial to its combination of good antibacterial activity and resistance to hydrolysis by virtually all beta-lactamases.

As a product of the streptomyces, this new family of antibiotics was of interest because it exhibited important biologic differences from the closely related cephalosporin antibiotics. As shown in Fig. 4, both the cephamycins and the cephalosporins share the basic cephem nucleus. However, the cepha-

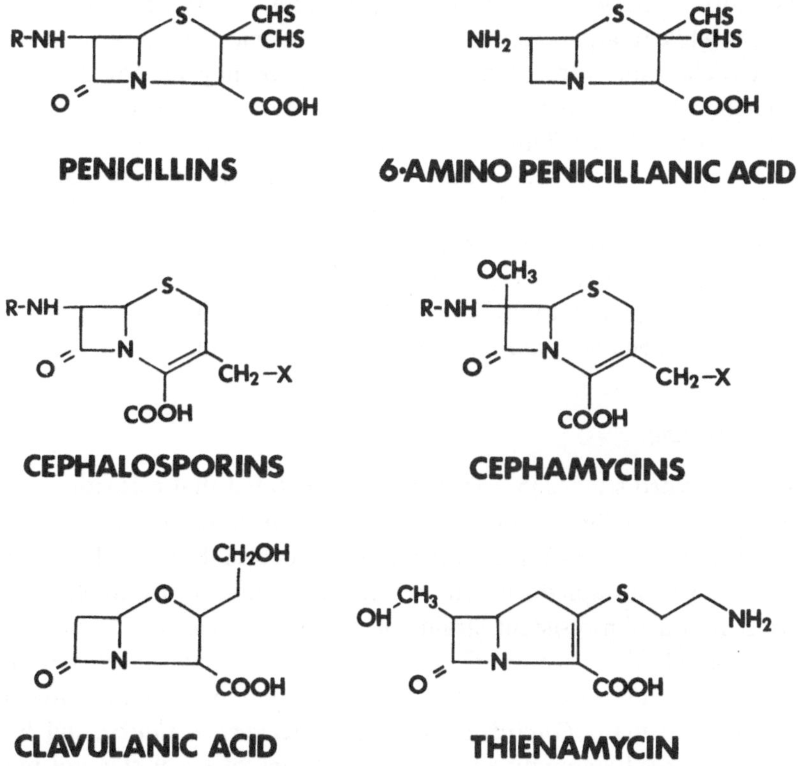

Fig. 4. Structures of beta-lactam antimicrobial agents.

mycins have a methoxy group in place of the hydrogen at the 7 position of the cephalosporins and as a consequence are resistant to degradation by beta-lactamase enzymes. Furthermore, any one of several substituents may be seen at the 3 position of the cephamycins, whereas the cetoxy group is found at this position on the natural cephalosporins. The presence of these changes in the side chain at the 3 position results in stability of cephamycin to enzymes that are capable of deacetylating cephalosporin C. Cephamycin A was found to be a broad spectrum antibiotic active both in vitro and in vivo against Gram-positive as well as Gram-negative pathogens [55]. Cephamycins B and C in contrast were narrow spectrum agents active against Gram-positive and Gram-negative organisms, respectively [55]. The potency and chemical stability of cephamycin C were excellent [55]. All three compounds were found to be highly resistent to beta lactamases. Miller et al. reported that cephamycin C was a remarkably non-toxic antibiotic [53]. Cephamycin C was clearly the most valuable compound in terms of potency and chemical stability, but lacked the breadth of spectrum that had been observed in the less stable substance cephamycin A.

The studies performed with the cephamycins indicated that it was desirable to develop a semisynthetic form of cephamycin C that would broaden its spectrum while retaining its characteristics of potency, stability, and activity against cephalosporin-resistant Gram-negative pathogens [55]. A series of new chemical reactions to permit the preparation of semisynthetic cephamycins were developed. This series of reactions was developed by Karady and co-workers [56] and resulted in the synthesis of cefoxitin from cephamycin C. The structure of cefoxitin shown in Figure 3 is comparable to that of cephalothin. The structural differences between cefoxitin and cephalothin are exactly the same as those between cephamycin C and cephalosporin C, that is cefoxitin has the 7-alpha-methoxyl and the 3-carbamoyl groups in the place of the 7-alpha-hydrogen and 3-acetoxy groups of cephalothin.

In Vitro Testing

Multiple in vitro studies [55–65] have demonstrated that cefoxitin is active against both penicillinase and non-penicillinase producing staphylococci, as well as beta hemolytic streptococci and pneumococci. In general, the drug is less active against staphylococci than most of the clinically available cephalosporins. Methicillin-resistant strains of *Straphylococcus aureus* are usually resistant to cefoxitin, as are enterococci. The drug is active in concentrations readily obtained in serum against most of the common Gram-negative bacteria, including many *Enterobacteriaciae*, *Neisseria gonorrhoeae*, and *Hemophilus influenza*. Its activity against many strains of *Klebsiella* and indole-positive *Proteus* and some strains of *Serratia* are of particular clinical importance. Cefoxitin has usually been inactive against *Pseudomonas aeruginosa* and most strains of *Enterobacter*.

The activity against a wide range of anaerobes is particularly notworthy [55–65]. Some 85–98% strains of *Bacteroides*, including most strains of *B. fragilis*, are inhibited usually by therapeutic concentrations of cefoxitin. Similarly, strains of *Peptococcus*, *Peptostreptococcus*, *Fusobacterium*, *Eubacterium*, and *Bifidobacterium* are generally inhibited by concentrations of cefoxitin that are obtainable in serum after the usual therapeutic dosage. Activity against clostridium species other than *C. perfringens* is less striking.

The antibacterial spectrum of cefoxitin has been presented in detail by Wallick and Hendlen [57]. They noted cefoxitin to be considerably more active than cephalothin against *E. coli*, *Proteus mirabilis*, and *Klebsiella*, which represents organisms normally considered sensitive to the cephalosporins. There was a very marked increase in susceptibility for the indol-positive *Proteus* species and *Providencia*, which represent Gram-negative organisms that normally are resistant to cephalothin. Cefoxitin showed some activity against *Serratia*. This early study suggested that cefoxitin was superior to cephalothin against Gram-negative pathogens. It also showed that the Gram-positive pathogens *Staphylococcus aureus*, *Streptococcus pneumoniae*, and *streptococci* (excluding the enterococcus and methicillin resistant staphylococcus) were sensitive to cefoxitin at MICs of 0.6 – 6 μg/ml, levels well within the susceptibility range for the Gram-negative bacteria. Thus, although less potent against Gram-positive bacteria, cefoxitin is sufficiently active against all organisms normally sensitive to cephalothin. Wallick and Hendlen noted that there was very little inoculum effect and that factors such as pH and medium had very little influence on the MICs of cefoxitin for Gram-negative bacteria [57]. It is characteristic of cefoxitin that the cidal activity is equivalent, or very close to the concentration that is inhibitory. Several workers have shown that cefoxitin is active against *Neisseria gonorrhoeae* in levels of less than or equal to 1 μg/ml [58, 59]. Cefoxitin is equally efficacious against non-penicillinase producing and penicillinase-producing gonococci [66]. Berg and co-workers demonstrated that 100% of penicillinase-producing *N. gonorrhoeae* were sensitive to 5 μg/ml of cefoxitin [66]. Cefoxitin has been reported to be active against *Hemophilus influenzae*, although not as active as some of the cephalosporins. Cefoxitin has not been shown to have much activity against *Pseudomonas aeruginosa* or the enterococci [55–65]. Its activity against Enterobacters is weak and sporatic [55–65].

Stapley et al. reviewed the susceptibility to cefoxitin of Gram-positive and Gram-negative bacteria isolated from hospitalized patients in the U.S. [55] This included 6715 Gram-positive nosocomial isolates and 17473 Gram-negative isolates. Overall, 81% of these isolates were sensitive to cefoxitin as compared with only 63% for cephalothin. Nearly 3000 Gram-negative isolates in the survey were susceptible to cefoxitin, but not to cephalothin. Three hundred and sixty-two isolates of Gram-negative anaerobes were also studied. Of these, 76% were sensitive to cefoxitin as compared to only 19% that were sensitive to cephalothin. The important pathogen *Bacteroides fragilis* was significantly more sensitive to cefoxitin than to cephalothin. In this survey, 99% of *Staphylococcus aureus* were susceptible to 16 μg/ml of cefoxitin, 100% of *Streptococcus pneumoniae*, 88–97% of *Streptococci*. Only 6% of the enterococcus were sensitive, 95% of *E. coli*, 91% *Klebsiella*, 96% *Proteus mirabilis*, 69% indole-positive *Proteus*, 97% *Providencia*, 41% *Serratia*, 51% *Citrobacter*, and 96% *Salmonella* were sensitive. Only 18% *Enterobacter* and 4% *Pseudomonas* were susceptible. Seventy-one percent of the *Bacteroides fragilis* strains, 100% *Bacteroides melaninogenicus* and 83% of *Bacteroides* species were sensitive.

Cefoxitin has been shown to have greater activity than the cephalosporins against the *Bacteroides fragilis* group of bacteria. Sutter et al. noted that Cefoxitin showed good in vitro activity at achievable peak levels in serum (32 μg/ml) against most anaerobic strains tested [60]. Cefoxitin is the most active of the cephalosporin type compounds against bacteria in the *Bacteroides fragilis* group. It is more active against other bacteroides species. Cefoxitin is the least active of the cephalosporin compounds against clostridium species other than *C. perfringens*. This group of investigators noted that 89% of *Bacteroides fragilis* group organisms were sensitive to cefoxitin at 32 μg/ml; this compared to 11% with cephalothin, 14% with cefamandole, and 13% with cefuroxime. Washington reported that at 16 μg/ml Cefoxitin inhibited 80% *B. fragilis* [16].

Data reported by Darland and Birnbaum [65], Sutter and Finegold [64], and Tally [63], showed that 81% of 340 strains of *bacteroides fragilis* were susceptible to cefoxitin (MIC 16 μg per ml) whereas only 7% of 299 strains tested were susceptible to that amount of cephalothin. It is obvious from these data that cefoxitin has activity against *Bacteroides fragilis*, a pathogen quite resistant to the cephalosporins.

Additional surveys of susceptibility of anaerobic organisms have been reported by Tally et al., who found that less than or equal to 16μg of cefoxitin/ml was active against most (82%) of 155 Gram-negative isolates [63]. Sutter, Kirby and Finegold reported the in vitro activity of cefoxitin against anaerobic bacteria [60]. They noted that at 32 μg/ml, 89% of the *Bacteroides fragilis* group were susceptible, 100% *Bacteroides melaninogenicus*, and 97% of other *Bacteroides* species. At this level, 100% of *fusobacterium neucleum*, other *Fusobacter* species, anaerobic Gram-positive, Gram-negative cocci, and *Clostridium perfringens* were sensitive.

The major loophole seemed to be other clostridium species with only 64% of isolates susceptible to 32 μg/ml of cefoxitin.

Washington has compared the in vitro susceptibility patterns of cephalothin, cefamandole, and cefoxitin [25]. Cephalothin was the most effective against *S. aureus*. Against *E. coli*, cefamandole was most active, followed by cefoxitin and then cephalothin; at 8 μg/ml cefamandole and cefoxitin inhibited 96% of *E. coli* strains. At 1 μg/ml levels cefamandole demonstrated greater activity against *Klebsiella pneumoniae*, but by 8 μg/ml cefoxitin and cefamandole inhibited 90%. Cefamandole was the most active agent *Enterobacter cloacae* and *E. aerogenes*, against which cefoxitin and cephalothin demonstrated no activity. Cefoxitin was five times more active against *Serratia marcescens* than cefamandole. *Proteus mirabilis* was equally sensitive to all three antimicrobials. Against *Proteus vulgaris* and *Proteus morganii* cefoxitin was most active. Cefamandole and cefoxitin demonstrated similar activity against *Proteus rettgeri* and *Providencia stuartii*. Cefamandole was substantially more active against *Citrobacter freundii*. Cefoxitin demonstrated greatest activity against *B. fragilis* with 80% inhibited at 16 μg/ml.

Other comparative in vitro studies [17, 18, 28, 31, 69, 70] demonstrate that similar high percentages of *E. coli, Klebsiella* species and *Proteus mirabilis* are susceptible to cefoxitin and cefamandole. With few exceptions, cephalothin-resistant (usually beta-lactamase-producing) strains of *E. coli* and *Klebsiella* species demonstrate that higher percentages of such isolates are susceptible to cefoxitin [17, 71, 73]. Almost all comparative studies [17 18, 28, 31, 69, 70, 71, 74] reveal that higher percentages of indole-positive *Proteus* are susceptible to cefoxitin.

The most likely explanation for the greater activity demonstrated by cefoxitin against *B. fragilis* and some of the Enterobacteriaceae is its resistance to beta-lactamase enzymes. While cefoxitin is only minimally hydrolyzed by different types of beta-lactamases from Gram-negative bacteria [9], cefamandole is hydrolyzed at a substantial rate by both type IIIA (R plasmid mediated) and type IVc (chromosomally mediated) enzymes [9].

Thus, in vitro studies with cefoxitin demonstrated a broad antibacterial spectrum against many clinically significant pathogens. Cefoxitin is active against virtually all of the clinically important Gram-negative facultative bacteria other than *Pseudomonas* and *Enterobacter* species. It exhibits activity against Gram-positive aerobic bacteria, except for enterococci. In addition, virtually all clinically important anaerobic organisms, including *Bacteroides fragilis* are sensitive to this drug. Like other beta lactam compounds, cefoxitin is a bactericidal agent that inhibits both Gram-positive cocci and Gram-negative bacilli [53, 57, 61]. By virtue of its resistance to hydrolysis by beta-lactamase, cefoxitin inhibits many organisms characteristically resistant to the cephalosporins, namely *Serrattia marcescens, Proteus vulgarius, Providencia* and *Bacteroides fragilis* [61–64].

Pharmacokinetics of Cefoxitin

Cefoxitin can be considered a non-metabolized drug because only 2%–4% of the parenteral compound is transformed in vivo into an inactive decarbamoyl form [67]. Thus, cefoxitin is excreted unchanged by the kidneys. Elimination of the drug occurs by both glomerular filtration and tubular secretion, and can be inhibited by the concurrent administration of probenecid.

The disposition of cefoxitin infused intravenously is best described by a linear two compartment open pharmacokinetic model [68]. Serum levels following IV administration show a biexponetial decline, with a rapid initial distribution phase followed by a slower elimination phase [68].

It has been estimated that 60–80% of cefoxitin is bound to serum proteins [67, 68]. After IV or IM administration, peak serum levels of cefoxitin are in the range 100–200 μg/ml after doses of 2 g. The level of cefoxitin rapidly declines over the next two to three hours to a range of 2–5 μg/ml. The serum $T\frac{1}{2}$ of cefoxitin after IV administration is 40 to 60 min. The urinary elimination of cefoxitin is rapid; 80% to 90% of injected dose is recovered from the urine during the first two hours after the start of infusion [67]. The drug penetrates poorly into the cerebro-spinal fluid, being present in high concentrations only if the meninges are inflamed [67].

Humbert and colleagues evaluated the pharmacokinetics of cefoxitin in normal patients and patients with renal insufficiency [67]. In subjects with normal renal function after a single IV dose of 30 mg/kg, serum concentrations were initially very high, but decreased rapidly and were approximately 10 μg/ml in 2 h. This is just above the MIC for most sensitive Gram-negative bacteria. These investigators made several observations in regard to the effect of renal failure on the pharmacokinetics of cefoxitin. The serum concentrations at the end of an IV infusion of 30 mg of cefoxitin/kg did not vary significantly according to the degree of renal insufficiently. Secondly, the elimination serum $T\frac{1}{2}$ of cefoxitin was correlated inversely with a rate of creatinine clearance and increased exponentially when the rate of creatinine clearance fell below 30 ml/min. Thirdly, there was no significant difference between the apparent volume and distribution for this central compartment in normal subjects than this value in patients with renal insufficiency. Fourthly, the decrease in urinary elimination of cefoxitin was parallel to the degree of renal insufficiency. Furthermore, it should be noted that urinary concentrations of cefoxitin remain above the MICs of susceptible organisms for greater than 24 hours in patients with renal impairment. Fifthly, the clearance of cefoxitin from serum may be increased five-fold by hemodialysis in patients with end-stage renal disease.

239

Clinical Studies

In view of the excellent microbiologic and pharmacokinetic properties of cefoxitin, clinical studies of its efficacy in the therapy of various infections were undertaken. Recent investigations have stressed the importance of mixed flora of aerobic/anaerobic bacteria in the pathogenesis of genital tract infections. There appears to be a definite pattern of isolation of these mixed infections. The commonly isolated aerobic organisms are Gram-negative facultative bacteria, especially *E.* coli. Commonly isolated anaerobes include *Peptostreptococcus*, *Peptococcus*, *Bacteroides* species, and *Bacteroides fragilis*. The in vitro studies, which demonstrated a broad antibacterial spectrum for cefoxitin, suggested that this agent may be an effective single antimicrobial agent for the treatment of these mixed aerobic/anaerobic infections encountered in the practice of obstetrics and gynecology. The high degree of the effectiveness of cefoxitin in the therapy of anaerobic infections including those caused by beta-lactamase producing strains of the *Bacteroides fragilis* group has been extensively documented [73–76]. Bartlet et al. have reported the results of studies utilizing cefoxitin in experimental intraabdominal sepsis produced in Wistar rats [50]. In the model used in these experiments, the rats were implanted intraperitoneally with capsules containing pooled rat cecal contents in preproduced peptonease glucose broth in 10% (weight/volume) barium sulfate. Previous studies in untreated animals receiving this challenge had shown a well-defined biphasic disease. During the first five days, there is acute peritonitis, *E. coli* bacteremia, and a mortality of approximately 40%. Animals which survive this acute peritonitis stage then develop intra abdominal abscesses in which the predominant flora is anaerobic bacteria, most commonly *Bacteroides fragilis*. This study indicated superior results with cefoxitin, which were comparable to a combination clindamycin/gentamicin regimen. The investigators felt that the increased in vitro activity of cefoxitin against *Bacteroides fragilis* was responsible for the greater efficacy of this agent as compared to cephalothin and cefamandole in the amimal model.

There are numerous reports of the high effectiveness of cefoxitin in daily doses of 4–8 g in the therapy of mixed aerobic/anaerobic infections encountered in predominantly medical patients, abdominal surgery, and obstetrics and gynecology. Weinstein and Eickhoff [77] evaluated 21 patients with respiratory tract infections treated with cefoxitin; all but one responded satisfactorily. The organisms isolated from this group included: *Streptococcus pneumoniae* (10), *Haemophilus influenzae* (4), *E. coli* (1), *Klebsiella* species (2), *Fusobacterium* species (1), and *Veillonella* species (1). Perkins and coworkers [78] demonstrated the efficacy of cefoxitin for the treatment of skin, soft tissue and bone infections; 25 of 27 (93)% of infections resolved with cefoxitin therapy. The etiologic agents included staphylococci, streptococci, Enterobacteriaceae, and anaerobes. Alford reported on the use of cefoxitin in a nosocomial outbreak of infections due to bacteria resistant to multiple antibiotics [79], most multiple resistant isolates of *Klebsiella pneumoniae, Serratia marcescens*, and *Proteus mirabilis* were sensitive to cefoxitin in vitro. *Cefoxitin therapy resulted in clinical and bacteriologic cure in seven of 11 patients. Pazin et al. summarized the use of cefoxitin in 135 bacteremic patients and concluded that cefoxitin was a suitable agent for use in septicemic patients* [80]. The organisms isolated included: *S. aureus*, streptococci, *S. pneumoniae*, *E. coli*, *K. pneumoniae*, *B. fragilis*, and *Bacteroides* species. These investigations reported an overall 83% cure rate with cefoxitin in these 135 bacteremic patients.

Cefoxitin has been shown to be highly effective in mixed aerobic-anaerobic abdominal infections [73, 74, 81–85]. In obstetric and gynecologic infections, cefoxitin has been demonstrated to be highly effective, with clinical cure occurring in 90–95% of cases [86–89]. Sweet and Ledger reported on the use of cefoxitin in109 patients – 68 with salpingitis, 25 with endomyometritis, nine with pelvic cellulitis, and seven with pelvic abscesses [89]. Overall, 100 of 109 (92%) of infections responded to treatment with cefoxitin alone. The major cause of treatment failure was the presence of abscsses which required surgical drainage. In addition, they noted the bacteriologic response to cefoxitin was excellent. Of the bacteria that could be evaluated by pre- and post-treatment cultures, 86 of 99 isolates were eradicated, four were suppressed, and nine persisted. No bacteria became resistant. They concluded that cefoxitin as a result of its resistance to beta lactamase and its broad spectrum of antimicrobial activity appears to be an effective antimicrobial agent for the treatment of pelvic infections. Ledger and Smith [87] noted that cefoxitin seemed to prevent progression to abscess formation; this good clinical result reflects the effectiveness of cefoxitin against anaerobes – especially *B. fragilis*.

The broad spectrum of activity demonstrated by cefoxitin in the treatment of mixed aerobic-anaerobic pelvic infections has led to its use as a peri-operative antibiotic. Mickal et al. [90], Hemsell et al. [91] and Harding et al. [92] have documented the efficacy of cefoxitin in the prevention of post operative pelvic infection in women undergoing vaginal hysterectomy. Mickal reported that cefoxitin decreased the incidence of major morbidity from 30% in their placebo group to 10% [90] Hemsell noted that only 8% of 50 women given cefoxitin had major post-operative infection, compared to 59% of 49 women given placebo. Harding et al. were able to decrease the post vaginal hysterectomy pelvic infection incidence from 39% in the placebo group to 7% in the cefoxiti group [92]. However, none of these studies revealed that cefoxitin was more effective than first generation cephalosporins for prophylaxis in vaginal hysterectomy. Several investigators have demonstrated that cefoxitin is an excellent peri-operative agent for Cesarean section [93–95]. Harger noted that cefoxitin decreased the inidence of endomyometritis from 22% in the placebo group to 10% [94]. Of special importance are the results of Ledger [93] and Polk [95] which demonstrate that not only did cefoxitin prevent endomyometritis, but was able to prevent the severe post-Cesarean section infections such as abscesses and septic pelvic thrombophlebitis. Thus, for Cesarean section prophylaxis an advantage may lie with cefoxitin over the first generation cephalosporins. Additional prospective comparative studies are needed to confirm this finding. The FDA has recently approved cefoxitin as a prophylactic agent for vaginal hysterectomy and Cesarean section.

Third Generation Cephalosporins

The continued emergence of antimicrobial resistance, particular among hospital acquired Gram-negative bacilli, has stimulated research to find new antimicrobial agents. Although the second generation cephalosporins – cefoxitin, cefamandole and cefuroxime – inhibit the majority of *Enterobacteriaceae*, they have little or no activity against *Pseudomonas aeruginosa*. Recently, several new cephalosporin – cephamycin compounds have been developed that have increased antibacterial activity, broader spectrum, or resistance to hydrolysis by beta lactamases. These drugs which are currently under in vitro and/or in vivo investigation have been called the third generation cephalosporins. Third generation compounds now being tested include cefoperazone (T1551) and cefotaxime (HR756). Moxalactam (LY127935) and another new beta lactam antimicrobial agent thienamycin, though not cephalosporins, resemble them in their spectrum of activity and are currently under study.

CEFOPERAZONE

Cefoperazone is a broad spectrum cephalosporin structurally similar to cefamandole (see Fig. 5). In vitro studies have demonstrated a wide antibacterial spectrum against aerobic and anaerobic Gram-positive and Gram-negative microorganisms [92–102]. Of particular note is its excellent antibacterial activity against *Enterobacter* and indole-positive *Proteus, Citrobacter and Serratia marcescens*. It also has very good activity against *Pseudomonas aeruginosa*. Jones et al. reported that cefoperazone demonstrated significantly increased antimicrobial activity against 5500 isolates of *Enterobacteriaceae* compared to cephalothin and gentamicin [96]. This agent was very effective against cephalothin and aminoglycoside resistant organisms – inhibiting 78% and 68% of strains, respectively. Cefoperazone

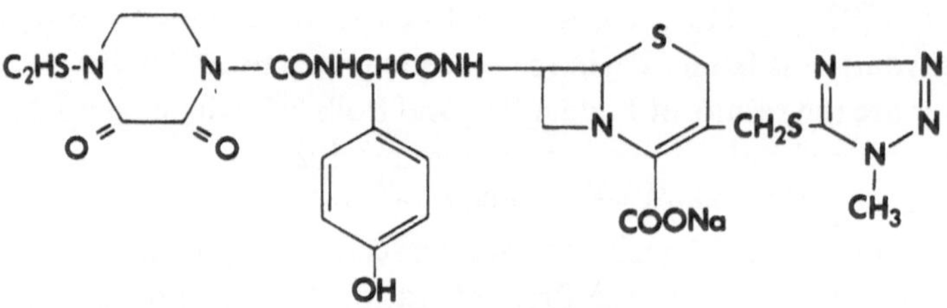

242

CEFOPERAZONE

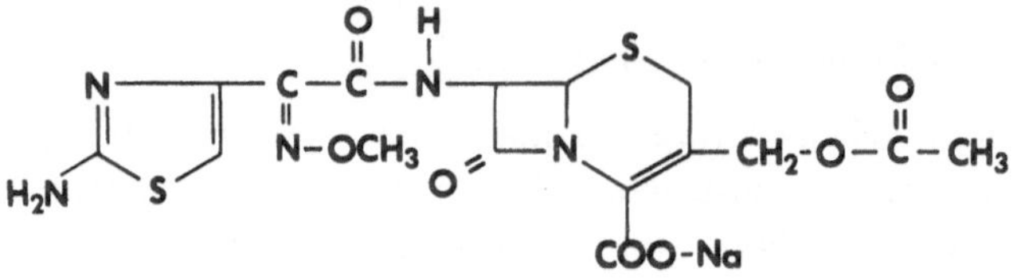

CEFOTAXIME

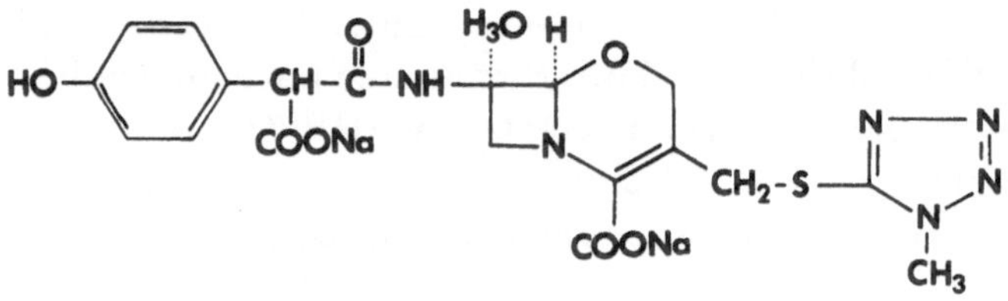

MOXALACTAM

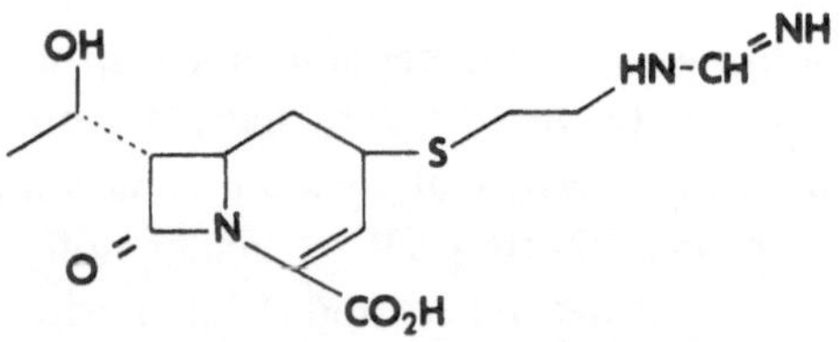

N·FORMIMIDOYL THIENAMYCIN

Fig. 5. Third generation cephalosporins.

inhibited 75% of *Bacteroides fragilis* group at less than or equal to 32 μg/ml [96]. The only uniformly resistant organisms detected were enterococci and Acinetobacters. The major advantage of cefoperazone over the other cephalosporins currently available is its antipseudomonal activity. However, Hinkle has noted that there is a considerable decrease in activity that results when the size of the inoculum was increased [97]. After intramuscular or intravenous administration, cefoperazone is absorbed rapidly and high serum levels are obtained. Thirty minutes after intravenous injections of 2 g, serum concentrations are approximately 175 μg/ml. One hour following intramuscular injection of 1 g the peak serum concentration is 85 mg/ml. Cefoperazone is stable in vivo and excreted unchanged in the urine and bile. In addition, it has a long plasma half-life.

To date, only limited clinical investigations have been performed with this agent. Ledger evaluated the results in 54 patients with gynecologic infections [103]. Cefoperazone was given at a mean dose of 2 g intravenously every 12 h. Fifty-one cases (94%) were judged as cures and two additional cases (4%) were called improved. Thus, there was only a single failure in these 54 cases. Side effects were extremely rare with the most common being phlebitis at the site of infusion, which occurred in two patients.

The role cefoperazone will play in the management of obstetric and gynecologic infections obviously must wait further clinical trials, including prospective comparative studies, evaluating its efficacy against older established regimens.

CEFOTAXIME

Cefotaxime is a third generation semi-synthetic cephalosporin (Fig. 5). It has demonstrated excellent activity against many of the Gram-negative and Gram-positive organisms [104–107]. It has excellent activity against *E. coli*, *H. influenzae*, indole-positive and negative *Proteus*, *Klebsiella*, *Enterobacter*, *Serratia*, *Providencia*, *Neisseria*, *Salmonella*, and Citrobacter. The MIC values are very low for the majority of strains tested. In addition, it has activity against *Pseudomonas aeruginosa*, which is greater than that of carbenicillin. At a concentration 12.5 μg/ml, this agent inhibited 86% of the isolates of *Pseudomonas aeruginosa* [108]. Cefotaxime is active against 84–95% of Enterobacteriaceae isolates resistant to cephalothin, cefamandole, and/or cefoxitin. Cefotaxime was an extremely active antibiotic against *Neisseria gonorrhoae*, and more than 90% of the isolates were inhibited by 0.008 μg/ml [109]. Cefotaxime is resistant to beta-lactamase enzymes of enterobacteriaceae. Against *Bacteroides fragilis*, cefotaxime was similar in potency to second generation cephalosporins. In general, cefotaxime showed good inhibitory activity against various species and strains of *Bacteroides*, Fusobacterium, peptococcus, peptostreptococcus, and clostridium. Neu et al. reported that cefotaxime inhibited only 60% of the isolates of *Bacteroides fragilis* at 25 μg/ml [104]. In addition, Enterococci are resistant to this agent.

Hemsell et al. reported that cefotaxime was an effective agent in patients with gynecologic infections [110]. One hundred and two women with obstetric and gynecologic infections were treated. Cefotaxime was effective in all 90 patients with gynecologic infections. Sixteen percent of the initial 55 women treated for post-Cesarean section infections, with 1 g IV q 8 h, after a 2 g loading dose, required the addition of chloramphenicol to effect clinical cure. The subsequent 28 post-Cesarean section infection subjects were treated with 2 g IV q 8 h; only 7% of these required the addition of chloramphenicol. Mild to moderate phlebitis at the infusion site that responded to conservative therapy was observed in 11 women. There were no significant alterations in hepatic or renal function or hemograms. These authors concluded that cefotaxime was a safe and effective single agent for the treatment of women with polymicrobial pelvic infections. Additional studies in a prospective randomized comparative manner will be needed before the final place in the armanentarium of the obstetrician/gynecologist for this agent is recognized.

MOXALACTAM

Moxalactam is a new semisynthetic 1-oxa-beta-lactam antibiotic (Fig. 5). The replacement of the sulphur atom by an oxygen atom at the 1 position of the cephem nucleus, enhanced antibacterial activity to a great extent. This finding stimulated efforts to modify the 1-oxa-cephem to confer beta-lactamase stability and to extend the Gram-negative spectrum. Hershida et al. reported that this agent had several characteristics features [111]. The antibacterial activity favored Gram-negative, rather than Gram-positive bacteria; high susceptiblility of organisms, almost independent of their beta-lactamase production; extremely extended antibacterial spectrum; a bactericidal effect that closely correlated to the MIC; high and sustained plasma levels after parenteral dosing; and potent in vivo efficacy. Jorgansen et al. noted that moxalactam possessed an extremely broad spectrum, which included aerobic Gram-positive cocci, enterobacteriaceae, *Pseudomonas aeruginosa*, *Hemophilus influenzae*, and anaerobes [112]. In addition, these authors noted that moxalactam had good activity against *Serratia marcescens* and that it acted synergistically with amikacin against the majority of *Serratia* isolates. Fass noted that although moxalactam was less active than cephalothin against Gram-positive cocci, it still was an active drug, and at concentrations easily obtained clinically inhibited 100% of strains of *S.* aureus, Streptococcus Pyogenes, and

Streptococcus pneumoneae [113]. Fass reported that all strains of *Bacteroides fragilis* tested were sensitive to obtainable levels of moxalactam. Moxalactam's activity against anaerobic cocci was less than first and second generation cephalosporins. When compared to cefamandole, cefoxitin, and cephalothin, moxalactam was the least active antibiotic against facultatively anaerobic Gram-positive cocci and the most active against aerobic and facultatively anaerobic Gram-negative baccilli. Reemer et al. also noted that moxalactam had excellent in vitro activity against all aerobiv Gram-negative organisms, including *Pseudomonas aeruginosa*.[114] They also concurred in the excellent activity against anaerobic organisms, especially the *Bacteroides fragilis* group. Against Gram-positive organisms, moxalactam showed less activity. All enterococci, *Listeria monocytogenes*, and corynebacterium species were resistant in vitro. These authors concluded that moxalactam did not have a sufficiently broad spectrum of in vitro activity to recommend safely alone for the empirical treatment of sepsis of unknown etiology.

Gibbs et al. have reported preliminary findings in 62 patients with post-partum or post-abortal genital tract infections who received moxalactam 6 g per day as a single agent [115]. They reported a good clinical response occurred in 56 of 62 (90%). Moxalactam was well tolerated with little irritation and minimal hepatic, renal, or hematological abnormalities. The six patients with poor clinical response all had endometritis after Caesarean section. These authors recovered 201 isolates from the uterine culture in these 62 patients. Eighty-four percent had anaerobes. None of the 30 aerobic Gram-negative rods tested were resistant to moxalactam. Among the anaerobes, only two isolates, *Clostridium leptum* and *Bacteroides disiens*, had MICs of greater than or equal to 32 μg/ml. Among the aerobic organisms, only the five enterococcal isolates were resistant. Future additional studies will be required to determine the role of moxalactam as a single agent in the treatment of pelvic infections.

THIENAMYCIN

The newest group of natural occurring betalactam agents to be identified include thienamycin [116] and the related clavulanic acids [117, 118]. Thienamycin, a novel betalactam antibiotic, was noted to have an unusually broad spectrum of antibacterial activity, with potency comparable to or greater than the penicillins against Gram-positive species and to the aminocyclotols against Gram-negative species, including *Pseudomonas aeruginosa*. Thienamycin was stable in the presence of beta-lactamase, and thus exhibited no cross-resistance with penicillins or cephalosporins. However, utility of theinamycin was hindered by its unacceptable degree of instability. This

246

problem was overcome by the synthesis of a anidene N-formimidoyl-thienamycin (MKO787). Kropp et al. have reported that MKO787 retains and, indeed, significantly improves upon the excellent in vitro antibacterial activity of the parent antibiotic [120]. These authors reported that the potencies of the thienamycin antibiotics far exceed those of other beta lactam antibiotics against both Gram-positive species, including *Enterococci* and Gram-negative species, including *Pseudomonas*. Twenty-nine *Bacteroides* isolates all showed a very high susceptibility to this agent; the median MIC for MKO787 (0.2 µg/ml) was comparable to clindamycin and far superior to that of cefoxitin. These authors evaluated 13 isolates of *Pseudomonas aeruginosa*, of which six were resistant to carbenicillin and reported that MKO787 had median MICs that were superior to moxalactam, cefotaxime, gentamicin, amakacin, piperacillin, and carbenicillin. These isolates were uniformly susceptible to MKO787.

Kesado et al. confirmed the findings that MKO787 has great activity against a broad range of bacteria, including Gram-positive and negative anaerobes [120]. They noted that it showed excellent activity against *Pseudomonas aeruginosa*, and Enterococci. The activity of this new agent against anaerobic bacteria was noted by Tally et al. to be greater than that of clindamycin, cefoxitin, and metronidazole [121]. The activity of MKO787 was similar to those of penicillin G, clindamycin and metronidazole against anaerobic Gram-positive cocci and clostridia and was superior to that of cefoxitin. All anaerobic organisms were inhibited by 2 µg or less of MKO787/ml. They noted that MKO787 was the most active antimicrobial agent tested against Gram-negative facultative bacilli, demonstrating superior results compared with gentamycin, amikacin, and carbenicillin. In comparing this new compound with other beta lactam antibiotics, its activity is superior to those of moxalactam and cefotaxime, especially against strains of *Enterobacter*, *Proteus*, *Serratia*, *Pseudomonas*, and *S. aureus*. This drug also inhibited *Bacteroides fragilis* strains that were highly resistant to other antibiotics, including strains known to produce high levels of beta lactamase, those with high resistance to clindamycin, and the only strain resistant to metronidazole so far isolated. These in vitro studies have demonstrated that thienemycin is a unique beta lactam antibiotic. Resistance appears to be rare. This lack of resistance has been correlated with the inability of either chromosomal or plasma associated beta lactamases to hydrolize the drug [122]. Second, thienamycin possesses a high degree of activity against Gram-negative species. It also is highly active against *Staphylococcus aureus*. Third, and as noted by others, it is highly active in vivo against both Gram-negative and Gram-positive species. All these properties suggest that this compound could play an important role in the management of clinical infections caused by susceptible organisms. To data, clinical studies have yet to be undertaken.

REFERENCES

1. Abraham EP, Loder PB: Cephalosporin C. In: Flyn EH (ed). Cephalosporins and penicillins. New York: Academic Press, 1972
2. Moellering RC: Cefamandole – a new member of the cephalosporin family. J Infect Dis 137:52–59, 1978
3. Moellering RC, Swartz MN: The newer cephalosporins. N Engl J Med 294:24–28, 1976
4. Silverblatt F, Harrison WO, Turck M: Nephrotoxicity of cephalosporin antibiotics in experimental animals. J Infect Dis 128 (Suppl): S367–S372, 1973
5. Maudell G: Cephaloridine. Ann Intern Med 79:561–565, 1973
6. Foord RD: Cephaloridine, cephaloth, and the kidney. J Antimicrob Chemother 1 (Suppl):119–133, 1975
7. Barza M: The nephrotoxicity of cephalosporins: An overview. J Infect Dis 137:560–573, 1978
8. Andriole VT: Pharmacokinetics of cephalosporins in patients with normal or reduced renal function. J Infect Dis 137:588–597, 1978
9. Richmond, MH, Wottin S: Comparative study of seven cephalosporins: susceptibility to B-lactamases and ability to penetrate the surface layers of *Escherichia coli*. Antimicrob Agents Chemother 10:219–222, 1976
10. Farrar WE, Jr, O'Dell NM: Beta-lactamases and resistance to penicillins and cephalosporins in *Serratia marcescens*. J Infect Dis 134:245–251, 1976
11. Nagarajan R, Boech LD, Gordon M, et al.: Beta-lactam antibiotics from streptomyces. J Am Chem Soc 93:2308–2310, 1971
12. Stapley EP, Jackson M, Hernanez S, et al.: Cephamycins, a new family of B-lactam antibiotics. I. Production by actinomycetes, including *Streptonyces* lactamdurans sp.n. Antimicrob Agents Chemother 2:122–31, 1979
13. Kass EH, Evans DA: Introduction. Rev Infect Dis 1:2–4, 1979
14. Wick WE, Preston D: Biological properties of three 3-heterocyclic-thiomethyl cephalosporin antibiotics. Antimicrob Agents Chemother 1:221–234, 1972
15. Webber JA, Ott JL: Structure-activity relationships in the cephalosporins. II. Recent developments. In: D. Perlman (ed). Structure/activity relationships among the semisynthetic antibiotics. New York: Academic Press, 1977, pp. 161–237
16. Meyers B, Leng B, Hirschman S: Cefamandole: antimicrobial activity in vitro of a new cephalosporin. Antimicrob Agents Chemother 8:737–741, 1975
17. Bodey GP, Weaver S: In vitro studies of cefamandole. Antimicrob Agents Chemother 9:452–457, 1976.
18. Washington JA, II: The in vitro spectrum of the cephalosporins. Mayo Clin Proc 51:237–250, 1976
19. Griffith RS, Black HR, Brier GL, Wolney JD: Cefamandole: in vitro and clinical pharmacokinetics. Antimicrob Agents Chemother 10:814–823, 1976
20. Neu HC: Cefamandole: a cephalosporin antibiotic with an unusually wide spectrum of activity. Antimicrob Agents Chemother. 6: 177–182, 1974
21. Shemonsky NK, Carrizosa J, Levison ME: In vitro activity and pharmacokinetics in patients of cefamandole, a new cephalosporin antibiotic. Antimicrob Agents Chemother 8:679–683, 1975
22. Eykyn S, Jenkins C, King A, Phillips I: Antibacterial activity of cefamandole, a new cephalosporin antibiotic, compared with that of cephaloridine, cephalothin, and cephalexin. Antimicrob Agents Cehmother 6:657–661, 1973
23. Jones RN, Fuchs PC: Comparison of in vitro antimicrobial activity of cefamandole and cefazolin with cephalothin against over 8,000 clinical bacterial isolates. Antimicrob Agents Chemother 9:1066–1069, 1976
24. Knothe H, Laver B: The microbiOlogical comparison of cephalothin, cephalexin, cephacetrile, cephradine, cefazolin, and cefamandole. Adv Clin Pharmcol 8:80–88, 1974
25. Washington JA, II: Differences between cephalothin and newer parenterally absorbed cephalosporins in vitro: a justification for separate discs. J Infect Dis 137 (Suppl):S32–S37, 1978

26. Meyers BR, Hirschman SZ: Antibacterial activity of cefamandole in vitro. J Infect Dis 137 (Suppl):S25–S31, 1978

27. Kaiser GV, Gorman M, Webber JA: Cefamandole – A review of chemistry and microbiology. J Infect Dis 137 (Suppl):S10–S16, 1978

28. Fu KP, Neu HC: A comparative study of the activity of cefamandole and other cephalosporins and analysis of the B-lactamase stability and synergy of cefamandole with aminoglycosides. J. Infect Dis (Suppl) 137:S38–S48, 1978

29. Weinrich AE, Del Bene VE: Beta-lactamase activity in anaerobic bacteria. Antimicrob Agents Chemother 10:106–11, 1976

30. Sutter VL, Finegold SM: Susceptibility of anaerobic bacteria to 23 antimicrobial agents. Antimicrob Agents Chemother 10:736–52, 1976

31. Ernst EC, Berger S, Barza M, Jacobus NV, Tally FP: Activity of cefamandole and other cephalosporins against aerobic and anaerobic bacteria. Antimicrob Agents Chemother 9:852–855, 1976.

32. Darland G, Birnbaum J: Cefoxitin resistance to beta-lactamase: a major factor for susceptibility of Bacteroides fragilis to the antibiotic. Antimicrob Agents Chemother 11:725–734, 1977

33. Eykyn S, Jenkins C, King A, Phillips I: Antibacterial activity of cefuroxime, a new cephalosporin antibiotic, compared with that of cephaloridine, cephalothin and cefamandole. Antimicrob Agents Chemother 9:690–695, 1976

34. Chow AW, Bednorz D: Comparative in vitro activity of newer cephalosporins against anaerobic bacteria. Antimicrob Agents Chemother 14:668–671, 1978

35. Wold JS, Joost RR, Black HR, Griffith RS: Hydrolysis of cefmandole nafate to cefamandole in vivo. J Infect Dis 137 (Suppl):517–524, 1978

36. Turner JR, Preston DA, Wold JS: Delineation of the relative antibacterial activity of cefamandOle and cefamandole nafate. Antimicrob Agents Chemother 11:105–109, 1977

37. Fong IW, Ralph ED, Engelking ER, Kirby WMM: Clinical pharmacology of cefamandole as compared with cephalothin. Antimicrob Agents Chemother 9:65–69, 1976

38. Meyers BR, Ribner B, Yancovitz S, Hirschman SZ: Pharmacological studies with cefamandole in human volunteers. Antimicrob Agents Chemother 9:140–144, 1973

39. Russell DG, Levine LR, McCain E: Cefamandole in the treatment of anaerobic infections. 17th Interscience Conference on Antimicrobial Agents anD Chemotherapy, New York, 12–14 October, 1977 (Abstract No. 1974)

40. Greenberg RN, Scalcine MC, Sanders CV, Lewis AC: Cefamandole therapy for anaerobic infections. Antimicrob Agents Chemother 15:337–341, 1979

41. Perkins RL, Fass RJ, Warner JF, et al.: Cefamandole nafate therapy of respiratory tract, skin and soft tissue infection in 74 patients. J Infect Dis 137 (Suppl): S110–S118, 1978

42. Plaut ME, Perlino CA: Cefamandole vs. Procaine Penicillin for treatment of pneumonia due to Streptococcus pneumoniae. J Infect Dis 137 (Suppl) S133–S138, 1978

43. Gentry LO: Efficacy and safety of cefamandole plus either gentamicin or tobramycin in therapy of severe Gram-negative bacterial infections. J Infect Dis 137 (Suppl): S144–W149, 1978

44. Stone HH, Guest BS, Geheb CE, et al.: Cefamandole in treatment of peritonitis. J Infect Dis 137 (Suppl): S103–S109, 1978

45. Levine LR: Cefamandole in the treatment of anaerobic infections. Contemp Surg 13:33–37, 1978

46. Cunningham FG, Gilstrap LC: Treatment of obstetrics and gynecologic infections with cefamandole. Am J Obstet Gynecol 133:602–610, 1979

47. Gibbs RS, Huff RW: Therapy of puerperal endomyometritis with intravenous cefamandole. Am J Obstet Gynecol 136:32–37, 1980

48. Leveine LR, MCCain, E: Clinical experieNce with cefamandole for treatment of serious bone and joint infections. J Infect Dis 137 (Suppl): S117–S124, 1978

49. Slama TG, Fass RJ: Comparative efficacy of prophylactic cephalothin and cefamandole for elective colon surgery. 18th Interscience Conference on Antimicrobial Agents and Chemotherapy, Atlanta, Georgia, 1–4 October, 1978. (Abstract 10)

50. Bartlett JG, Louie TJ, Gorbach SL, et al.: Comparative efficacy of three cephalosporins and cefoxitin in experimental intra-abdominal sepsis. *Current Chemotherapy*: Proc. 10th International Congress Chemotherapy. Siegenthaler W, Luthy R (eds.) Washington, D.C.: American Society Microbiology, 1978, pp. 298–299

51. Kreutner AK, Del Bene VE, Delamar D, et al.: Perioperative cephalosporin prophylaxis in cesarean section: effect on endometritis in the high-risk patient. Am J Obstet Gynecol 134:925–933, 1979

52. Long WH, Rudd EG, Dillon MB.: Intrauterine irrigation with cefamandole nafate solution at cesarean section: a preliminary report. Am J Obstet Gynecol 138:755–758, 1980

53. Miller AK, Celozzi E, Pelak BA, et al.: Cephamycin, a new family of Beta-lactam antibiotics. III. In vitro studies. Antimicrob Agents Chemother 2:281–286, 1972

54. Onishi HR, Daouse DR, Zimmerman SB, et al.: Cefoxitin, a semisynthethic cephamy n antibiotic: Resistance to Beta-lactamase inactivation. Antimicrob Agents Chemother 5:38–48, 1974

55. Stapley EO, Birnbaum J, Miller AK, et al.: Cefoxitin and cephamycins: Microbiological studies. Rev Infect Dis 1:73–89, 1979

56. Karady S, Pines SH, Weinstock LM, et al.: Semisynthetic cephalosporins via a novel acyl exchange reaction. J Am Chem Soc 94:1410–1411, 1972

57. Wallick H, Hendlen D: Cefoxitin, a semisynthetic cephamycin antibiotic: susceptibility studies. Antimicrob Agents Chemother 5:25–32, 1974

58. Jones RN, Thornesberry C, Barny AL, et al.: BL-5786, a new parenteral cephalosporin II. In vitro antimicrobial activity in comparison with six related cephalosporins. J Antibiot (Tokyo) 30:583–587, 1977

59. Phillips I, King A, Warren C, et al.: The activity of penicillin and eight cephalosporins on *N. gonorrhoeae*. J Antimicrob Chemother 2:31–39, 1976

60. Sutter VL, Kriby B, Finegold SM: In vitro activity of cefoxitin and parenterally administered cephalosporins against anaerobic bacteria. Rev Infect Dis 1:218–222, 1979

61. Neu HC: Cefoxitin, a semisynthetic cephamycin antibiotic: Antibacterial spectrum and resistance to hydrolysis by Gram-negative beta-lactamases. Antimicrob Agents Chemother 6:170–176, 1974

62. Moellering RC, Jr, Dray M, Kunz LJ: Susceptibility of clinical isolates of bacteria to cefoxitin and cephalothin. Antimicrob Agents Chemother 6:320–323, 1974

63. Tall FP, Jacobus NV, Bartlett JG, Borbach SL: Susceptibility of anaerobes to cefoxitin and oTher cephalosporins. Antimicrob Agents Chemother 7:128–132, 1975

64. Sutter VL, Finegold SM: Susceptibility of anaerobic bacteria to carbenicillin, cefoxitin, and related drugs. J Infect Dis 131:417–422, 1975

65. Darland G, Birnbaum J: Cefoxitin resistance to beta-lactamase: a major factor for susceptibility of Bacteroides to the antibiotic. Antimicrob Agents Chemother 11:725–734, 1977

66. Berg SW, Kilpatrick ME, Harrison WO, McCutchan JA: Cefoxitin as a single-dose treatment for urethritis caused by penicillinase-producing *Neisseria gonorrhoeae*. N Engl J Med 301:509–511, 1979

67. Humbert G, Fillaster JP, Leroy A, et al.: Pharmacokinetics of cEfoxitin in normal subjects and in patients with renal insufficiency. Rev Infect Dis 1:118–126, 1979

68. Schrogie JJ, Rogers JD, Yeh HC, et al.: Pharmacokinetics and comparative pharmacology of cefoxitin and cephalosporins. Rev Infect Dis 1:90–98, 1979

69. Adams HG, Stilwell GA, Turck M: In vitro evaluation of cefoxitin and cefamandole. Antimicrob Agents Chemother 9:1019–1024, 1976

70. Eickhoff TC, Ehret JM: In vitro comparison of cefoxitin, cefamandole, cephalexin, and cephalothin. Antimicrob Agents Chemother 9:994–999, 1976

71. George WL, Lewis RP, Meyer RD: Susceptibility of cephalothin-resistant Gram-negative bacilli to piperacillin, cefuroxime, and other selected antibiotics. Antimicrob Agents Chemother 13:484–489, 1978

72. Lewis RP, Meyer RD, Kraus LL: Antibacterial activity of selected beta-lactam and aminoglycoside antibiotics against cephalothin-resistant Enterobacteriaciae. Antimicrob Agents Chemother 9:780–786, 1976

250

73. Busch DF, Hesltine PNR,. Meyer RD, et al.: Cefoxitin sodium therapy of anaerobic infections. J Antimicrob Chemother 4 (Suppl. B):197–202, 1978
74. Gorbach SL, Miao PVW, O'Keefe JP, Tally FP: Treatment of anaerobic infections with cefoxitin. In: Current chemotherapy. W. Siegenthaler and R. Luthy (eds). Washington, D.C.: American Society Microbiology, 1978, pp. 300–302.
75. Heseltine PNR, Busch DF, Meyer RD, Finegold SM: Cefoxitin: clinical evaluation in thirty-eight patients. Antimicrob Agents Chemother 11:427–434, 1977
76. McCloskey RV: Cefoxitin sodium treatment of anaerobic and polymicrobial aerobic infections. J Antimicrob Chemother 4 (Suppl. B): 223–225, 1978
77. Weinstein MP, Eickhoff TC: Clinical evaluation of cefoxitin in the treatment of respiratory tract and other acute bacterial infections. Rev Infect Dis 1:158–164, 1979
78. Perkins RL, Slama TG, Fass RJ, et al.: Therapy of skin, soft tissue, and bone infections with cefoxitin sodium. Rev Infect Dis 1:165–169, 1979
79. Alford RH: Infections Due to endemic, multiple resistant Gram-negative rods: sensitivity to and therapy with cefoxitin. Rev Infect Dis 1:175–182, 1979
80. Pazin, GJ, Schwartz SN, Ho M, et al.: Treatment of septicemic patients with cefoxitin: pharmacokinetics in renal insufficiency. Rev Infect Dis 1:189–194, 1979
81. Rambo WM, Del Bene VE, Delamar DK: Cefoxitin therapy for surgical patients. Rev Infect Dis 1:195–198, 1979
82. Laplante L, Bastienn E, Giroux Y, Girard R: Intravenous treatment of systemic infections in 20 patients with cefoxitin sodium. J Antimicrob Chemother 4 (Suppl.B): 219–222, 1978
83. Nair SR, Cherubin CE: Use of cefoxitin, new cephalosporinlike antibiotic in the treatment of aerobic and anaerobic infections. Antimicrob Agents Chemother 14:866–75, 1978
84. Schumer W, Nichols RL, Acharya A: Use of cefoxitin sodium in moderate to severe surgical infections. J Antimicrob Chemother 4 (Suppl B): 231–233, 1978
85. Wilson P, Leung T, Williams JD: Antibacterial activity, pharmacokinetics and efficacy of cefoxitin in patients with abdominal sepsis and other infections. J Antimicrob Chemother 4 (Suppl. B): 127–141, 1978
86. Gonzalez-Enders, R, Calderon J, Trelles J: Treatment of postpartum endometritis with cefoxitin. In: Current chemotherapy. Proceedings of the 10th International Congress of Chemotherapy, Zurich, Switzerland, 1977. 11:768–770, 1977
87. Ledger WJ, Smith D: Cefoxitin in obstetric and gynecologic infection. Rev Infect Dis 1:199–201, 1979
88. Sweet RL, Hadley HW MIlls J, et al.: Cefoxitin in the treatment of pelvic infections. In: Current Chemotherapy. ProceedIngs of the 10th International Congress of Chemotherapy, Zurich, Switzerland, 1977. 11:767–768, 1977
89. Sweet RL, Ledger WJ: Cefoxitin: Simple-agent treatment of mixed aerobic-anaerobic pelvic infections. Obstet Gynecol 54:193–198, 1979
90. Mickal A, Curole D, Lewis C: Cefoxitin sodium: doubleblind vaginal hysterectomy prophylaxis in premenopausal patients. Obstet Gynecol 56:222–225, 1980
91. Hemsell DL, Cunningham FG, Kappus S, Nobles B: Cefoxitin for prophylaxis in premenopausal women undergoing vaginal hysterectomy. Obstet Gynecol 56:629–634, 1980
92. Harding GKM, Yuen CK, Thompson MJ, Lank B: A prospective randomized comparison of cefoxitin, cefazolin, and placebo in premenopausal women undergoing vaginal hysterectomy. 20th Interscience Conference Antimicrobial Agents Chemotherapy, New Orleans, La., September 2–24, 1980. Abstract #228.
93. Ledger WJ: Personal communication.
94. Harger J, English D: Perioperative cefoxitin prophylaxis in Cesarean section at high risk for infection. 20th Interscience Conference Antimicrobial Agents Chemotherapy, New Orleans, La., September 22–24, 1980. Abstract #229
95. Polk F: Personal communication.
96. Jones RN, Fuchs PC, Barry AL, et al.: Antimicrobial activity and spectrum of cefoperazone against recent clinical isolates. Clin Therapeutics, 3 (Suppl):14–23, 1980
97. Hinkle AM, LeBlanc BM, Bodey GP: In vitro evaluation of cefoperazone. Antimicrob Agents Chemother 17:423–427, 1980

98. Kurtz TO, Winston DJ, Hundler JA, et al.: Comparative in vitro activity of moxalactam, cefotaxime, cefoperazone, piperacillin, and aminoglycosides against Gram-negative bacilli. Antimicrob Agents Chemother 18:645–648, 1980

99. Kaye D, Kobasa W, Kaye K: Susceptibility of anaerobic bacteria to cefoperazone and other antibiotics. Antimicrob Agents Chemother 17:957–960, 1980

100. Matsubara N, Minami S, Muraoka T, et al.: In vitro antibacterial activity of cefoperazone (T-1551), a new semisynthetic cephalosporin. Antimicrob Agents Chemother 16:731–735, 1979

101. Neu HC, Fu KP, Aswapokee AN, et al.: Comparative activity and B-lactamase stability of cefoperazone, a piperazine cephalosporin. Antimicrob Agents Chemother 16:150–157, 1979

102. Hall WH, Opfer BJ, Gerding DN: Comparative activities of the oxa-B-lactam LY127935, cefotaxime, cefoperazone, cefamandole, and ticarcillin against multiply resistant Gram-negative bacilli. Antimicrob Agents Chemother. 12:273–279, 1980

103. Ledger WJ: Cefoperazone in the treatment of patients with gynecological infections. Cefoperazone Symposium. New Orleans, 1980, Excerpta Medica.

104. Neu HC, Aswapokee N, Aswapokee P, Fu KP: HR756, a new cephalosporin active against Gram-positive and Gram-negative aerobic and anaerobic bacteria. Antimicrob Agents Chemother 15:273–281, 1979

105. Greenwood D, Pearson N, Eley A, O'Grady F: Comparative in vitro activities of cefoTaxime and ceftizoxime (FK749): new cephalosporins with exceptional potency. Antimicrob Agents Chemother 17:397–401, 1980

106. Drasar FA, Farrell W, Howard AJ, et al.: Activity of HR756 against *Haemophilus influenzae. Bacteroides fragilis*, and Gram-negative rods. J Antimicrob Chemother 4:445–450, 1978

107. Hamilton-Miller JMT, Brumfitt W, Reynolds AV: Cefotaxime (HR756) a new cephalosporin with exceptional broad-spectrum activity in vitro J Antimicrob Chemother 4:437–444, 1978

108. Sosna JP, Murray PR, Medoff G: Comparison of the in vitro activities of HR756 with cephalothin, cefoxitin and cefamandole. Antimicrob Agents Chemother 14:876–879, 1978

109. Murray PR, Christman JL, Medoff G: In vitro activity of HR756, a new cephalosporin, against *Neisseria gonorrhoeae*. Antimicrob Agents Chemother 15:452–454, 1979

110. Hemsell DL, Cunningham FG, DePalma SS, et al.: Treatment of obstetric and gynecologic infections with cefotaxime. 20th Interscience Conference of Antimicrobial Agents and Chemotherapy. Abstract No. 19, New Orleans, La., September 22–24, 1980

111. Yoshida T, Matsuura S, Mayama M, Kameda Y, Kuwahara S: Moxalactam (6059-S), a novel 1-oxa-β-lactam with an expander antibacterial spectrum: laboratory evaluation. Antimicrob Agents Chemother 17:302–312, 1980

112. Jorgensen JH, Crawford SA, Alexander GA: In vitro activities of moxalactam and cefotaxime against aerobic Gram-negative bacilli. Antimicrob Agents Chemother 17:937–942, 1980

113. Fass RJ: In vitro activity of LY127935. Antimicrob Agents Chemother 16:503–509, 1979

114. Reimer LG, Mirrett S, Reller LB: Comparison of in vitro activity of moxalactam (LY127935) with cefazolin, amikacin, tobramycin, carbenicillin, piperacillin, and ticarcillin against 420 blood culture isolates. Antimicrob Agents Chemother 17:412–416, 1980

115. Gibbs RS, Blanco JD, Castaneda YS, St.Clair PJ: Therapy of obstetrical infections with moxalactaM. Antimicrob Agents Chemother 17:1004–1007, 1980

115a. Gall S, Addison WA, Hill GB: The use of moxalactam in the therapy of obstetric and gynecological infections. 20th Interscience Conference on Antimicrobial Agents Chemotherapy. New Orleans, La., Sept. 22–24, 1980, Abstract #373

116. Kahan JS, Kahan FM, Goegelman R, et al.: Thienamycin, a new B-lactam antibiotic. I. Discovery and isolation. 16th Interscience Conference on Antimicrobial Agents and Chemother. Chicago, Ill., 1976, Abstract #227

117. Brown AG, Butterworth D, Cole M, et al.: Natural occurring B-lactamase inhibitors with antibacterial activity. J Antibiotics 29:668–669, 1976.

252

118. Reading C, Cole M: Clavulanic acid a B-lactamase-inhibiting B-lactam from *Streptomyces clavuligerus*. Antimicrob Agents Chemother 11:852–857, 1977
119. Kropp H, Sundelof JG, Kahan JS, et al.: MK0787 (N-Formimidoyl Thienamycin): evaluation of in vitro and in vivo activities. Antimicrob Agents Chemother 17:993–1000. 1980
120. Kesado T, Hashizume T, Ashai Y: Antibacterial activities of a new stabilized thienamycin, N-formimidoyl Thienamycin, in comparison with other antibiotics. Antimicrob Agents Chemother 17:912–917, 1980
121. Tally FP, Jacobus NV, Gorbach SL: In vitro activity of N-Formimidoyl Thienamycin (MK0787). Antimicrob Agents Chemother 18:642–644, 1980
122. Neu HC, Labthavikul P: Comparative activity and β-lactamase stability of N-formimidoyl thienamycin. 20th Interscience Conference Antimicrobial Agents Chemotherapy, New Orleans, La., Sept. 22–24, 1980, Abstract # 260

Author's address:
Department of Obstetrics and Gynecology
San Francisco General Hospital
1001 Potrero Avenue
San Francisco, California 94110
U.S.A.

INDEX

254